Principles of Clinical Practice

An Introductory Textbook

Principles of Clinical Practice

An Introductory Textbook

Edited by

Mark B. Mengel, M.D., M.P.H.

Edmond, Oklahoma

PLENUM MEDICAL BOOK COMPANY • NEW YORK AND LONDON

Library of Congress Cataloging-in-Publication Data

Principles of clinical practice : an introductory textbook / edited by
Mark B. Mengel.
p. cm.
Includes bibliographical references and index.
ISBN 0-306-43847-X
1. Clinical medicine. 2. Physician and patient. I. Mengel, Mark
B.
[DNLM: 1. Clinical Medicine. 2. Physician-Patient Relations. W
62 P957]
RC48.P74 1991
616--dc20
DNLM/DLC
for Library of Congress 91-21149
CIP

ISBN 0-306-43847-X

233 Spring Street, New York, N.Y. 10013

Plenum Medical Book Company is an imprint of Plenum Publishing Corporation

Printed in the United States of America

To Laura and Sally
whose support made this textbook possible

and

To those dedicated practitioners who taught us that the central core of clinical practice remains the doctor–patient relationship

Contributors

Gregory H. Blake, M.D., M.P.H., Assistant Professor and Residency Director, Department of Family Medicine, University of Mississippi Medical Center, Jackson, Mississippi 39216

Alvah R. Cass, M.D., Associate in Family Practice, Guthrie Medical Group, Corning, New York 14830

William M. Chop, Jr., M.D., Clinical Assistant Professor, Department of Family Practice, University of Oklahoma, College of Medicine—Tulsa, Tulsa, Oklahoma 74129

Steven A. Crawford, M.D., Chairman, Department of Family Medicine, Oklahoma City Clinic, Oklahoma City, Oklahoma 73104

Daniel S. Marley, M.D., Clinical Decision-Making Fellow, Division of Clinical Affairs, Department of Family Medicine, University of Oklahoma, Health Sciences Center, Oklahoma City, Oklahoma 73190

Mark B. Mengel, M.D., M.P.H., Assistant Professor and Course Coordinator, Introduction to Clinical Care, Department of Family Medicine, University of Oklahoma, Health Sciences Center, Oklahoma City, Oklahoma 73190

James W. Mold, M.D., Associate Professor and Director, Geriatrics Division, Department of Family Medicine, University of Oklahoma, Health Sciences Center, Oklahoma City, Oklahoma 73190

Michael L. Parchman, M.D., Assistant Professor and Medical Director, Department of Family Medicine, University of Oklahoma, Health Sciences Center, Oklahoma City, Oklahoma 73190

Kathryn E. H. Reilly, M.D., Assistant Professor and Associate Director, Residency Program, Department of Family Medicine, University of Oklahoma, Health Sciences Center, Oklahoma City, Oklahoma 73190

L. Peter Schwiebert, M.D., Assistant Professor, Department of Family Medicine, University of Oklahoma, Health Sciences Center, Oklahoma City, Oklahoma 73190

Stephen J. Spann, M.D., Chairman, Department of Family Medicine, University of Texas Medical Branch—Galveston, Galveston, Texas 77550

Garth L. Splinter, M.D., M.B.A., Assistant Professor and Director of Strategic Planning, Department of Family Medicine, University of Oklahoma, Health Sciences Center, Oklahoma City, Oklahoma 73190

Howard F. Stein, Ph.D., Professor, Department of Family Medicine, University of Oklahoma, Health Sciences Center, Oklahoma City, Oklahoma 73190

Richard A. Wright, Ph.D., Director, Center for Biomedical and Health Care Ethics, University of Oklahoma, Health Sciences Center, Oklahoma City, Oklahoma 73190

Foreword

As we move into the 21st century it is becoming increasingly difficult to offer appropriate introductory clinical experiences for medical students. Many schools offer clinical experiences in the first year of medical school, when the learner has little background in the traditions and origins of the doctor–patient interaction. Others begin this process in the second year, after a professional language base has been established, but concise educational materials are scarce that integrate the meaning of the privileged clinical encounter with the process and content of interviewing and examining patients. In the tertiary hospitals, where most medical schools are based, the educators must provide an orientation to the clinical encounter, an intensely personal experience, in the midst of glittering technological marvels that easily distract both the novice physician and the wizened teacher. Understanding the context and historical basis for the privilege of interviewing and examining another person about intimate matters relating to health and disease is essential to this process. Considering these factors, this textbook is written to assist medical educators and medical students involved in early clinical training.

As the demand for "high-tech" medicine has accelerated, so has the public concern over the loss of "high-touch" or compassionate, humane interactions with physicians. Physicians are perceived as more concerned with readouts from machines and fiberoptic views of the patient than with understanding and caring about the people we have labeled as patients. This text is offered to improve the integration of human meaning and connectedness in the training of new physicians. The context of the medical encounter is reviewed from four different domains: purposes, processes, relationships, and values.

For generations we have trained physicians in the "art" of medicine in a haphazard manner and have reaped the predictable consequences. As our profession sprints into the next century on the shiny wheels of technology, we must regain our human spirit and professional esteem.

Within this text are essays, case presentations, and study questions that can stimulate small and large group discussions, which are needed to process the topic thoroughly. By stimulating collaborative and lively involvement of both teacher and student, this approach can model appropriate interactions with patients for the future physician, interactions that are respectful, questioning, creative, and enjoyable.

From the first chapter's historical review of the basis of the doctor–patient relationship to the vision of the final chapter on patient-centered care, the text orients the reader to the complexities and opportunities of clinical practice. Newcomers to medicine and seasoned veterans will enjoy this exploration of the clinical, historical, and personal dimensions of our professional interactions with patients.

Macaran A. Baird, M.D., M.S.

Chairman, Department of Family Medicine
SUNY at Syracuse

Preface

> . . . the secret of the care of the patient is in caring for the patient.
>
> Francis W. Peabody, M.D., 1927

Principles of Clinical Practice is an introductory textbook focusing on the doctor–patient relationship. Formerly closeted behind closed doors, this most intimate of relationships is coming under increasing scrutiny not only because of scientific interest but because of widespread public dissatisfaction with the care patients receive from physicians. This dissatisfaction has been reflected in many recent societal trends, including the rise in the medical self-help movement, particularly among women, the increased incidence of malpractice suits, and the increased assertiveness of patients toward physicians in expressing their needs and demanding input into medical decisions that affect their health. This dissatisfaction cannot be entirely blamed on the poor relations some patients have with their physicians; however, it is clear that a "good" doctor–patient relationship will ameliorate many of these dissatisfactions.

The difference between a poor and a good doctor–patient relationship has only recently been the subject of scientific scrutiny. Even though it clearly is a plea for more compassionate treatment of ill patients by physicians, Peabody's famous article, a quote from which begins this preface, also reflected his feeling that the doctor–patient relationship can be subjected to scientific scrutiny and taught to medical students, the results of which would benefit both the doctor and the patient. Unfortunately, the tools to study and teach the doctor–patient relationship were not available in Peabody's time. Tape recorders, video cameras, and elegant statistical analyses are necessary to study this most intimate of relationships. Even though this research is clearly in its infancy, it has progressed to a point where the difference between a good and a poor doctor–patient relationship is becoming evident. This book examines that evidence in the hope that future physicians will be able to establish more good than poor relationships with their patients.

This evidence has been organized into four main sections: purposes, processes, relationships, and values inherent to patient care. Issues from each of these areas have been clearly shown to affect clinical care. A concluding section attempts to integrate the many themes developed in the four main sections into a coherent whole by describing a new emerging approach to clinical practice: patient-centered care.

The purpose section of this text reviews the reasons why patients come to physicians, both historically and currently. It may surprise students to learn that the nature of the doctor–patient relationship has not remained static but has changed dramatically through the years. The philosophical and ethical foundations of the doctor–patient relationship are then described. This chapter concludes with a description of a framework for clinical decision making, many of the components of which are described in more detail in later chapters.

The process section examines the methods and tools physicians use when caring for patients. These processes, including interviewing, history taking, physical examination, laboratory testing, clinical decision making, clinical management, and health promotion, not only help doctors gather clinical data but enable doctors to decide on treatment, an often difficult task given the uncertainty inherent in clinical practice.

The relationship section discusses how emotions, behaviors, dynamics, and cultural norms affect the care physicians provide patients. In this section, chapters are organized outward from the doctor–patient relationship beginning with the doctor–patient relationship itself, proceeding through the patient's family and the patient's culture, and finally ending with a discussion of the physician's culture, the health care system.

The values section discusses those beliefs, rules, and incentives that affect clinical practice. Although some may find it surprising that a discussion of medical economics occurs within this section, the amount of money we spend as a nation on health care and what we buy with those dollars are very clear indications of what we value as a people and as a society.

Educationally, we hope that these chapters will not simply be read and forgotten but will be the focus of spirited discussion. In our own course for first-year medical students, the cases for discussion at the end of each chapter serve as a focal point for small group discussion. We hope that these cases for discussion will stimulate others to form such discussion groups, not only within existing introductory clinical practice courses but outside of the structured medical school curriculum as well. Additionally, we find that the educational experience is enhanced if students can actually observe doctors treating patients in offices and hospitals. In our course, students spend 16 half-day sessions with physicians of various specialities during their first year. Although this can in no way serve as an in-depth exposure to clinical medicine, it does help to stimulate discussion, as real-life examples can be used for the students' own experience.

Patients are demanding more from physicians not only in terms of their health but from the doctor–patient relationship as well. To many, it is not clear whether past injuries to the doctor–patient relationship can be healed. However, because of ongoing research and the renewed dedication we see in students of medicine today, we feel that the doctor–patient relationship can once again flourish and be the source of professional satisfaction for physicians and therapeutic benefit for patients. This textbook is offered as an attempt to convince those just starting their medical careers that the doctor–patient relationship, as the center of clinical practice, is vitally important and should be the subject of continued study. Gains from such study will enable future physicians to continue to crack the secret of patient care by truly caring for their patients.

Mark B. Mengel, M.D., M.P.H.

Oklahoma City, Oklahoma

Acknowledgments

Without the aid of many people, this textbook simply would not have been possible. Jim Mold and Howard Stein deserve mention for their support of this work throughout its development. Jim was instrumental in the development of the initial organization of the text and served as an early editor for many of the chapters. Howard provided moral support by emphasizing that his work should be not only a description of knowledge in the area but an opportunity to synthesize that knowledge through faculty discussion into a workable conceptual framework. Richard Wright and Michael Parchman, both of whom joined this effort in its later stages, also deserve special mention, not only for the contributions they made in the form of specific chapters but for the support and encouragement they provided as the text was being readied for publication. Finally, all the authors deserve mention for the time and effort each put into his or her own chapters and into the course that stimulated the development of this text. As teaching is not a well-rewarded activity at most medical schools, their efforts in this area are even more noteworthy, representing a true "labor of love."

Although many department secretaries contributed to this work, one stands out: Debbie Isham. For the past 2 years she has worked tirelessly, not only on the text but on coordinating Introduction to Clinical Care. Debbie has decided to obtain a graduate degree in public health, and her efforts in this area are going to be sorely missed.

Our students and our patients also deserve special praise. Early drafts of this work have been used during the past 3 years of Introduction to Clinical Care. First-year medical students in that course have been very helpful in suggesting revisions and new topic areas that should be covered in this introductory work. Also, our patients, on whom we actually practice patient-centered care, have been a continual source of support and feedback and in many ways have served as our best teachers.

Last, the University of Oklahoma Department of Family Medicine also deserves praise not only for its commitment to teaching medical students the important principles of clinical practice early in their careers but also because of their early support of this work.

Contents

PART I

Purposes of Clinical Practice

Although the answer to the question "Why are there doctors?" seems obvious—to care for the sick—the components of that care and the definition of the sick have changed throughout history and are even today hotly debated. This section reviews the historical and philosophical underpinnings of physicianhood in an attempt to prepare the student to intelligently enter the debate by beginning to form his or her own conceptual framework of what it means to be a physician.

CHAPTER 1

A Historical Overview of Patient Care

Michael L. Parchman

Case 1-1. In Abdera, Anaxion, who was lodged near the Thracian Gates, was seized with an acute fever; continued pain of the right side, dry cough, without expectoration during the first days, thirst, insomnolency; urine well colored, copious and thin. On the seventh, in a painful state, for the fever increased, while the pains did not abate, and the cough was troublesome and attended with dyspnea. On the eighth, I opened a vein at the elbow, and much blood, of a proper character, flowed; the pains were abated, but the dry coughs continued. On the twenty-seventh the fever relapsed; he coughed and brought up much concocted sputum; sediment in urine copious and white. Explanation of the characters: it is probable that the evacuation of the sputum brought about the recovery on the thirty-fourth day (Hippocrates, 1979).

INTRODUCTION

Throughout history, mankind has sought relief from pain and suffering by seeking out those perceived to have a special knowledge of disease states and an ability to cure them. The relationship between patients and physicians is largely shaped by this help-seeking process and by the quality of medical care delivered by physicians. However, the nature of the relationship is also shaped by societal forces; as those forces have changed, the relationship has changed. Indeed, the history of the doctor–patient relationship is best understood by tracing the technological advances in medical diagnosis and treatment in the context of societal forces existing at the time. The interplay of these factors has produced a doctor–patient relationship whose qualities have changed dramatically, particularly during the past few centuries.

The doctor–patient relationship is even now undergoing a transformation as a result of further pressures exerted by societal expectations and technological advances. As with any relationship, its nature will continue to be defined by the expectations brought to the encounter by both parties, the values and belief systems that give rise to those expectations, and the ability of both parties either to meet or to change those expectations in the process of the encounter. This chapter seeks to review the societal forces, medical advances, and the physician's and patient's expectations and values that have exerted such a profound impact on the doctor–patient relationship.

THE AGE OF HIPPOCRATES

The doctor–patient relationship in the Western world was profoundly influenced by the Greek view of health and disease well into the early 19th century. Hippocrates believed that all bodily functions could be related to four humors: blood, mucus, yellow bile, and black bile. Illness resulted from a lack of equilibrium among these four bodily fluids. Usually one humor became too strong and overwhelmed the other three. Hippocrates was convinced that the body was usually able to restore humoral balance on its own; thus, most of his notes consist of descriptions of the nature of these four bodily humors within a given patient, as in Case 1-1. Medicine was viewed as a descriptive science, not one of intervention. Treatment modalities were implemented to assist the body in its effort to restore humoral balance. These interventions consisted mostly of removal of excess humors, such as by bleeding. In Case 1-1, recovery was attributed to the eventual coughing up of excess sputum. Death ensued if this equilibrium was not restored.

The contrast between Hippocrates and the typical New England physician of 1755 is not very great. Like Hippocrates, the New England physician had four basic treatment modalities according to one chronicler of the times: bleeding, vomiting, blistering, and purging (inducing diarrhea, usually with enemas). The patient's symptoms were regarded as the disease itself, not as a sign of the disease (Starr, 1982). Thus, the descriptive phrases commonly employed during that time: "consumption" for tuberculosis, "dropsy" for congestive heart failure, and "yellow fever" for any form of hepatitis.

This symptom orientation was indicative not only of a lack of scientific medical knowledge but also of the powerful position occupied by the patient in the doctor–patient relationship. Physicians came to their patient's homes to attend to them. Patients often requested particular treatments and chose physicians who would agree with their assessments and plans. A natural result of this arrangement was a high degree of social intimacy between the physician and the patient as well as the patient's family. The physician was often expected to sit at the patient's bedside through a portion of the illness.

Patient authority was further reinforced by the conditions of agrarian life existing before the late 19th century, which prohibited dependence on professional medical authority (Starr, 1982). Most care of the sick was undertaken by family members or relatives. If any outside advice was sought, it was usually obtained first from local midwives, wise women, or other nonregular medical practitioners. One such lay practitioner in Illinois in the late 19th century, known as Aunt Glory, explained her treatment of poliomyelitis as follows:

> Why, I'd take and I'd bile me a big yellow yam, then strain off the bilin's an' mix it with corn meal. I'd then sprinkle it with sheep drippin's an let it stand out one night . . . in the dark of the moon. Then I'd say certain words over it, which I ain't a-gwine to tell ye. An' then I'd give the patient a whole tablespoon o' that there liquid every single hour, an in a day he'd be plumb well (Shastid, 1944).

If a physician was consulted it was often done only to obtain what the lay public perceived as stronger cathartics (to purge or induce diarrhea) or emetics (to induce vomiting). Thus, the name physician came from the ability of doctors to prescribe "physics" or drugs.

THE AGE OF ENLIGHTENMENT

Case 1-2. In Mount Meigs . . . a women in the last stages of consumption [tuberculosis] . . . called Dr. Childers to her. Dr. Childers believed in bleeding patients when any signs of fever were present. Presently, the blood came trickling down from the elbow . . . and the poor little woman fainted and fell over. Ah, said Dr. Childers, that is just what I wanted. Now she will be better. She died very soon after he left (Sims, 1889).

Although medicine in the 17th and 18th centuries was strongly influenced by Hippocratic concepts, several philosophical developments occurred that had great importance for the doctor–patient relationship. Medicine during this period was perhaps most influenced by René Descartes' mind–body dualism. This concept encouraged practitioners to view the body as a separate entity and ignore the mind's effect on bodily symptoms. Disease was then viewed as either "organic," meaning that all symptoms originated from a purely biological basis, or "functional," meaning that no biological cause could be found for the patient's symptoms.

The introduction of the concept of scientific reductionism, in which a problem is best solved by reducing it to its component parts, also had a profound effect on medicine. Physicians began applying this framework of science to their profession both in research and in the way they treated their patients. Disease models based on separate organ systems were developed and eventually led to specialization in the diagnosis and treatment of diseases of each organ system. Physicians in the late 17th and early 18th centuries also became much more aggressive in their treatment approaches, leaving behind the Hippocratic tradition of gentle intervention to restore equilibrium to the body. Often the very mention of a fever was equated with frequent copious bloodletting, as in Case 1-2, or purging by use of strong cathartics to induce diarrhea. Mercury was popular because it also caused salivation, believed to be beneficial in relieving the body of bad humors or poisons. Unfortunately, this medical aggressiveness was extremely detrimental for some patients, as in Case 1-2 and in the case of George Washington, who died of bleeding instituted because of his sore throat, but it no doubt encouraged practitioners to delve deeper into the etiology of disease and make advances not allowed by the traditional Hippocratic method.

Aggressive intervention dominated American medical practice in the early 19th century, encouraged by Benjamin Rush and others who greatly influenced several generations of physicians at the University of Pennsylvania. He told his students in 1796: "Be not startled, gentlemen, follow me and I will say there is but one disease in the world." He described this disease as a "morbid excitement induced by capillary tension." He advised but one treatment approach: deplete the body of blood until the patient faints and empty the stomach and intestines by using powerful emetics and cathartics (Starr, 1982). This approach was a far cry from the gentle efforts of the Hippocratic tradition to restore balance and equilibrium to the body.

Despite medicine's heroics, indeed perhaps because of them, the patient still dominated the relationship. This dominance was maintained by the fact that very few physicians in reality had any formal training, and all sorts of people took up the title of Doctor. Only a few had served a 1-year apprenticeship with an experienced physician. Patients would often reject the recommendations of a physician out of hand, and often directly to his face. A young Hungarian physician arriving in New York in 1870 remarked that

> . . . the rank and file of the profession were, as far as general education went, little, if any, above the level of their clientele. And the clientele not only felt this but knew it (Sims, 1889).

The suspicion and mistrust with which most people viewed physicians continued through most of the 19th century bolstered by the growth of democratic rationalism, which supported the idea that every man should be his own doctor, lawyer, carpenter, etc. Any appearance of complexity in medicine was viewed by the public as an imposition by a self-interested class of physicians in order to mystify, deceive, and monopolize. This belief was reflected in the almost uniform rescinding of state medical practice laws by most states in the mid-19th century (Starr, 1982).

Thus, the relationship between physician and patient was dominated by mistrust and skepticism well into the late 19th century. Ironically, this mistrust reached its height during a period when remarkable advances were occurring, advances that would radically change medicine and the doctor–patient relationship.

THE RISE OF SCIENTIFIC MEDICINE

Case 1-3. A woman, fifty years of age, who had been affected with cough and expectoration for several years, and which had gotten much worse within a few months past, came to the hospital on the thirteenth of April, having for the first time been obliged to desist from her ordinary occupation. She looked much older than she was and was very thin. The pulse was quick, skin slightly hot, and the expectoration, which was in moderate quantity consisted of thick yellow sputa, intermixed with much transparent ropy mucus. The stethoscope applied to the anterior and upper part of the right side and to the right axilla detected distinct pectoriloquism [clear transmission of the patients voice]; and in the same places when the patient coughed

> or spoke and still more during respiration, there was heard a tinkling, like that of a small bell which had just stopped ringing, or of a gnat buzzing within a porcelain vase. A mucous rattle, or a strong gurgling, existed in the same points; in all, these phenomena were distinctly perceptible over the whole space from the top of the shoulder to the fourth rib, being only more distinct anteriorly and under the axilla than behind. From these various signs, I made the following diagnosis: Vast tuberculous cavity occupying the whole of the superior lobe of the right lung and containing a small quantity of fluid; tubercles especially at the top of the left and the root of the right lung (Laennec, 1827).

Two discoveries occurred in the 19th century that were to change forever the face of medicine and eventually dispel the mistrust and skepticism held by the public toward physicians. The first was a broadening acceptance of the germ theory of disease made possible by the use of the microscope. The second was the introduction of pathological anatomy in Paris in the mid-19th century. The former helped link changes in the internal organs with specific causative agents. The latter for the first time allowed physicians to correlate outward signs and symptoms of disease with underlying pathological changes in the body. These advances prompted physicians to begin performing "hands-on" physical examinations in an attempt to identify changes in the internal organs and their causes. Prior to this a physician only catalogued a patient's symptoms in the descriptive Hippocratic method and at most examined the tongue or urine.

The advent of a more thorough physical examination of the patient had a profound impact on the doctor–patient relationship. This intimate physical contact between physician and patient created a different sort of relationship, one that placed the physician in a special position of prominence and privilege, as a searcher for hidden clues to the nature of the disease process. Physicians began listening with a new device known as the stethoscope (from the Greek words "chest" and "I view"), invented in 1819 by the French physician René Laennec.

Case 1-3 illustrates the application of this new technology. The Hippocratic method would have concluded with the description of the mucus. In fact, it strongly resembled Case 1-1 up to that point, a reflection of how little medicine had advanced in over 2000 years. With the application of the stethoscope to the patient, however, a door opened to an entirely new world as Laennec proceeded with a detailed description of the inner workings of his patient's lungs as perceived through his new instrument. Even more remarkable is the connection of these physical findings with a diagnosis. The physician could now see and hear things a patient could not. A plethora of devices for elucidating internal clues of disease ensued: the ophthalmoscope, used to visualize the inner eye, in 1850 by Helmholtz; the x ray in 1895 by Roentgen; the sphygmomanometer, used to measure blood pressure, in 1896 by Riva-Rocci; and the electrocardiogram, for tracing the electrical activity of the heart, in 1901 by Einthoven.

People increasingly turned to physicians for assistance as this idea of disease caused by the malfunctioning of internal bodily systems captured their imagination. The symptoms they brought to physicians as recorded in medical records of the turn of the century were increasingly related to the malfunctioning of certain internal organs. This new sensitivity to the inner workings of the body also greatly increased the number of symptoms for which people would seek medical care (Shorter, 1985).

The scientific revolution in medicine was accompanied by profound societal changes. As society became less agrarian and more urban, the distance between physician and patient made consultation increasingly available. This further supported a growing dependency on physicians for medical care and advice. Physician accessibility was markedly improved by the development of the telephone, car, and paved roads. The railroads brought far-away patients to specialists for consultation, allowing physicians to prosper by narrowing their focus.

Simultaneously, the advent of the progressive movement in the late 19th century saw a decline of confidence in the ability of people to diagnose and treat themselves. The progressive movement encouraged acceptance of occupational licensing, as independent professionals and small businessmen fought back against large corporations by gaining protection through licensing of all sorts of professionals: plumbers, barbers, horseshoers, pharmacists, and others (Starr, 1982). This soon included physicians.

At the same time, people increasingly accepted the legitimate complexity of the world around them. As a result, they were more likely to accept the need for expert professionals, including physicians. As the demand for services increased, a physician's dependence on a handful of wealthy patients decreased. Just as the patient was the dominant figure in the doctor–patient relationship in the 18th century, the physician began to occupy that position of prominence in the late 19th century. People were converted into patients.

A change in the locations of patient care also began to affect the doctor–patient relationship. Treatment in offices and hospitals had generally been regarded as a mark of lower status through most of the 19th century (Starr, 1982). By the turn of the century, however, the home was less frequently the site of medical care. As the physician's position and authority began to rise, the patient was expected to come to the physician, a reflection of the belief that the physician's time was more valuable than that of the patient. Urbanization, the transportation revolution, and the rise of hospitals all worked together to reinforce this change in location of care.

By the early 20th century the physician had less and less contact with people in their homes and thus was no longer exposed to the families or the living conditions of the patients they treated. The loss of information from the social and environmental milieus of the patient made the doctor–patient relationship less personal. It also created less opportunity for an understanding of disease processes in a broader context and further promoted a narrowing of interest to the biological aspects of disease only, ignoring family, social, and environmental factors.

Despite their new-found authority, physicians still felt insecure because of competition from a variety of other kinds of medical providers. Eclectic medical movements grew as a result of bitter feuds and divisions within the medical profession itself, resulting in the formation of competitive sects. Patent medicine companies and the large volume of new physicians produced by proprietary medical schools, which operated merely to profit the physicians who operated them, also provided more competition for the practicing physician. Physicians were largely dependent on a lay referral network rather than referral from colleagues and thus were preoccupied with the image they projected to patients.

Medical books of the late 19th century advised physicians to project an image of competency first rather than to concentrate on actual competency itself (Shorter, 1985). Physicians were encouraged to avoid errors in diagnosis and prognosis at all costs, as those errors were felt to be far more damaging to one's reputation than errors in treatment. They were also encouraged to be bold and prompt in their diagnosis and treatment of ordinary disease in order to impress, especially since there were only a handful of truly effective treatments. Thus, physicians were further drawn to active and "heroic" intervention to bolster their image. Less dramatic preventative measures were not even considered. This trend began to dominate the doctor–patient relationship as patients were encouraged to seek medical care for their acute illnesses rather than preventative interventions. Patients came to their physicians expecting prompt and dramatic cures, usually as a result of some new "miracle drug." Rising patient expectations of a cure for their acute illnesses no doubt further encouraged physicians to search for truly effective cures using their new-found scientific tools.

THE ADVENT OF MODERN MEDICINE

Case 1-4. The surgeon's voice was deep, calm and authoritative. It was not raised at any time. . . . I developed a very disagreeable pain in the right calf during the operative procedure. . . . I remember that several times I moved the leg, seeking to ease its position—not exactly an appropriate behavior in the situation. I recall very distinctly the surgeon's voice saying quietly but definitely, "Don't move your leg, Dr. Wertham." My emotional response to this remark is difficult to describe. From that moment on it was unthinkable that I should move my leg, however it felt. The remark had such an authoritative effect on me that—pain or no pain, impulse or no impulse—the idea of moving my leg did not come up again (Pinner & Miller, 1952).

As physicians became more confident in their diagnostic abilities, and as patients came to them with more trust, confidence, and rising expectations, the ability of physicians to successfully treat many diseases increased. This success often had little to do with new treatments or medicines, because truly effective medicines were still largely unavailable in the early 20th century. The success in treatment was more often based on the new trust and confidence patients placed in their doctors. By inspiring confidence and trust in their treatment, many physicians discovered the power of the "placebo effect." Placebo pills became quite popular, and many physicians often concocted their own, both to prevent the pharmacist from "spilling the beans" and to increase the perceived potency of the pill by increasing its bitterness.

The few real treatments that were available supported the physician's new-found claim of authority. Diphtheria antitoxin, made available in the mid-1890s, dramatically reduced the case–fatality ratio of diphtheria. Few parents could resist the impulse to take their child with a sore throat to a physician after the advent of the diphtheria antitoxin, even if the probability of diphtheria was low. This generated a dependence that was easily generalized into other areas where physicians had less ability to treat. Thus, the stature and social position of physicians rose quite rapidly during the early part of this century. Physicians did little to discourage this change, since much of their ability to cure was based on their new-found authority. They often had little else at their disposal.

Reforms in medical education and licensure also had an effect on the doctor–patient relationship. With the growing acceptance of occupational and professional licensure in the 1870s came new state medical practice laws. Over the following decades these laws required stiffer training qualifications for licensure. This produced fewer physicians and distributed more of them into urban settings. Licensing also legitimized physicians and the practice of medicine in the eyes of the public: a group with specialized knowledge that could be trusted to dispense and use this knowledge for the benefit of their patients.

The early 20th century also saw the beginning of a radical change in medical education. As alluded to earlier, most 19th-century medical schools in America were "proprietary" in that they operated largely to profit the physicians who ran them. At the turn of the century approximately 160 such schools existed, with over 25,000 students (Starr, 1982). Most schools offered 2-year programs with no organized curriculum, no laboratories, and no exposure to patients. The most radical departure from this approach to medical education occurred when Johns Hopkins opened its doors in 1893. Built from monies donated by a wealthy Baltimore merchant, it opened with a 4-year course of study and the unheard of admission requirement of an undergraduate degree. A hospital was attached to the school, combining research with clinical practice for the first time. Students spent 2 years studying laboratory sciences, then finished their last 2 years on the hospital wards. Students who once learned their clinical skills in the office of a local practitioner or in the homes of their patients now saw clinical medicine entirely from the perspective of the teaching ward of a hospital.

This marriage of scientific research with hospital practice further removed the locus of medical care from the patient's environment and contributed to the development of a biomedical disease-oriented model that excluded psychosocial factors. This model was supported by basic science research transferred from the laboratory onto the hospital ward. René Descartes' mind–body dualism became thoroughly entrenched as a result of this development. This model of medical education was widely replicated by medical schools throughout the country after the Flexner report of 1910.

Abraham Flexner was the man chosen by the Carnegie Foundation to conduct an investigation of then existing medical schools at the invitation of the American Medical Association's (AMA) Council on Medical Education. He was met with open arms at most schools, as administrations assumed he was on a scouting mission for the philanthropist who would supply desperately needed money to some schools. Flexner's report was full of details and uncovered the false claims made by many if not most of the weaker proprietary schools: libraries with no books, laboratories with no equipment, and admission requirements waived for those with the required fee. Flexner went even further and made very specific recommendations largely based on the model created by Johns Hopkins. His report was more successful in limiting the number of medical schools and graduates than any action the AMA could have taken. By 1915 the number of medical schools dropped to 95, and the number of graduates to 3556 (Starr, 1982). Most schools closed, and the few remaining adopted the Johns Hopkins model of clinical practice, teaching, and research. Academic medicine drew away from an emphasis on private clinical practice. Medical research began to take center stage. The doctor–patient relationship was now secondary to the emerging science of medical practice.

THE REIGN OF TECHNOLOGY

Case 1-5. Mrs. J. was a 41-year-old housewife with a husband on disability from diagnosed coronary artery disease, a 16-year-old son with a delinquent record, and a 5-year-old mentally retarded daughter with inoperable congenital heart disease. Mrs. J. was admitted to the hospital in severe respiratory distress. She had neglected her own medical needs over the past several years because she was caring for her disabled husband and daughter. Two months prior to admission her symptoms worsened, and by the time of admission she was no longer able to preform her household duties.

On physical exam she was breathing quite rapidly. The patient was told by the doctor that it was necessary to insert a nasal trachea tube to control her ventilation with a volume-cycled ventilator, to begin intensive respiratory therapy, and to transfer her to the intensive care unit. The patient pleaded, "Please let me go home. We have no money to pay you. I have to go home to take care of my daughter and husband." The physician considered her behavior inappropriate, the result of a mental state created by the low oxygen and high carbon dioxide levels indicated by laboratory tests. Ventilatory support of the patient was complicated by several episodes of pneumonia. It became apparent that unless an operation was performed to correct large bullae (empty lung cavities that impair oxygen exchange) in both upper lung fields, the patient would have no improvement in gaseous exchange and would be unable to care for her family and home.

The patient underwent surgery, and the operation was successful. During the postoperative period a dispute arose between the respiratory therapist and the physician concerning the appropriate time and manner of weaning the patient from the ventilator. They finally reached a mutually satisfactory decision, but the dispute troubled the staff and the patient, who was aware of the dispute. The patient's recovery was gradual, and she was ready for discharge after 90 hospital days, still requiring supplemental oxygen, suction equipment, and ventilation assistance four times a day. For these needs, equipment was placed in her home to maintain her there. A visiting nurse called on the family weekly.

The total hospital bill was $250,798, and the husband signed the house mortgage and his life insurance policy over to the hospital. The family would live on welfare and Medicaid assistance. The average monthly bill for oxygen in the home alone was $275. Nine months after the patient's discharge from the hospital, her husband died of a heart attack. Her son, who needed money to support the family, was arrested for armed robbery 1 month later. The daughter died 6 months after the father. One year after her operation the respiratory crippled woman was able to pursue her activities of daily living. However, 4 years after surgery, Mrs. J. finally succumbed to the complications of her illness. The cause of death was respiratory failure (Reiser & Anbar, 1984).

The increasing use and dependency on instruments to provide information concerning health and disease had a great impact on the doctor–patient relationship. As one medical chronicler observed, their use not only required the physician to "isolate himself in a world of sounds inaudible to the patient," but also encouraged him to "move away from involvement with the patient experiences and sensations, to a more detached relation, less with the patient but more with sounds from the body" (Reiser, 1978). The net effect was to reduce reliance on the patient's recounting of symptoms.

Patient acceptance of new technology, and indeed even expectation that it must be used to correctly diagnose and adequately treat any symptom, allowed physicians to occupy a more powerful position of authority in the relationship. Physicians spent more time "backstage" with the result of tests and procedures, usually in conference with other specialist colleagues. This added further credence to their opinion by buttressing it with the opinions of other specialists. This reliance on new-found technology reduced the strong emphasis on history and physical exam skills needed at the turn of the century. The physician's traditional "hands-on" physical exam was seen as less reliable than available x-ray and laboratory tests. Thus, the relationship between patient and physician became less intimate. Dr. William Osler, a physician known as a clinician's clinician, bemoaned this new trend in 1905 by stating:

> And finally every medical student should remember that his end is not to be made a chemist or physiologist or anatomist, but to learn how to recognize and treat disease, how to become a practical physician (Osler, 1985).

This new style of medical practice gathered "steam" in the 1940s with the revolution in drug therapy begun by the discovery of penicillin. Infections were once considered a terrible calamity often resulting in the loss of toes, feet, or entire limbs in an effort to save a patient's life. Following the advent of penicillin came a deluge of truly effective drugs, not only for infection but for inflammation, heart disease, and diseases of the central nervous system. The effect of this revolution in therapy was to reinstill a relentless enthusiasm for treating organic disease based on an increasingly reductionistic view of the human body. No longer were there specialists who just dealt with organs such as lungs or the heart; there now arose specialists who dealt with disease at the microscopic level such as immunologists, who studied the body's ability to fight disease, and endocrinologists, who studied physiological regulatory mechanisms mediated by hormones.

During this time it was recognized by some that this emphasis on technological medicine was perhaps deficient in some ways. An associate dean of the London Medical School in 1956 stated:

> It is not that American medical students take poor histories and make poor examinations, it is that they appear to suffer from a lack of balance between their knowledge of medicine and their knowledge of diseased people (Ellis, 1956).

An attending physician recounts the story of a student presentation of a case submitted to the medical service after a suicide attempt. The medical student's workup included the following: "Social history: noncontributory" (Feldman, 1978).

Is it any wonder that patients in the 1960s felt more alienated from their doctors than those in the 1920s? By the end of the 1960s physicians found themselves facing an entirely new kind of patient no longer willing to accept physician's authority. Cases like Case 1-5 made this lack of acceptance more common as the indiscriminant use of technology saved lives but often had an adverse effect on the quality of the patient's life. Patients demanded greater input into the selection of therapy and diagnostic tests. They also obtained more sophisticated information about their medical problems through the mass media, especially television and magazines. Because of this new knowledge, patients were much more likely to seek alternative sources of health information as well as alternative therapies, much as the patient of the 18th century once sought alternative healers. A veritable explosion of alternative health movements ensued, many of them critical of the monopoly by physicians over the control and release of prescription medication. A survey in the late 1970s of 98 arthritic patients revealed that 93 had tried some alternative remedies such as liniments, copper jewelry, special diets, and self-dosing of medications acquired from foreign countries that were not allowed on American drug store shelves (Shorter, 1985).

Recently, physicians seem to have drawn their "medical wagons into a circle" as a result of attacks by patients on their motivation, integrity, and even their ability to help. The doctor–patient relationship at times seems to be more like a battleground than a relationship where healing can take place. As a result there has been a reexamination of the current reductionistic biomedical model that has dominated Western medical care for the last half-century. Increasing attention is being paid to new paradigms of medical care. A rallying cry was issued by psychiatrist George L. Engel (1977). Engel states:

> To provide a basis for understanding the determinants of disease and arriving at rational treatments in patterns of health care, a medical model must also take into account the patient, the social context in which he lives, and the complementary system devised by society to deal with the disruptive effects of illness, that is, the physician's role and the health care system. By evaluating all the factors contributing to both illness and patienthood rather than giving primacy to biologic factors alone, a biopsychosocial model would make it possible to explain why some individuals experience as "illness" conditions which others regard merely as "problems of living," be they emotional reactions to life circumstances or somatic symptoms.

Ian R. McWhinney (1986) reinforces this call for a new model:

> The transformed clinical method will be patient-centered rather than doctor-centered. The essence of the patient-centered method is that physicians try to enter the patient's world and to see the illness through the patient's eyes. In the traditional doctor-centered method physicians try to bring the patient's illness into their own world and to interpret the illness in terms of their own pathologic frame of reference.

CONCLUSION

The doctor–patient relationship was dominated by the Hippocratic model until very recently. This traditional approach emphasized a disease model based on a loss of equilibrium between bodily humors. The physician was relegated to a descriptive style of practice, and intervention was a gentle attempt to restore balance to the body. The patient occupied a position of prominence in the relationship, and medical authority was limited, largely because of a lack of effective treatments. Physicians usually visited patients in their home and thus had the advantage of developing insight into the psychosocial and environmental conditions existing during a patient's illness.

The Enlightenment introduced the concepts of mind–body dualism and scientific reductionism to medicine. Patients eventually became known as "the gallbladder case" or "the lady with the functional bowel syndrome" as a result of an emphasis on purely organic illness. The effect of the mind on bodily symptoms was virtually ignored. A new medical aggressiveness was instituted in order to bolster the image of the doctor by emphasizing heroic interventions rather than preventative strategies.

With the advent of pathological anatomy and the germ theory of disease, physicians and their patients developed a more intimate encounter through a more complete physical examination. The use of medical instruments placed the physician in a more prominent position as the one searching for hidden clues of disease states. Growing acceptance of professional medical authority by the patient was reflected in the passage of state medical practice laws in the 1870s. The change from rural to urban life along with the telephone and improved roads and rail travel completed the development of a growing dependency on medical professionals for advice and treatment. The locus of medical care moved from the home to the office or hospital. The stature of the physician in the relationship continued to rise as a result, but doctors lost some insight into the context of their patients' illnesses.

The changes in medical education brought about by the Johns Hopkins model of medical education and Flexner Report of 1910 not only limited the supply of physicians through closure of many medical schools but also forever bound medical research to clinical practice. The physician's view of medical practice was dominated by the hospital ward experience instead of the office or the patient's home. The doctor–patient relationship became secondary to the emerging science of medical practice.

The veritable explosion of new drugs and technology since the 1940s has moved the physician farther away from the patient's bedside and into the laboratory, x-ray suite, or procedure room. Patients have felt more disenfranchised from their medical care than ever before. As a result, they have demanded more information and more input into decision making. The doctor–patient relationship has begun to resemble a battleground as demands are made and expectations of instant cures are raised to an all-time high. Alternative health movements have grown in popularity. A cry for a new model of medical care has been heard, one that takes into consideration the patient, the context in which he or she lives, and the impact of that context on the patient's disease. These developments are summarized in Table 1-1.

Table 1-1
The Development of the Doctor–Patient Relationship

Era/time period	Disease model/ characteristics of the doctor–patient relationship	Location of care	New developments	Problems
Age of Hippocrates/ before 1700s	Humoral balance/descriptive home medicine, no intimacy or contact, gentle interventions, patient dominant	Home	Emphasis on observing and describing illness	Inability to diagnose, no truly effective treatments available
Age of Enlightenment/ 1700s to mid-1800s	Still mostly Hippocratic/ increased aggressiveness in treatment, patient dominant	Home	Mind–body dualism, scientific reductionism	Inability to diagnose, no truly effective treatments available
Rise of scientific medicine/mid-1800s to early 1900s	Biomedical/hands-on physical exam increases intimacy, physician dominant	Office, hospital	Pathological anatomy, germ theory, diagnostic instruments	Few effective treatments, loss of insight into patient's home and family life with changing loci of care
Advent of modern medicine/early 1900s to 1940s	Biomedical/patient dependence on medical authority, placebo effect	Office, hospital	Medical education reform, emphasis on medical research with development of many effective treatments against infectious diseases	Biomedical disease model achieves predominance with continued loss of insight into the patient's context, growing dominance of medical research over clinical practice
Reign of technology/ 1940s to present	Biotechnical/technology creates distance between patient and physician; patients question and often reject medical authority	Office, hospital, laboratory, procedure room	Dominance of technology, proliferation of effective drugs and treatments against many diseases	Attacks by consumer groups on organized medicine, no insight into psychosocial aspects of care, medical care becomes very expensive

The doctor–patient relationship is entering a challenging era because of a mismatch among our technological abilities, societal expectations of what medical technology can offer, and the limited resources available to meet those expectations. At the center of this controversy remains the quite personal, usually overlooked, intimate relationship between patients and physicians as they seek not only to cure diseases but to optimize quality of life and discover hope through the process of relationship.

CASES FOR DISCUSSION

Case 1

I called on Mistress Paradine of Bedford, a linen draper, who on the 26th of that month [June, 1637] had returned from London (but this fact the messenger concealed from me). She fell ill on the journey and when she reached home on the 27th she collapsed, felt pain all over her body, [and] could not sleep. On the 28th she vomited much and was prostrated by a very bad headache, yet she got up for the greater part of the day. Along with the vomiting she was racked by a hiccough, together with a flux of blood from the nose which was thought to be up to ten ounces.

A surgeon of the name of Rowland, a resident of that town, applied dry cupping glasses to the stomach and umbilicus and left them for some time, but they had no effect on the hiccough. Her pulse was hard, deep, swift, and tumid, and I thought it a bad sign that a sweat broke out over her whole body. She was very thirsty and asked for drink; we gave it to her, but the cold drinks made the hiccough, which had stopped for some time, start again. She was still unable to sleep.

On July 1st, Mr. Woodcock of Ampthill, who had arrived long after me on the previous night, accompanied me on my visit to the patient. The urine, as on the preceding days, was turbid, highly colored, and appeared to be slightly blackish in spots. The pulse was fast, jumpy and occasionally intermitting. Mr. Woodcock wanted to let blood; I was against it, but he was importunate and I assented only on condition that no more than five ounces was taken, it was agreed. The blood was drawn; nobody was at fault. The pulse then became weaker and frequently intermitted; advice was given about diet, medicine and other things required for the future, and everything was entrusted to Rowland.

We left the bedside and were just about to leave for breakfast when the woman made a sign to her husband to enquire about the pain in her abdomen. Straightway he urged Rowland to see what it was and to look and see if any plague bubos were coming up. The latter did so and asserted most emphatically that a bubo had broken out in her groin. There was little for us to advise in this case (Poynter & Bishop, 1951).

1. The physical exam of this patient is limited to what one item?
2. The treatment modalities used were based on what dominant medical viewpoint of the time?

3. What three treatments were attempted?
4. The correct diagnosis was made at the insistence of which party, the physician or the patient? Who was the dominant figure in this relationship?

Case 2

The patient whom we shall discuss today is an example of the more severe form of stomach dyspepsia. She is an Irish servant girl, forty years old. About two years ago she began to have pain and vomiting after her meals. After nine weeks these symptoms ceased, and she enjoyed tolerable health until eight months ago. At that time, she again began to vomit about fifteen minutes after eating. At the same time, there was a dull boring pain in the epigastric region and extending into the back. She has never vomited blood. The pain and vomiting continued; she became much emaciated and was so feeble as to remain in bed much of the time. Her appetite continued to be good; her bowels were somewhat constipated. I saw her for the first time five months after the commencement of her illness. She was then very feeble and emaciated. She had been put under a variety of medical treatment and had been kept on a milk diet for some time, but without relief. The pain and vomiting would cease for a few hours or a few days and then return.

In the epigastric region was a globular tumor, tympanitic on percussion, which I supposed to be the dilated stomach. At that time, three months ago, I stopped all drugs and washed out her stomach with the stomach pump everyday. This treatment was continued, with occasional intermissions, for two months. The pain and vomiting became less frequent and then ceased entirely. She has steadily recovered her strength and flesh and is now able to work. For the past month the pumping has been discontinued, and her health has continued good (Delafield, 1885).

1. What is the most striking feature of this narrative?
2. What period was characterized by this aggressive form of treatment?
3. What impact did this type of therapy have on the physician-patient relationship?

Case 3

. . . We describe a condition—“liquor lung”—in which hemoptysis was produced by the aspiration of Bucca. . . .

A 22-year-old healthy nonsmoking man presented after coughing up a cup of bright red blood. The initial history and physical examination were unrevealing.

1. What period of medicine does this case resemble thus far? Why?

A chest roentgenogram, arterial blood gas levels, the complete blood count, indexes of coagulation, the platelet count, and the blood urea nitrogen concentration were all normal.

2. Now what period does this case appear to represent? Why?

Bronchoscopy with a flexible fiberoptic instrument was performed within 24 h, since the hemoptysis totaled 75 ml of blood. The trachea and right mainstem bronchus were erythematous and friable and contained a small quantity of fresh blood. No infectious organisms or neoplastic cells were found in the tracheobronchial specimens submitted for analysis. The bronchoscopic findings prompted additional questioning of the patient. He revealed that he had experienced a coughing paroxysm the previous evening. He had been at a party and had "guzzled from a bottle of Bucca." While drinking in this manner he began to choke and cough repeatedly. A few hours later frank hemoptysis began (Conetta, Tamarin, Wogalter, & Brandstetter, 1987).

3. Why is dialogue, as a method of scientific inquiry, bypassed in favor of diagnostic procedures in our current model of health care, as illustrated in the above account?

Case 4

T.J. is a premature infant born 10 weeks before the mother's due date and only weighed 1100 g at birth. Normal birth weight for a full-term baby is about 2500 g. T.J. was born to an 18 year old mother at a community hospital, 3 h outside of Oklahoma City. At 2 hours of age, T.J. began to experience difficulty breathing from a condition known as hyaline membrane disease in which the lungs are not mature enough to provide adequate oxygen to the blood. The parents were informed that the infant is critically ill and must be transferred to the neonatal unit in Oklahoma City in order to receive proper care. Oxygen was administered, and a decision was made to transfer to the medical center via helicopter to save precious time.

On arrival at the local hospital, the flight team expertly assessed the infant's rapidly deteriorating condition by measuring the amount of oxygen in the blood, and a decision was made to pass an endotracheal tube into the infant's windpipe to assist the infant's breathing ability. This was attached to a ventilator. Next, a small tube, or catheter, was passed into a vessel in the infant's umbilical stump in order to obtain access to the circulatory system in case special drugs were needed. This tube also allows blood to be taken so that the oxygen content can be measured.

Once stabilized the infant was transferred in a self-contained incubator into the helicopter, and the flight was made in less than an hour back to the city. The parents were not able to see T.J. until 2 days later, when the mother was able to travel. Both are unemployed. The hospital social worker is actively involved in analyzing the needs of the young teenage couple but has doubts about their ability to cope with this grave situation. T.J. does well for 5 days and then suddenly takes a turn for the worse. All the evidence points to intercranial bleeding, a common complication of extremely premature infants. A special type of ultrasound test is performed on the head and confirms the diagnosis. Permanent brain damage almost certainly exists, and this new development makes that even more certain. The parents feel overwhelmed in the large medical center and passively accept whatever recommendations are made. The neurology consulting team is unable to provide definitive answers about the extent of the damage, and so the decision is made to continue to support the infant.

1. What expectations does our current society have concerning the outcome of pregnancy?
2. How do these expectations impact on the doctor–patient relationship in this case?
3. With whom should the decision lie to both apply and remove lifesaving technology? How does one define the role of the physician, the parents, and "expected standards of care" in this decision-making process?

Case 5

Mrs. ______ with her daughter, after an opinion by myself that the daughter's trouble was purely "bronchial." "Sure," says the mother, "Doctor, you didn't try the little glass thing that goes in the mouth? Sure, Mrs. Mc______ told me that you would put a little glass thing in her mouth, and that would tell just where the disease was, entirely." I used the "little glass thing" and thereby suited the interested mother at once; and I dare say, that while my opinion was taken as absolute after using the thermometer, it would not have been taken had I not used it; but a doctor would have been found who used the "glass thing." Again, where will it end? Shall we practice regular deceit, or shall we bulletin at each visit the exact condition to friends and patient (Reiser, 1978)?

1. Thermometry developed as a highly regarded technique in the 18th century. What is the mother suggesting about the physician's credibility as it relates to use of the thermometer?
2. What do patients place similar faith in today as methods of diagnosis?
3. How do these expectations affect physician behavior?

RECOMMENDED READINGS

Starr, P. (1982). *The social transformation of American medicine.* New York: Basic Books.

Perhaps the most comprehensive, in-depth examination of the history of medicine in America. It provides a depth of perspective and insight into the social trends and development that resulted in our current system of medicine that no other work can provide.

Shorter, B. (1985). *Bedside manners: The troubled history of doctors and patients.* New York: Simon and Schuster.

Shorter weaves anecdote, history, and science into a thorough examination of the evolution of the doctor–patient relationship. Although critical of the current status quo, he provides needed insight into the historical forces leading up to our present system of care.

Reiser, S. J. (1978). *Medicine and the reign of technology.* Cambridge: Cambridge University Press.

A remarkable exploration of the history of technological advances from the 17th and 18th centuries to the present day. Reiser also goes beyond a new descriptive approach and explores the implications of each new development and its effect on the doctor, the patient, and the medical care establishment.

CHAPTER 2

Philosophical and Ethical Foundations of the Physician–Patient Relationship

Richard A. Wright

Case 2-1. A second-year resident was called to the emergency room at 2 A.M. to care for a 21-year-old insulin-dependent diabetic (IDDM) who came in with acute diabetic ketoacidosis (DKA). The patient was J.S., a noncompliant, unemployed high school dropout with frequent DKA admissions, so the resident got up slowly and ambled down to see J.S.

On arrival in the emergency room, the resident found J.S. nearly comatose although able to answer a few questions coherently. It appeared that J.S. had not been injecting himself with insulin over the past 2 weeks and had not been following his diet. After examining laboratory data, the resident reluctantly admitted the patient to the intensive care unit.

Once J.S. was in the intensive care unit and initial treatment had begun, the resident knew a complete physical exam was necessary. The resident was tired, did not particularly like J.S. or his dirtiness, and had just received a page to admit a patient with a myocardial infarction. There was time to perform the physical exam, however, since the patient with the myocardial infarction was stable, so, reluctantly, he began the examination.

Having completed everything but a rectal examination, the resident stopped. He didn't particularly like performing rectals, and J.S.'s personality and odor did not make it any easier.

After thinking about it, the resident decided to perform the rectal exam because he knew a rectal infection could precipitate DKA. To the resident's amazement, the exam revealed a very tender 4×5-cm perirectal abscess. The resident then requested a surgical consultant who agreed that the abscess should be incised and drained.

After the incision and drainage of the perirectal abscess, J.S.'s diabetes was brought under rapid control, and he was discharged 5 days later. Two months later the resident was once again called to the ER in the middle of the night to care for J.S., once again in DKA.

INTRODUCTION

Throughout the history of medicine the physician–patient relationship (PPR) has been of great importance. In fact, the success of medical practice, as well as the nature of the practice itself, depends entirely on how the physician understands and utilizes the PPR.

Although physicians think frequently about this relationship, they have generally not thought through the various dimensions of this most important element of their practice. Unfortunately, everyone has an idea of what medicine is all about and how it should be practiced. Changes in the structure and values of society (Engelhardt, 1983) and changes in the way medicine is practiced (Veatch, 1983) add significant diversity to these ideas. However, since people's ideas about the PPR are most often unconscious or poorly articulated, a consistent general understanding of the relationship is not easy to identify. This chapter is designed to give a general outline of the PPR that will allow physicians to better understand the PPR and how they, their patients, and their colleagues may understand it. For there *is* diversity, and there *is* some disagreement about how the relationship should be structured.

Because the PPR affects all of the physician's interactions, it must be understood in a general way, not based on unique situations (Bayles, 1989). Fortunately, some significant components of the PPR are agreed on and understood. Learning about these components allows an understanding of the PPR that is abstract enough to cover the whole of one's practice yet specific enough to be useful in particular cases.

The application of medical science, the clinical practice of medicine, embodies the multifaceted relationship between the physician and the person receiving care. Those who come together in that relationship are unique individuals with little or no interaction except through the PPR. Guided almost exclusively by the clinical needs of the patient, the interaction is not only occasional, it is highly specific and quite selective. Thus, in Case 2-1, we cannot imagine J.S. and the

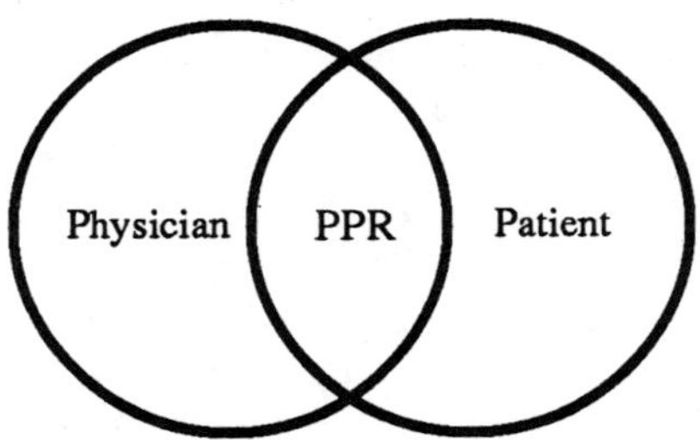

Figure 2-1. Spheres of Interaction.

resident coming together except through the PPR. Moreover, their relationship is fully defined by the clinical needs of the patient at the time.

The diagram in Fig. 2-1 portrays this relationship; by representing each participant by a circle, we see that the PPR forms an intersecting set of concerns.

Consideration of the PPR does not end with noticing that the physician's and patient's spheres of life intersect in that relationship; rather, it is important to fully analyze and understand all the components of that intersecting relationship. The first thing that must be understood is that the PPR is not simplistic and, moreover, has important components of ethics as its fundamental base. As Beauchamp and McCullough (1984) have shown in their book *Medical Ethics: The Moral Responsibility of Physicians,* a complete understanding of the practice of medicine has four basic elements:

1. The general *moral end* of medicine to promote the patient's best interest.
2. A *principle* that provides the moral significance of distinct perspectives on the patient's best interest.
3. *Obligations* (or duties) that derive from this principle.
4. *Virtues* that derive from this principle.

Any attempt to understand the PPR must focus on these four elements. The basic premise of this text is that the moral end of medicine **is** promoting the patient's best interest. This chapter thus deals with the basic principles of medical practice and the obligations of the practitioner. The ethical foundations of practice (the virtues) are discussed in Chapter 12.

The most important thing to recognize, however, is that the PPR is, above all else, a social interaction. Physicians thus have the same basic obligation toward their patients as each human being has to one another (Clouser, 1983). Additionally, aspects of the PPR either are unique to medical practice or are significant to medical practice in ways that may be different from other professions. Development of the characteristics of the PPR in this chapter involves not only the historical basis for the relationship as it is now understood but also some of the alternative ways in which the relationship can be structured and the underlying structure of the medical decision making on which it is based.

Oath of Hippocrates. I swear by Apollo Physician and Asclepius and Hygieia and Panaceia and all the gods and goddesses, making them my witness, that I will fulfil according to my ability and judgment this oath and this covenant:

To hold him who has taught me this art as equal to my parents and to live my life in partnership with him, and if he is in need of money to give him a share of mine, and to regard his offspring as equal to my brothers in male lineage and to teach them this art—if they desire to learn it—without fee and covenant; to give a share of precepts and oral instruction and all the other learning to my sons and to the sons of him who has instructed me and to pupils who have signed the covenant and have taken an oath according to the medical law, but to no one else.

I will apply dietetic measures *for the benefit of the sick* according to my ability and judgment; *I will keep them from harm and injustice.*

I will neither give a deadly drug to anybody if asked for it, *nor will I make a suggestion to this effect.* Similarly, *I will not give a woman an abortive remedy.* In purity and holiness I will guard my life and my art.

I will not use the knife, not even on sufferers from stone, but will withdraw in favor of such men as are engaged in this work.

Whatever houses I may visit, I will come *for the benefit of the sick,* remaining *free of all intentional injustice,* of all mischief and in particular of sexual relations with both female and male persons, be they free or slaves.

What I may see or hear in the course of the treatment or even outside of the treatment in regard to the life of men, which on no account one must spread abroad, I will keep to myself holding such things shameful to be spoken about.

If I fulfil this oath and do not violate it, may it be granted to me to enjoy life and art, being honored with fame among all men for all time to come; if I transgress it and swear falsely, may the opposite of all this be my lot (Edelstein, 1943, p. 3; italics added).

PRINCIPLES OF PRACTICE

The history of medicine, not only in our own culture but in other cultures as well, contains significant writing and discussion focused on how the physician and the patient should interact. The Oath of Hippocrates has been the most important Western influence on the development of the physician–patient relationship, including the practice of medicine in the 20th century. This oath, although not taken as an oath by many physicians today, still contains important elements of the physician–patient relationship as it is now known.

Careful examination of this oath shows two different components: first, discussion of appropriate and inappropriate types of treatment; and, second, specific guidelines regarding ways of interacting with others. This chapter focuses almost exclusively on the ways of interacting, because the types of treatment that are discussed may not be appropriate in all situations. Recognize, however, that accepting a treatment prohibition affects the PPR by eliminating certain kinds of actions that a physician may be willing to perform within a patient care situation.

The most widely recognized component of the PPR to arise from the Hippocratic Oath is the injunction against doing harm. With this single statement, the Hippocratic Oath has done more to influence our understanding of health care than anything else. For on the basis of this statement, physicians are enjoined from any action that would intentionally harm the individual being given care. Notice, however, that this prohibition against harm does not prevent medical practices, since some practices can be harmful in the sense of causing pain and suffering. For example, we now know that bleeding a person is harmful and generally without therapeutic benefit. Yet the physicians who used bleeding were not intentionally harming their patients because they *thought* it was beneficial. If a physician today were to bleed a person, except in very specific situations (e.g., hemachromatosis), it *would* be harmful, because he or she should know better.

The important point here is that a physician is enjoined from ever undertaking those actions that will, to his or her best knowledge, do nothing but harm the person. The physician's requirement then is to do good if at all possible and to studiously and carefully avoid intentional harm. The doing of good and the avoidance of harm have throughout history been articulated via two basic principles: the principle of beneficence (doing good) and the principle of nonmaleficence (the prevention of harm) (Beauchamp & Childress, 1989).

Although these two principles have been applied throughout the history of medicine, their emphasis has changed (Duffy, 1983). In Great Britain and the United States, both principles became crucial components of the codes of practice for health care professions. Thus, for example, Thomas Percival asserts that medicine should be "founded on principles of the purest beneficence." Accordingly, the physician

> . . . should be the minister of hope and comfort to the sick; that by such cordials to the drooping spirit, he may smooth the bed of death, revive expiring life, and counteract the depressing influence of those maladies which rob the philosopher of fortitude, and the Christian of consolation (Percival, 1803).

Because Percival's writings became the basis for the code of practice of the British Medical Association, this rendition of the Hippocratic tradition was carried forward into 19th century British medical practices. Similarly, because the British medical codes were almost wholly transferred to American medicine, we see a similar emphasis in the United States. The first code of the American Medical Association thus says:

> . . . His counsels, or even remonstrances, will give satisfaction, not offence, if they be proffered with politeness, and evince a genuine love of virtue, accompanied by a sincere interest in the welfare of the person to whom they are addressed. . . . Equally derogatory to professional character is it, for a physician to hold a patent for any surgical instrument, or medicine; or to dispense a secret nostrum, whether it be the composition or exclusive property of himself, or of others. For, if such nostrum be of real efficacy, any concealment regarding it is inconsistent with beneficence . . . (AMA, 1848).

The Oath of Hippocrates is also the origin of a third principle of the PPR, the principle of justice. The oath enjoins physicians to protect the patient from injustice and to prevent "intentional" injustice. Although there might be a difference between these two, the importance lies in the specific injunction to uphold justice.

In this context, as subsequently developed, the term "justice" has several meanings. First, as a legal term, its use attributes compliance with the rules and guidelines of an existing legal system. Second, as a term prevalent in the study of ethics, its use attributes an understanding of how our resources will be distributed. The second sense is the focus for our understanding of the PPR, because the PPR is essentially an ethical relationship (despite its legal overtones).

Justice requires that the PPR be structured so the physician not only does good for the patient, and as much as possible prevents harm, but accomplishes these ends according to basic principles of equality and fairness (Rawls, 1971; Arthur & Shaw, 1978; Barrow, 1982). It is thus inappropriate for a physician to intentionally discriminate against patients in the quality or type of care that they receive. Thus, in Case 2-1, for example, the resident cannot refuse to care for J.S. despite disapproval of J.S.'s lifestyle, lack of compliance, and middle-of-the-night care pattern. To do so would be unjust and unacceptable.

This does not mean that a physician is required to care for everyone, nor does it mean that the physician must care equally for everyone. Rather, the principle of justice means that those for whom the physician does care will be treated in an equally caring way (Noddings, 1989). It further means (at least in the context of the Hippocratic Oath) that the physician has a social responsibility to assure that this level of equality pervades the system. The exact nature of this responsibility to justice, both at the individual and the societal level, is not yet fully developed but has become increasingly important in the 1990s as health care funding problems have emerged.

The final principle that is important to the physician–patient relationship does not arise essentially from the Hippocratic tradition but instead from the interaction among patients, physicians, and the legal system of contemporary society. The principle of autonomy, also known as the principle of self-determination, was first formally introduced into medical practices by a court decision in 1914. In the now famous case of *Scholendorff v. The Society of New York Hospital*, Judge Benjamin Cardozo applied the force of law to the principle of autonomy in medical practices when he ruled that:

> . . . every human being of adult years and sound mind has a right to determine what shall be done with his own body; and a surgeon who performs an operation without his patient's consent commits an assault for which he is liable in damages (*Scholendorff v. The Society of New York Hospital*, 1914).

Judge Cardozo's statement was directed toward surgery because the case being tried was a surgical case. That case, nonetheless, formed a basis for several other cases and, through our system of legal precedent, expanded gradually but surely to nonsurgeons as well. It is important to note that the judge is not *giving* a patient the right of self-determination; rather, the judge is recognizing that such a right *already exists* and is applying the law as a force to uphold that right. More recently, court rulings have consistently upheld not only this basic right to autonomy but a correlative right to informed consent and the right to refuse treatment, including life support.

In addition to the court rulings just noted, the American Hospital Association in 1972 put forward for the first time a document entitled *The Patient's Bill of Rights*. Although this document has only 12 stipulated rights, eight of those relate to the patient's right to knowledge and informed consent, i.e., to the patient's right to autonomous decision making. This document, plus others that were issued subsequent to it, together with the growing consumerism and increased education of persons about their rights in health care, has made autonomy not only an important factor in health care, but an important factor in medical malpractice as well. As a result, the role of patient autonomy has become a crucial factor in considering the physician–patient relationship.

These four principles—beneficence, nonmaleficence, justice, and autonomy—underlie the practice of medicine. However, all the principles are not necessarily utilized at the same time, especially when a course of action involves a conflict between principles. As a result, each physician usually focuses on one or two of the principles to guide his or her practice, with the others subordinated to the primary ones.

The problem, of course, is to determine which of the principles should take precedence. Beauchamp and McCullough (1984), for example, focus on beneficence and autonomy as the primary principles underlying practice. They point out how medical practice changes depending on whether physicians are trying to produce the greatest amount of good or trying to promote autonomous decisions, and argue for a balance between both principles. Veatch (1972), on the other hand, argues that only by respecting autonomy and promoting justice can a medical practice be morally sound; and most recently, Pellegrino and Thomasma (1988) focus solely on beneficence as the basic principle according to which medicine should be practiced. This variation in adoption of a basic principle may appear inconclusive and frustrating. However, as Beauchamp and McCullough (1984) point out:

> A central task of medical ethics is thus to fix the limits of [competing] models in light of the demands of [each] other. Because [different] perspectives merit consideration, discretion is required in clinical decision making (p. 51).

Thus, each physician must understand the basic principles and how their application affects his or her practice. When this understanding has been reached, a basic model of practice can be formulated.

It is important to note, however, that none of the four principles is self-sufficient. *Together* they form a foundation on which the PPR will be built. That foundation, which grows out of the historical traditions of health care practice, enables physicians to look in more detail at various ways to establish their framework of practice.

FRAMEWORK OF PRACTICE

Case 2-2. Karen Rebikov, a 16-year-old high school junior, was diagnosed as having an oat-cell cancer of the leg. Although chemotherapy may be of some help, amputation plus chemotherapy has an excellent 10-year survival rate. Karen agrees to the chemotherapy; however, she refuses surgery because, she says, "I would rather die than lose my leg." Her surgeon is quite upset about this, as she believes Karen's refusal is unreasonable. From the surgeon's perspective, it is not acceptable to refuse surgery, which is relatively uncomplicated, with a low mortality rate and a high cure rate. As a means of helping Karen change her mind, she arranges for Karen to visit with Mark Williams, a handsome 17-year-old football player who had an amputation, although not for cancer. Mark comes and talks with Karen, after which the surgeon again visits. Karen changes her mind and agrees to the surgery. Her comment to the surgeon is, "Well, if the amputation can cure Mark's cancer, and he can still do everything he wants except play football, I guess it is dumb for me to refuse." The surgeon does not challenge her misunderstanding of Mark's condition; she believes that the surgery is in Karen's best interests. The surgery is scheduled and performed the next day.

At the beginning of the 20th century, medicine began a significant turn toward what we now know as medical science. This change encouraged a refocusing of medical practice from the individual person who was receiving care to the disease process itself. This meant that there was a shift in the conceptual framework within which medicine was practiced. This section discusses two different versions of that framework and shows how each significantly affects the PPR.

Paul Ramsey (1970) was a strong proponent of moving away from the growing medical–scientific framework of practice established in the early 1900s. His book, *The Patient as Person,* articulated an understanding of the need to treat patients not as objects of medical science but as persons with feelings, hopes, desires, and ideas of their own. The two frameworks for medical practice were not consistently articulated, however, until "Two Philosophies of Caring" by Gary Benfield (1979). In that article, Benfield does not focus on the operant principle of medicine but rather on the nature of medical care itself, identifying two distinct approaches to medical care: disease-oriented and person-oriented care. These are not new, having been articulated in various ways through history (Amundsen & Ferngren, 1983). However, the transition to scientific medicine, which was historically most important in the 1960s and early 1970s, emphasized the specific disease or disease process that the patient exhibited, bringing forward once again the disease-oriented approach. Disease-oriented medical practice is intended to prevent or cure some specific, identified disease process. This approach generally uses beneficence and nonmaleficence as primary principles and relies heavily on scientific and technical elements of medicine (Pellegrino, 1983a).

In contrast, person-oriented medical practice focuses on the person as a whole, recognizing the disease but seeing its treatment as only one part of medical care. This approach utilizes autonomy as the primary principle of health care and focuses on the person receiving care as a part of an entire environment. As a result, medical practice may be seen to involve decisions to withhold or withdraw care and to decide to ignore disease "cure" in favor of other goals that may be legitimate in the patient's larger "life framework."

The contrast between these two approaches is that one focuses narrowly (on the disease) and the other steps back and focuses broadly (on the whole person, her environment, and the significant activities and elements of her life). Case 2-2, for example, is a clear instance of a disease-oriented approach. The failure to correct Karen's misunderstanding is little more than a type of manipulation

Table 2-1
Frameworks of Medical Practice[a]

	Disease-oriented	Person-oriented
Main concerns	(1) Medical science (2) Disease process	(1) Application of science (2) Patient and family
Priority	Eradication of disease	Wellness of the person
Life/death orientation	(1) Life is all that matters (2) Death is the enemy to be fought and avoided	(1) Quality of life is as important as life itself (2) Death is a natural end to life
Primary principle	Beneficence, nonmaleficence	Autonomy
Communication	Physician knows best and makes all the decisions	Patient and family are partners in the decision process

[a]Based on Benfield (1979).

intended to achieve a disease-cure end, this despite requirements for consent and without a real attempt to inform Karen's decision. The patient-centered approach might have achieved the same end without the manipulation by paying attention to Karen's needs, feelings, self-image, fear, etc., and working to overcome those in a way that recognized Karen as an autonomous person.

Obviously, the focus of a person's understanding of the practice of medicine will influence how he or she will interact with patients, as Table 2-1 shows.

As a result, we cannot fully understand medical practice without recognizing the distinctive differences between these two frameworks of medical practice. Moreover, understanding these two frameworks is important to developing models of the PPR.

MODELS FOR THE PHYSICIAN–PATIENT RELATIONSHIP

Case 2-3. A.P., a 45-year-old woman with urinary incontinence, was very embarrassed about her symptoms, as they limited her social activities, and so decided to discuss her problem with her physician.

The physician evaluated the patient, diagnosed stress incontinence secondary to bladder relaxation, and reassured A.P. that this was a common problem in women her age. Even though the physician believed surgery to be the treatment of choice in this case, he believed it was best to mention all the options to his patients before recommending surgery. He therefore described "Kegel" exercises, estrogen cream therapy, and finally concluded with the advantages of surgery. The patient had many questions, but the physician felt good when he could fully inform his patient about all of the options in the hope that the patient would be more comfortable with the decision process.

The patient elected to try a combination of "Kegel" exercises and estrogen cream therapy. Unfortunately, 3 months later the symptoms had not improved. The physician rediscussed the surgical option, the patient consented, the appropriate operation was performed, and the patient's incontinence vanished. Even though the patient had spent 3 more months with her incontinence, utilizing therapies that ultimately did not work, she was grateful to the physician for not performing surgery immediately and for allowing her a role in the decision-making process.

Once the basic principles and frameworks of practice are understood, it is necessary to combine them with other elements to form a "model" for practice. For regardless of which principles and framework are accepted as appropriate for the practice of medicine, there remains the problem of identifying and articulating the physician–patient relationship itself. The principles give the basic "rules" to be followed, the framework gives the overall approach to practice, but neither alone is sufficient to delineate the PPR adequately. Development of a model thus allows the physician to understand clearly how these components work together.

The PPR is at base a relationship between two persons, the defining characteristic of which is that one person is seeking assistance from the other. Moreover, the person seeking assistance has generally done so voluntarily and in a way that establishes a personal and private relationship between the two individuals. Of equal importance is the fact that the person seeking assistance is in some sense dependent on the assistance to be rendered, a psychological position of dependency that may even be understood as a form of weakness. The goal of an acceptable PPR is thus to render the assistance that is required while still retaining an appropriate relationship between the two persons. Physicians have long been concerned with the PPR, as illustrated by Hippocrates' concern with patient visits, sexual relations, confidentiality, use of drugs, styles of living, etc. Although much has been written on this over the years, the most influential contemporary work on the PPR originated in two articles: the first is by Robert Veatch (1972), "Models for Ethical Medicine in a Revolutionary Age," and the second is by William F. May (1975), "Code, Covenant, Contract or Philanthropy." Because these two articles have framed the current discussion of the PPR, we focus on the ideas that originate with them, using Veatch's schemata as outlined in Table 2-2.

Each of the four models is not necessarily exclusive of the others but instead focuses on a particular set of PPR characteristics. For example, the priestly model emphasizes the traditional role of the physician as a healer. According to this model, the physician acts in the relationship as one who is in charge, not only through the status of office but also through the complexity and mysticism of medical knowledge. The priestly physician takes a comforting, all-knowing, and fully directive role in patient care, using either a disease-oriented or person-oriented framework. Of crucial importance is the fact that the physician is totally, unquestionably in charge, and the patient simply accepts and follows whatever the physician prescribes with the understanding that the physician knows what is best. This model of practice is shown in Case 2-2 by the fact that the physician is solely concerned that Karen acquiesce to medical advice. The patient's role in this model is then only one of giving information and following directions.

Table 2-2
Models for the Physician–Patient Relationship[a]

Model	Principles utilized	Practice framework utilized	Patient role
Priestly	Beneficence, nonmaleficence	Disease or person	Information giving, passive
Engineering	Beneficence, nonmaleficence	Disease	Information giving, passive
Collegial	Beneficence, nonmaleficence, autonomy, justice	Person	Co-decision maker, active
Covenant/contract	Whatever the contract stipulates	Whatever the contract stipulates	Whatever the contract stipulates

[a]Based on Veatch (1972).

The second model, the engineering model, characterizes the physician as the ultimate technician, a highly specialized, highly skilled, technically trained expert. The engineering physician's role is very focused, utilizing the disease framework of practice. The physician in this model is the ultimate technician to whom the patient goes to have his specific problem fixed; once it is fixed, there is no further need for the relationship. For example, the orthopedic surgeon "fixes" a hip fracture, or the cardiologist "fixes" an MI. As with the priestly model, the engineering model assigns the patient a role as the information giver who passively follows physician directives.

The third model, the collegial, also known as the "team" model, places the physician as one of a set of collaborators in the patient's care. In this model the patient and other health professionals are active collaborators at some level in the decision-making process, although it leaves open the exact role and level of each participant. Usually, however, the physician is the chief collaborator, or the "captain" of the team, and everyone else is a member of the team, with varying levels of authority. Case 2-3 is a good example of this model in action; because of the interaction between physician and patient, they worked *together* to resolve the medical problem. The physician and patient were *partners* in the problem solving that led to alleviation of the patient's medical problem.

Whereas the priestly and engineering models place the physician as the sole decision maker, the collaborative model assigns some elements of decision making to other participants in the collaboration. In a simple PPR, for example, an office practice, the collaborators will most likely be only the physician and the patient. In a complex PPR, for example, during inpatient hospital care, the set of collaborators will grow with the needs of patient care. The greater the number of collaborators, however, the more care the physician must take with the coordination of care and communication of information to the patient.

The fourth model, the covenant/contract, is similar to the business or legal model of a contract. The covenant or contract may be either explicit or implicit, defined through interaction between the physician and the patient, depending on the circumstances. May (1975, 1983) and others have argued that the physician always has some form of contractual relationship with the patient, regardless of operant model, because the patient employs the physician and the physician receives remuneration from the patient. This exchange of remuneration then, in a legal sense, implies a specific contract, although the details of that contract may be determined by further discussions and negotiations.

As part of establishing this contract, the physician becomes an "employee" of the patient, and the care that is given to the patient by the physician is a function of the agreements on employment. One important part of this contract would be whether the physician and patient would have a priestly, engineering, or collegial relationship. Thus, during contract formation, the patient and physician may agree that the physician will act totally in a priestly manner, with the physician deciding what is best for the patient and acting on that decision without further collaboration from the patient. Alternatively, the contract could establish the relationship to be collegial, wherein the physician would be a source of information for the patient, but the patient would be the ultimate decision maker. The important point of the covenant or contractual relationship is that the principles utilized, the practice model utilized, and the patient role in that model are all determined at the time the contract is established. On the other hand, the other three models (the priestly, the engineering, and the collegial) assume without question what relationship will exist between the physician and the patient.

Recent concern over which model of the PPR is most appropriate has arisen for several reasons: first, the business relationship that occurs in a remunerative practice is being scrutinized; second, our understanding of how individuals should treat each other in a very special, but still social, interaction is changing; and third, most importantly, the ethical dimensions of the healing relationship are being explored in greater depth. For example, recent writing urges a move away from the priestly model because it cannot accommodate the autonomy of the patient as an important factor (Gadow, 1980; Goldman, 1989). As Table 2-2 shows, the priestly model utilizes beneficence and nonmaleficence as primary principles that, though important in themselves, do not adequately account for either autonomy or justice. Similarly, the engineering model is frequently criticized on the same basis, although if the engineering model is functioning as a subset of the collegial model, this criticism could be avoided. The important thing to note, however, is that as each physician develops his or her model of the PPR, the aim must always be to fulfill the basic moral obligation of medical practice—to benefit the patient.

OBLIGATIONS OF THE PHYSICIAN–PATIENT RELATIONSHIP

Case 2-4. Dr. J. had cared for 55-year-old L.P. for 3 years. Although troubled by hypercholesterol, she had been very compliant with the expensive cholesterol-lowering medication he had prescribed and had done very well in lowering her cholesterol into the normal range. L.P. was also pleased with her care and so convinced her husband to come in for a physical exam. The husband, B.P., was recovering from a severe heart attack 3 years earlier, but his primary cardiologist had recently retired.

After Dr. J. finished his exam, he ordered a series of tests to evaluate B.P.'s risk factors and then asked him to come back for a follow-up appointment. At the follow-up appointment, Dr. J. noted that BP's cholesterol was 300 mg/dl, 100 mg/dl over normal, and so prescribed the same expensive cholesterol-lowering agent that L.P. was taking. Unfortunately, B.P. was not covered by the same insurance policy as his wife and so had to pay for the expensive cholesterol-lowering agent. After 1 month of therapy, B.P. asked Dr. J. to prescribe enough cholesterol-lowering medicine for L.P. so that B.P. could take it also but not have to pay for it. L.P. and B.P. explained that all the physician would have to do is prescribe a double dose for L.P., the insurance company would never know, and their finances wouldn't be so strained.

Dr. J. was upset with this request. He really enjoyed taking care of L.P. and B.P. but also realized that to honor their request he would have to deceive the insurance company. He explained his dilemma to the patients, stated that he could not in good conscience deceive their insurer, but would explore other options for B.P. so that he could continue to lower his cholesterol. The physician eventually discovered that B.P. was eligible for care at the local Veteran's Hospital and could obtain his cholesterol-lowering agents there. Even though B.P. and L.P. were initially displeased with the physician for not honoring their request, they were happy that another option was found for B.P. that would lessen their financial burden.

Regardless of how one structures the PPR, within whatever framework for practice is selected, utilizing any set of the various principles, there remains for each professional a common set of basic obligations that arise solely by virtue of engaging in medical practice. As Scribonius Largus, a second-century Roman physician made clear,

> . . . a central question is whether it is still possible to define some set of moral commitments common to the profession. . . . If such commitments are to be found, they will reside in the one medical reality that does not change with time—the need of the sick person for the physician's help and the promise the physician makes when he or she offers to provide that help (Pellegrino & Pellegrino, 1988).

There are no doubt dozens of obligations that could be specifically articulated; however, Bayles (1989) has identified six obligations as primary:

1. Honesty.
2. Candor.
3. Competence.
4. Diligence.
5. Loyalty.
6. Discreetness.

The intention here is not to establish a list of obligations that is either a maximum or a totality. Rather, these six obligations are inherent and essential to any professional practice. The listed obligations thus form a minimum set, so that if one wishes to establish a professional practice, these six obligations will need to be consistently met. The priority of these obligations, and other obligations that may be imposed on the physician, will be directly dependent on the principles of practice, the framework of practice, and the model of relationship that is incorporated into that practice.

The six obligations actually form three sets. The first set, honesty and candor, pertain to the way in which the professional communicates with the patient; the second set, competence and diligence, describe the way in which the physician practices; and the third set, loyalty and discreetness, establish basic parameters for the physician's handling of the patient's problems. With a recognition of these obligations, and the general areas of their grouping, the physician will then be able to structure each interaction with a patient. Moreover, these obligations provide a set of defining characteristics for the physician–patient relationship *regardless* of model.

There is another dimension to these obligations that is also very important, namely, that the establishment of a professional relationship requires that the person seeking the relationship, in this case the patient, be able to have trust and confidence in the professional. As Case 2-4 shows, this concern with trust and honesty also extends beyond the PPR to the physician's interactions with other members of the care-giving team or with society at large. This concern with trust is especially important in light of recent studies showing that physicians regularly use deception in resolving ethical problems (Novak, Detering, Arnold, & Farrow, 1989).

Although it should be the case that every licensed, established professional will be trustworthy, that is obviously not the case. Each professional then has the job of establishing his or her own trustworthiness, thereby establishing the legitimacy of his or her professional practice. By consistently adhering to these six obligations and practicing within a framework that recognizes the four basic principles of practice, the professional will be able to develop that trust.

As with the four basic principles of practice, professional obligations are not simplistic. For example, information exchange is a primary consideration in the PPR. Honesty and candor both affect information exchange and involve important elements of consent and truthtelling. Since professional obligations are so complex and yet so crucial (Bayles, 1989), it is important to explore these obligations and their relationship to the principles of practice and the models of the PPR already discussed.

The principle of autonomy recognizes an individual's right to self-determination. Although self-determination applies equally to physician and patient, the physician–patient relationship is such that the autonomy of the patient is at significantly greater risk than the autonomy of the physician. This is especially true if the relationship is structured under the priestly or engineering models, because both of those models rely on the primacy of the physician. From the patient's perspective, the principle of autonomy has its pivotal focus in the issues of information exchange. This is because the exercise of autonomy, via a decision process, requires that the individual making the decision have truthful and relevant information on which to base that decision (Wright, 1987). Insofar as the physician is not honest or candid with the patient, the information base on which the patient's autonomy rests is incomplete. As a result, any decision the patient might make under the principle of autonomy will automatically be deficient because of that lack of information.

The obligations of competence and diligence are different from the obligations of honesty and candor in that they speak directly to the way in which a physician practices, and they add to the dimension of trust within the PPR that honesty and candor are intended to help establish. When a person seeks out a physician, there needs to be an assurance that the physician is competent to practice. This does not simply mean having the M.D. degree from an accredited institution but means in addition that the physician will have appropriate expertise in his or her area of practice, will be able to recognize when that expertise is surpassed by the case being handled, and be willing and able to call on other professionals for assistance in such cases. Moreover, the obligation for competence requires that the physician maintain as current a level of education as possible, keeping up with the new developments in his or her area of practice.

Diligence, on the other hand, is a requirement that the physician devote appropriate efforts, not just expertise, to the care of the patient. In this regard, the physician who schedules 5-minute office visits so that the largest number of patients possible may be crammed into each hour of office time is not practicing with diligence. Although some cases may be adequately handled within 5 minutes, a large majority of cases cannot be, and thus the physician's attention to the needs of the particular patient will necessarily be diluted.

The physician's diligence may also be diluted because of feelings toward the patient or because of untoward circumstances under which the patient is being seen. Case 2-1 is an example of this problem, given the late hour of the visit, the patient's history of noncompliance, and the physician's dislike of performing certain procedures. If the resident had not gone ahead and done the rectal exam or had not seen the patient in the first place, the obligation of diligence would have been violated. Thus, although dilution of attention is the focal point of the obligation for diligence, other factors are also important. Each person who enters into a PPR has a legitimate expectation of adequate attention, i.e., diligence from the physician.

The final set of obligations, loyalty and discreetness, have to do with the way in which the physician handles the information that is received in the PPR. The long-time concerns with privacy and confidentiality, expressions of which go back at least to the Hippocratic Oath, become of paramount importance. A physician who is loyal to his or her patient will be an advocate for that patient and act on the patient's behalf in all appropriate ways. However, discreetness imposes the maintenance of privacy and confidentiality in doing so as a funda-

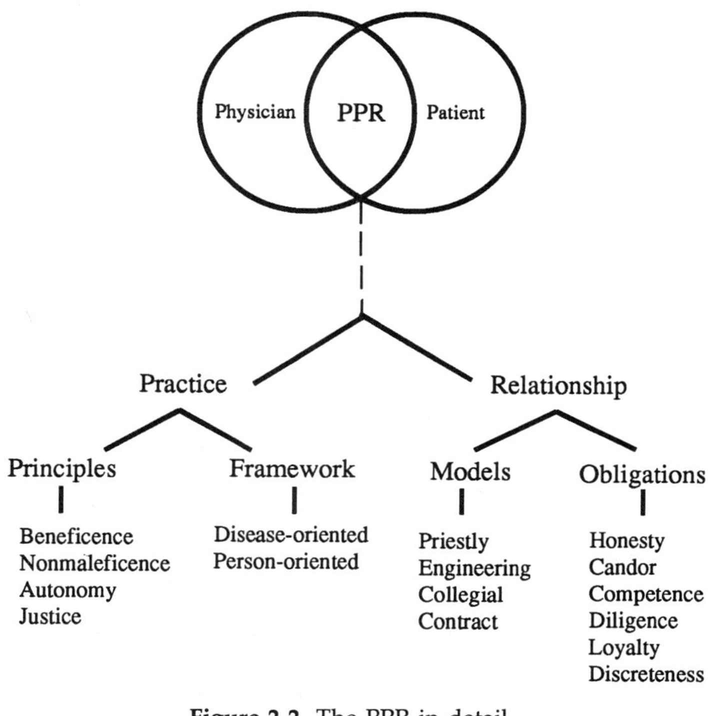

Figure 2-2. The PPR in detail.

mental moral requirement. Although the law and other professional responsibilities may on occasion require that the obligation for discreetness and loyalty be mitigated, for example, in the reporting of communicable diseases, the basic requirement is to maintain loyalty and discreetness.

Although this discussion of professional obligations, as with the other discussions in this chapter, has been brief, it should be clear how important these obligations are, not only to the PPR but to the practice of medicine as a whole. It is thus incumbent on each practicing physician to become more familiar with the requirements of these obligations and come to understand how they function within the PPR. These obligations, together with the relationship model, the framework for practice, and the principles of practice, *together* describe the physician–patient relationship, as shown in Fig. 2-2.

DECISION MAKING AND THE PHYSICIAN–PATIENT RELATIONSHIP

Case 2-5. A 6-week-old infant is admitted to the ICU with a diagnosis of pneumonia, complicated by the fact that the child's lungs are not well developed as a result of premature delivery. For 2 days the child does well on medication but on the third day after admission develops chicken pox. The pox are severe and, when combined with pneumonia, cause respiratory arrest. The child is intubated and put on a respirator. The parents are contacted and indicate they want "everything possible" done for the child. The respirator is continued. Again the child does well initially, but within 24 h P_{O_2} (level of oxygen in the blood) begins to fall, P_{CO_2} (level of carbon dioxide in the blood) begins to rise, and blood pressure begins a steady decline. The parents are again contacted and request that all available means be used to save their child. An IV cutdown is thus done for administration of medications and plasma. On day 5, while an arterial blood gas is being done, the cutdown is damaged, necessitating yet another. Several attempts are made at cutdown, and it is determined that only a very deep artery is accessible. The child is sent to surgery, and a central line is inserted. On day 6 new blood gas tests show a P_{O_2} of 23, a P_{CO_2} of 70, and a pH of 7.1 despite 100% O_2 and mechanical ventilation. The child's heart continues to beat on its own until early on day 7, when it suffers cardiac arrest. After 20 min of resuscitative efforts, the physician wonders whether to continue or not. He knows that the parents want "everything" done but believes that the child has suffered enough and has no real hope of recovery. After one more round of drugs, the team agrees that the code is having little visible effect. The process is halted, and the child is pronounced dead.

Now that the PPR has been more carefully detailed, it becomes important to see how that relationship and the practice of medicine come together into a coherent whole. This is done by first showing the key components of the medical decision-making process and then showing how those components relate to the PPR.

While the medical decision-making process is extremely complex, involving multiple components and interactions, it may nonetheless be understood as containing five key components:

1. Data base.
2. Values.
3. Action constraints.
4. Decision theory.
5. Ethical theory.

Each element of the medical decision-making process can be roughly categorized as falling under one of the five basic components of the decision-making process (Wright, 1987).

It may be a surprise to see this listing, since people frequently believe that the only concern of medical decision making is data collection. Although data are important—no good medical decision can be made in the absence of good data—the other components of the decision process each play a role as well. Granted, the role of each will vary from situation to situation, with one being more important than another in different cases; however, they are each always operative at some level in the process.

To see this more clearly, consider first of all the well-known data component. Here the physician attempts to obtain all relevant data from the case at hand. The data include not only information about the presenting problem but also information from the medical history, physical examination, and laboratory results, which aid understanding the presenting problem. Background knowledge and understanding of the data-gathering physician are also relevant components of the data process. There are, however, two important caveats: first, we never have all the data we want, and the certainty of what we have is always in doubt (Kassirer, 1989); and, second, there can be no utilization of these data without some component of decision theory. Decision theory encompasses the logic and structure of the decision process according to which the data are analyzed and a diagnostic conclusion is reached.

This interaction between the data and decision theory components does not finish our story, for the values that we impose on the situation, the action constraints that impose themselves on us, and the ethical theory on the basis of which we morally justify our decisions also play a role. For example, a decision process based on the given data may indicate a specific course of action as optimal for the patient's current complaint. Nonetheless, in some cases the optimal course of action cannot be taken because there is some action constraint in place. The most common action constraint is time; in many instances, the time it would take to exercise a certain decision is simply not available. This is particularly true in emergency situations where action must be taken immediately to save the life of the patient. Economics is another action constraint. For example, if optimal treatment entails a $4.00-per-tablet antibiotic three times a day for 10 days, but the patient is uninsured and unemployed, the physician's choice of antibiotic is limited.

The values the physician and the patient each bring to a medical situation are also important factors in the decision process. It is a simple fact of human nature that each person is who he is because of the values that he holds and exercises. These values not only frame the way in which a situation is perceived and thus the problems that situation presents, but they also make possible a selection of options for handling that problem and are instrumental in the choice of one option to resolve the problem. Even the scientific information that is utilized in the decision-making process, flowing out of the data base, is heavily influenced by values. For example, in different hospitals the "normal" range for laboratory "values" is different. Thus, there may be disagreements between physicians as to whether or not a specific numerical report for a given test is "within normal limits." This is a value judgment. In addition, economic, social, political, legal, religious, and ethical values accompany problem situations that the decision-making process is intended to resolve. These values influence the decision-making process, playing a role commensurate with their importance to the individual who holds the values.

Finally, ethical theory plays a role in the decision-making process because each of us utilizes ethical theory, usually without realizing it, to order the basic set of values that influence our decisions. Historically, people have traditionally used three different theoretical frameworks for ordering their ethical values:

1. Consequences.
2. Duties.
3. Rights.

The person utilizing consequences, for example, would order her values so that they would support production of the best possible set of consequences in any situation. The principles of beneficence and nonmaleficence are primary within a consequences-based ethical theory. A person who utilizes a duty framework would order his values so that it would be possible to achieve what he believed his duty required. Thus, if preservation of life is perceived as a duty, the physician will place high priority on values that promote the preservation of life, for example, refusing to perform abortions or to discontinue life support. The principle of justice is primary within a duty-based ethical theory. Finally, the rights-based theory would be reflected in an ordering of values that promoted the protection and exercise of individual rights. For example, upholding the right to privacy would require ordering values so that confidentiality of medical information could be adequately maintained. The principle of autonomy is primary within a rights-based theory. These ethical theories vary between individuals only in their frequency of use. What does vary significantly between individuals is how specific values are ordered within the operant theory.

The medical decision-making process is influenced by the ethical theory of the individual decision maker in the same way that it is influenced by the values of the individual. Each individual's ethical theoretical framework, i.e., how he or she views matters of morality, also affects seeing the problems, selecting alternatives to resolve those problems, and resolving the problem. Thus, a person working within a consequences-based theory will approach some problems differently than will the person working within a duty- or rights-based theory. Interestingly, however, the different approaches do not necessitate mutually exclusive considerations, so that persons utilizing different theories and different values may nonetheless reach agreement in a problem resolution situation.

The five components of the medical decision-making process may be schematized to show how they influence each other in that process. Figure 2-3 shows each of these five components as having a direct bearing on the resolution of the clinical problem.

Case 2-5 is a good example of how these components come together in a decision-making situation. To begin, the physician must make clinical determinations based on clinical data. The blood gases, ventilator settings, etc. are all part of the information needed for those determinations. In addition, however, the values of the physician and parents come into play. The parents, for example, have asked that "everything" be done; for them, the value of their child's life is most important. The medical team, on the other hand, has serious concerns about this request, since they see the deterioration of the infant's condition and are concerned that they are passing from beneficence to maleficence in treating the child. After all, high-tech intensive care is not benign, and when results continue to deteriorate, the relative value of that care also declines in comparison to its benefits.

Whenever care is initiated, however, as in Case 2-5, it is difficult to discontinue. Some might argue that care should have been discontinued on day 5, rather than inserting the central line, because it was already apparent by then that there was minimal hope for the child's recovery. Notice, however, that this is also an expression of values in this case. Moreover, the possible legal implications of discontinuing care may have served as an action constraint, keeping the team from withdrawing to a "comfort only" level of caregiving.

There are also questions in this case about the decision-making process. What role should the parents have in the decisions that were made to continue maximum efforts? If the medical team truly believes that it is not in the child's best interests to continue maximum efforts, why ask the parents what they want done? Why not simply tell them that all reasonable means have been exhausted and there is nothing more that can be done that will benefit their child? Were that done, the child could still have comfort care without being subjected to futile

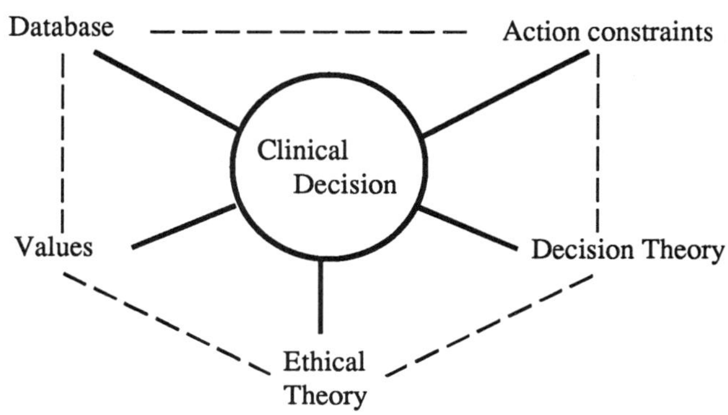

Figure 2-3. Interaction of decision-making factors.

aggressive care. Moreover, there would have been no pseudorole for the parents in the decision process. In any case, note that all these matters are a function of the decision theory component.

Finally, Case 2-5 presents important considerations of ethical theory. For example, one reason to continue maximal efforts, despite apparent negative results, is that a duties-based ethical theory would require such action. For example, if one assumes that a physician has an absolute duty to preserve life at all costs, regardless of the effort required, the physician could be seen as having a duty to continue, regardless of poor outcome. On the other hand, the final cessation of CPR so that death may finally have its way can be legitimate-

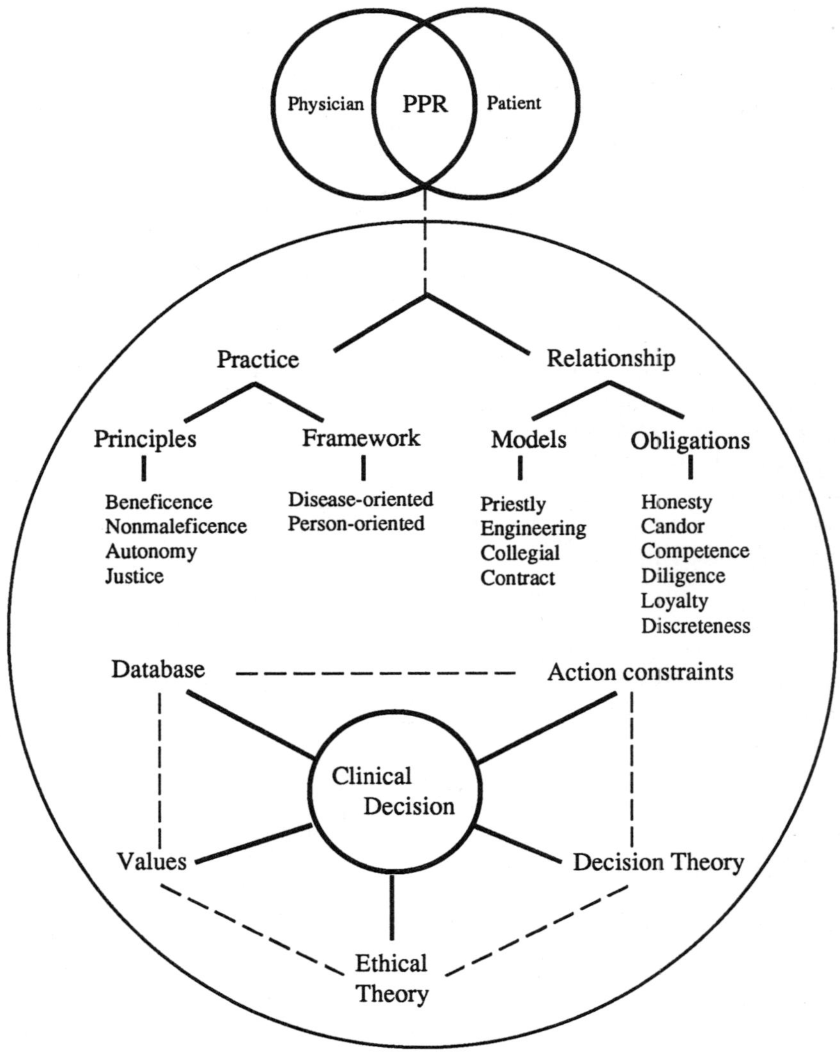

Figure 2-4. The complex PPR.

ly seen in the understanding that each person has a right to die with dignity in the absence of interventions that do no more than prolong the dying process. A consequences-based theory would also permit cessation of CPR on the grounds that the consequences of continuing did not outweigh the consequences of stopping, since the best hope was for recovery of a seriously impaired infant.

Although the above is only a brief analysis, it is intended to show how the decision components each come into play in a given case decision. At the same time, because this medical decision-making process, with its five major components, functions within the PPR, it is important to understand how all various factors that have been discussed in this chapter come together. In Fig. 2-4 we see the original diagram of the PPR as the intersection of the spheres of life for a physician and a patient. That PPR is then seen to consist of the four major components that are developed in the tree diagram, whereas the decision-making process is seen to function within the sphere of life that is defined by that PPR.

CONCLUSIONS

Although this all may seem very confusing, the remainder of the textbook is intended to discuss and delineate components of the decision-making process and further explicate elements of the PPR. Through a discussion of the PPR as an outgrowth of the intersection of two human lives, we hope that considerations of the PPR's complexity may be seen as important. Moreover, the PPR, because of this importance, should be understood as the keystone element in the overall development of the physician.

As described in this chapter, the PPR is an elaborate mixture of considerations about the principles and framework within which the physician will practice. It is also an understanding of the models and obligations that affect the relationships that develop as a function of that practice. Accordingly, the PPR must develop from these elements, although within the context of the value system of the physician.

When seen in its broader context, the PPR is also recognized as the influencing factor for a physician's overall attitude toward each aspect of his or her practice. Thus, the coupling of the multiple components of decision making with the practice and relationship characteristics of the PPR then encompasses an overarching structure that is itself the practice of medicine.

Because it is difficult to understand all of these components and their interactions in practice, they are referred to in different ways throughout the text. The concluding chapter then brings all these elements back together again into a coherent view of medical practice. The materials in this chapter are thus presented as a schematic, as an outline of ideas into which the remaining materials of the text may be structured. It is within this schematic that the PPR, and the practice of medicine itself, occurs. It is within this schematic that the physician must come to understand the various components of his or her practice, so that the development of that practice might be directly determined in a thoughtful, consistent manner that will result in the best possible patient care.

CASES FOR DISCUSSION

Case 1

Jennifer L. is a 19-year-old who has been admitted to the medical service of City Hospital for treatment of thrombosis and resulting pulmonary embolism. She is in severe distress from the emboli, thus requiring medication for pain as well as heparin to prevent further blood clots. She was started on intravenous fluids containing the appropriate dosages of heparin. On the second day of treatment, the patient pulled the IV and refused further treatment that requires injection or intravenous infusion. Jennifer is clearly too sick to leave the hospital, since the release of emboli continues, and such release would be seriously life-threatening. In staff conference, the following courses of action are suggested: (1) increase the dosage of pain medication, thus effectively reducing her ability to object, and then continue with the required life-saving treatment; (2) treat her refusal of prescribed treatment as equivalent to her signing out of the hospital against medical advice and have her transported back to her home; (3) call for a psychiatric consultant to determine whether Jennifer is considered competent: if she is not, then obtain a court order for her treatment; if she is, then decide between choices 1 and 2.

1. Discuss these alternatives and propose a solution to this problem. For purposes of discussion, assume that the IV heparin is the only treatment available with any hope of alleviating Jennifer's thrombotic disease. How will the solution be different with the disease-oriented or patient-oriented framework?
2. Assess the application of the principles of practice and determine which is most important in this case.
3. Determine which ethical theory approach you are utilizing to resolve this situation.

Case 2

You are seeing as a new patient an 18-year-old girl who is approximately 3 months pregnant. She has been in psychotherapy because of feelings of inadequacy. In her relationships with men she has frequently been exploited, but she repeatedly engaged in such relationships because sexual intercourse gave her a feeling of acceptance and seemed to prove to her that she possessed adequacy as a woman. She did not use birth control pills because she never planned to have intercourse.

She is undecided about marrying the father of the child because she is not sure that she loves him. He has offered to marry her, but his interest appears to be mainly one of duty. She is also undecided about whether or not to have the child. She has spoken to friends, some of whom advised one course of action and others the opposite.

She is mildly depressed about her state and feels that this is just another in a lifelong series of mistakes. She wants advice on what to do and so comes to you because her friend told her you are "a great doctor and really understanding."

1. What elements of the PPR are most important here?
2. Which decision-making factors are most crucial to the advice you will (or won't) give?

Case 3

John and Marsha are both 23 years old and have been married for 5 years. Although Marsha has been pregnant seven times, she has been unable to maintain a pregnancy, with spontaneous abortion having occurred in each case. Now she has carried to term and successfully delivered a baby girl; however, the baby is severely affected by Down's syndrome. In addition, it is discovered that the child has a duodenal obstruction that could be easily corrected with surgery. Without the surgery, the baby will surely die; with the surgery, there is no question but that it will live and be healthy.

After the physician explains the baby's problems, she requests consent to perform the surgery, but John and Marsha refuse. Although they have been trying to have a baby, they say they don't want one who won't be "normal" and so will keep trying. The physician carefully explains that the baby will die without surgery, but they still refuse.

State law allows the physician to request a court order for the surgery to save the infant's life, but the physician wonders whether she should honor the parents' wishes, since it is their child, not hers.

1. How, if at all, does the PPR affect the physician's decision?
2. Do any of the principles of practice justify the parents' decision?
3. Would any of the principles justify the court order? Would any of the ethical theories justify a court order?

Case 4

The police bring a patient into the ER for minor injuries following an auto accident. While he is being cared for, the officer requests both a blood alcohol test and a blood barbiturate test on the patient. In addition, the officer asks the nurse to check the patient's pockets to see if he is carrying any narcotics or other controlled substances. The law is such that an officer may request that a blood alcohol test be drawn, but he may not request that only a blood barbiturate be drawn. Also, the law is such at the time that the officer may not search without cause, but anything that is discovered by the nurse could be used as evidence, since the police did not do the search.

1. As the ER resident in charge of this case, would you permit the nurse to do the search? Why or why not, on the basis of the PPR?
2. Discuss each of the six relationship obligations in the context of this case.

Case 5

A third-year resident on call was paged to come to the emergency room at 3 A.M. to take care of a 2-year-old who was brought in by her mother because the child was "scratching at her bottom." When the resident arrived the mother said she became very concerned about the child's scratching when she saw little "worm-like" things around the child's rectum. The resident quickly diagnosed a pinworm infection and then excused himself from the room saying that he had to talk with another physician about the case, but inside being furious that the patient woke him from a sound sleep for such a minor medical problem.

As he was cooling off, the resident debated whether he should actually prescribe treatment for the pinworm infection or ask the mother to bring the child back during daytime office hours to reinforce the fact that this was an inappropriate use of ER facilities. He also knew that no pharmacy would be open in the middle of the night to supply the patient with medication anyway, the emergency room didn't have the necessary medicine, and so there would be no significant delay in treatment if he required the patient to come back during daytime office hours. He soon realized, however, that if he handled the problem tonight the patient and her mother wouldn't be a burden on office staff during the day, and his real reason for making the patient return was not so much as a reinforcement of what he wanted the patient to do but more revenge for waking him up in the middle of the night.

The resident went back into the room and prescribed appropriate therapy. He then gently stated to the patient that as pharmacies were not open and as this was a relatively minor medical problem, it would probably be best for her to take care of such problems during daylight hours. The patient became extremely angry at the resident's suggestions and left in a huff. The next day the resident learned that this was a frequent occurrence with this patient and that the whole practice was struggling with her inappropriate use of the emergency room.

1. Analyze this case using each component of the PPR discussed in this chapter.

RECOMMENDED READINGS

Goodman, A. H. (1980). *The moral foundations of professional ethics.* Totowa, NJ: Rowman and Littlefield.

This carefully thought out, well-written book examines the ethical basis for any professional practice. Utilizing examples from medicine as well as other professions, the authors tries to show the common moral content of any professional practice. In so doing, this book helps to enlighten one's understanding of the entire PPR, seen then as an instance of a greater vision of professional practice.

Katz, J. (1984). *The silent world of doctor and patient.* New York: Free Press.

Devoted to the discussion of the doctor–patient decision-making process, this book brings the physician's perspective to bear on the ethical issues of the PPR. Dr. Katz presents a strong argument in advocacy of an informed dialogue between physician and patient that respects the rights and needs of both sides.

Pellegrino, E., & Thomasma, D. (1988). *For the patient's good: The restoration of beneficence in health care.* New York: Oxford University Press.

This collaborative work of a physician and a philosopher tries to address the PPR from the perspective of the principles of practice. It does so, however, in the context of the PPR as a whole as well as the function of the PPR within an overall philosophy of medicine. Though dealing with difficult topics, the book is well written, with excellent use made of cases and their analysis. The book will help one's understanding of the conceptual components of the PPR.

PART II

Processes of Clinical Practice

How physicians can best care for patients is also a source of surprising controversy. Whereas traditionalists advocate a more formal exhaustive approach, new research is beginning to support a more collaborative, goal-oriented, process model of interviewing, examining, decision making, and managing. This section describes both sides of this controversy in the hope that exploring the tension between the two approaches can develop a new, more workable synthesis.

CHAPTER 3

Interviewing and History Taking

Alvah R. Cass and L. Peter Schwiebert

Case 3-1. It is July 1, and K.M. is a third-year student preparing for his first day on an inpatient service. The second-year resident with whom he is working tells K.M. about a patient just admitted with chest pain, saying, "This should be a good patient for you. Take a medical history from him." The resident then walks off, leaving him, starched white coat, spanking new stethoscope, and all, standing at the door of the patient's room. This is the moment for which he has been waiting, "real clinical medicine," but he can't help also feeling somewhat anxious. What should he ask? How can he put the patient and himself at ease? How can he get appropriate information so that he can "shine" on rounds?

INTRODUCTION

K.M. has been asked to obtain a medical history. To obtain this history, K.M. will have to *interview* his patient. Although many physicians feel that interviewing and obtaining a medical history are the same, the interview *process* is much more than simple data gathering; it includes the physician–patient interaction that occurs during data gathering. For instance, a questionnaire completed by a patient while waiting to see a physician or dentist is a medical history. Clearly, there is no interpersonal interaction involved in completing this task. On the other hand, an interview taking place between K.M. and the patient with chest pain concerns itself not only with data gathering but also with biases, body language, nuances in speech, and how questions are phrased. All these subtle communication processes can have a profound impact not only on how successful K.M. is in obtaining the necessary medical history for rounds but also on how successful K.M. is in establishing a relationship with his patient.

What is effective interviewing? It involves putting the patient at ease, getting to the heart of the patient's concerns, gathering accurate data, and arriving at an appropriate assessment of the patient's problems. Later phases of the interview process involve negotiating with patients over treatment plans and implementing those plans. Thus, effective communication facilitates the process of clinical decision making and management.

FUNDAMENTAL CONCEPTS

A skillful interviewer must understand several basic concepts. First, the medical interview is a scientific method that "measures" the patient's signs and symptoms. The medical interview should therefore reflect all of the desirable characteristics of any scientific test, including objectivity, precision, accuracy, sensitivity, specificity, and reproducibility (Feinstein, 1967).

The second concept is that the physician is the instrument that quantifies the patient's signs and symptoms through his or her interviewing skills. Taking this a step further, the physician not only "measures" the signs and symptoms but also analyzes them (Coulehan & Block, 1987). Analysis influences further data gathering, data gathering influences analysis, and so on. Thus, the interview is a circular process in which the physician, as both a test instrument and an analysis instrument, is a source of error in the measurement process. He or she can readily and unexpectedly introduce bias into the process. The physician's clinical knowledge, skills, values, beliefs, prejudices, family-of-origin issues, and past experiences are sources of bias that can undermine the scientific basis of the medical interview. For example, a physician who comes from a family that forbids alcohol, is a proponent of fitness, and believes obesity is a result of inadequate willpower is unlikely to be objective when interviewing an overweight, alcoholic man with chest pain.

The patient also influences the scientific basis of the interview process. The patient, having experienced various signs and symptoms, must try to accurately relate them to the physician. As with the physician, the patient's account of the situation will be influenced by his or her knowledge, values, beliefs, prejudices, family-of-origin issues, and past experiences with the health care system. For example, a patient who has seen several doctors without getting better, doesn't like professional women, and is worried about having cancer is unlikely to be entirely open and candid with a female intern in an ambulatory clinic.

Therefore, although only two people may be present in the medical interview, the interview process can be quite complex and is prone to many types and sources of error. Three common types of errors that produce inaccuracies in the histories obtained from the interview process include failure to clarify confusion, failure to delve into denial, and rating the reliability of information provided during the interview too quickly (Riegelman, 1981).

Interviewers and patients can introduce confusion into the interview process. The interviewer can add confusion by using technical terms or medical jargon. Patients inadvertently add confusion when using common terms to describe symptoms and illnesses. Phrases such as, "I have a cold," "I feel sick," or "I think I have a stomach flu" can mean many different things to different people. Failure to clarify the confusion introduced by various terms or phrases can lead to misdiagnosis and inappropriate advice or treatment.

Conscious or unconscious denial is a major impediment to accurate history taking. The interviewer should always keep in mind that denial is a common coping mechanism and be alert to cues that may indicate that the patient is denying important aspects of his or her presenting problem. Vague or confusing descriptions of problems or information that does not fit well with the rest of the findings can be cues to denial. The effective interviewer must be willing to delve into denial in a nonjudgmental manner.

Rating reliability too quickly refers to categorizing patients as good historians or poor historians. Prematurely judging the patient as a poor historian leads the interviewer to mistrust or disregard the information the patient is providing. The effective interviewer will continually suspend judgment while seeking ways to help the patient provide the most accurate description of his or her problem.

These biases can be minimized by careful application of clinical knowledge and close attention to the essential attitudes and communication skills described below.

INTERVIEWING SKILLS

A medical interview, like any form of dialogue, depends on the participants' abilities to articulate their points of view clearly and to correctly understand and comprehend each other's perspective. Therefore, the success of the medical interview process is directly related to the interpersonal and communication skills of the participants. For the purpose of this discussion, three broad categories of interpersonal and communication skills are considered: essential attitudes, nonverbal skills, and verbal skills.

Essential Attitudes

Carl Rogers (1961) and others have identified several essential attitudes necessary to the effective interviewer. These include unconditional positive regard, genuineness or congruence, and empathy.

Unconditional Positive Regard

Unconditional positive regard or respect is the ability to view the patient as a unique person, suspend critical judgments, and accept the patient as he or she is (Coulehan & Block, 1987). This requires that the physician not measure patients against his own values and beliefs. Just as the physician's personal values and beliefs help him deal with the rewards and tragedies of life, similarly the patient's values and beliefs, even though they may be at odds with the physician's, are methods for coping with life events. Accepting that people cope effectively in different ways is the first step to developing unconditional positive regard. Remembering that all people experience emotions, have pride, and need nurturing relationships is also essential to developing a respectful attitude.

Congruence

Genuineness or congruence is the ability to be oneself in a relationship, not hiding behind a role or creating false pretenses (Coulehan & Block, 1987). Congruence requires honesty, but brutal honesty must often be tempered by good judgment. Congruence means being precise about one's role in the health care team, not encouraging or promoting misconceptions on the part of the patient, and, importantly, being able to say, "I don't know." Developing an acceptance of one's own limitations, fallibility, and vulnerabilities is an essential ingredient of congruence. Incongruence in a doctor–patient relationship will usually be discovered and lead to feelings of betrayal and anger in the patient.

Empathy

Empathy is the ability to sense the patient's experience and feelings accurately and to communicate to the patient that you understand the types of feelings he is experiencing and the intensity with which he is experiencing them (Coulehan & Block, 1987). Empathy in the medical interview means being receptive to all forms of input from the patient including content, feelings, emotions, and behaviors. Secondly, it means being able to process that information and demonstrate to the patient that he or she was heard and understood. The intensity of feelings and emotions must also be accurately identified. Understating or overstating an experience can be as distracting to the interview process as ignoring the emotions entirely. Empathy requires the physician to be a skilled observer and listener and to respect the patient's feelings and vulnerability.

Nonverbal Skills

Nonverbal communication skills are those behaviors and utterances that facilitate effective communication independent of the verbal content of the communication.

Attending Skills

Attending skills are those behaviors that communicate nonverbally to the person being interviewed that the interviewer is ready to listen, interested in him, and regards him in a positive manner. Three basic behaviors are important to attending skills: eye contact, posture, and setting a positive environment.

In most western cultures maintaining comfortable **eye contact** with the person being interviewed is important for communicating readiness, interest, and respect. Maintaining eye contact can be viewed on a spectrum from no eye contact to uninterrupted staring. Obviously, the extremes are equally distractive to effective communication. Therefore, eye contact should be comfortable to both the interviewer and the interviewee. There should be natural breaks in eye contact. Eye contact should be maintained at a comfortable distance, somewhere between 3 and 4 feet.

Posture refers to the positioning of the interviewer's body in relation to the person being interviewed. Generally, the interviewer's posture should be an open posture, with the arms and legs uncrossed. The interviewer should be facing the patient or at a slight angle, preferably seated at a comfortable distance from the patient and at the same eye level. If the patient is seated on an examining table, the interviewer should position himself at the same eye level. Similarly, the interviewee should be positioned in a comfortable manner to meet his or her personal needs.

Setting a positive environment means that the interviewer takes responsibility for making the interview milieu comfortable and free of interruptions. A positive environment is physically and emotionally comfortable. The setting should provide privacy, and distractions should be minimized from both external and internal sources. For example, the room should be at a comfortable temperature with good lighting and appointed in soft colors. The door should be shut, with a minimum of sound from the exterior coming into the room. Other personnel in the setting should know not to interrupt the interview unless it is absolutely necessary. Internal sources of distractions, such as leafing through a chart, daydreaming, or nervous habits that distract the interviewee from the interview process should be eliminated if possible.

Facilitative Cues

Facilitation skills are those utterances or movements that encourage the patient to continue talking. They also communicate interest or concern. These include such behaviors as gentle nodding of the head periodically as the patient is speaking and careful use of utterances such as "uh-huh" or "mm-hm." A period of silence can serve as encouragement for the patient to continue to speak. Various types of hand motions can also encourage the patient to continue talking, and subtle behavior such as leaning forward or leaning back while the patient is speaking can encourage him to talk or be silent. On the other hand, inappropriate or too frequent use of facilitative cues can disrupt the interview process.

Verbal Skills

Verbal communication skills are those skills that are related to speaking and are directly dependent on the content and structure of speech. Verbal skills can be divided into three broad categories: questioning skills, responding skills, and sharing skills.

Questioning Skills

Questioning skills are a group of verbal communication skills that assist the interviewer in gathering information. A question not only constitutes a request for a response from another person but can also guide the respondent to give a certain type of response. Questions can also be divided into four broad types.

Open-ended questions are questions or directive phrases that do not have a simple yes, no or other preconceived correct answer. Open-ended questions tend to facilitate communication by encouraging the patient to tell his or her story in his or her own words. Open-ended questions can serve several functions in the medical interview, including description, explanation, or evaluation. A **descriptive** open-ended question may take the form of a request such as "Please, tell me more about the symptoms you have been experiencing during the last few days?" An **explanatory** open-ended question asks the patient to explain his or her understanding of a situation. For example, the physician may ask the patient, "What do you understand about high blood pressure" Finally, **evaluative-type** open-ended questions are useful in helping the patient describe the significance of a situation or to explain his or her opinion. For example, a patient may be asked, "How effective has the nicotine gum been in helping you stop smoking?" Open-ended questions are frequently used early in the interview process to expand the dialogue and encourage the patient to tell his or her story. On the other hand, extensive use of open-ended questions can become frustrating to the patient, prolong the interview process, and detract from effective data gathering.

Focused or **closed-ended questions** are questions that direct the patient to a specific answer. These questions can frequently be answered by yes or no or have a simple definitive answer. Focused questions are frequently used to fine-tune the physician's understanding of a problem and to clarify details that the patient may not have addressed in response to an open-ended question. An example of a closed-ended question is, "Does the pain ever radiate into your neck?" This type of question is directing the patient to consider a specific possibility and could be answered yes or no. If the preceding questions have been open and facilitative, closed questions may result in a more expanded answer. For example, the patient may say, "It never radiates into my neck, but I had noticed that it moves into my back and shoulders." An interview full of focused questions will tend to limit the participation of the patient and put the interviewer or physician at risk of creating a story different from what the patient truly has experienced.

A British study of 2000 consultations in general practice (Byrne & Long, 1976) showed that 75% of interviews were "doctor-centered" and made use almost exclusively of closed-ended questions about the patient's first complaint. The interviews were also characterized by frequent brushing aside of hints of other problems and ignoring important clues to other significant patient problems. Byrne and Long's study also described the "patient-centered" interview in which effective use of open-ended questions occurred, which left patients free to answer questions from their own perspective.

The use of **circular questions** is a more sophisticated type of information-gathering skill that asks the patient to provide information from a different perspective or from someone else's perspective. Circular questions are often very effective for gaining an understanding of the subtle nuances of a problem. For example, a 4-year-old child is being seen by a physician. In reviewing the child's past medical history, the parents state that the child had drowned in a swimming pool, was resuscitated, and was comatose on a respirator for 3 days before regaining consciousness. The physician, thinking that brain damage could have occurred, causing growth or developmental delays, asks the parents if the child has had any problems in growth and development. The parents reply no. The physician, suspicious that this might represent denial, could ask a question such as "If Sally's grandmother were here, how would she describe Sally's growth and development?" or the physician might say, "What have other people said about Sally's verbal maturity?"

A **leading question** is a question that suggests an answer. Door-to-door insurance salesmen are highly skilled at the use of leading questions. For example, a salesman in a customer's home with perhaps his wife and children present may ask "You wouldn't want to leave your family unprotected in case of your unexpected death, would you?" The answer is obviously no. Similarly, a medical interviewer can ask leading questions of a patient and put him in the same uncomfortable position of having to give the "right answer." For example, in talking to a patient with chest pain, the doctor may say, "You haven't experienced this pain with exertion, have you?" Even if the patient does have exertional chest pain, there is a possibility that he may minimize this particularly important symptom or actually agree with the physician out of respect and to avoid a conflict. In general, leading questions should be avoided or kept to an absolute minimum.

Questioning skills are useful for gathering information about the patient and the patient's problem. Open-ended questions, nonjudgmental focused questions, and circular questions encourage the patient to tell his or her story in his or her own way. They also indirectly communicate the interviewer's interest in hearing what the patient has to say and thus create a positive environment for the medical interview.

Responding Skills

Responding skills are a set of communication skills that enable the interviewer to demonstrate to the patient that he or she has been heard and understood. Responses can be made to content, feelings, or both.

The simplest responding skill is parroting or paraphrasing. **Parroting** simply means repeating the last few words that the patient said. This demonstrates that the interviewer is listening to the patient and frequently encourages the patient to continue. **Paraphrasing** is slightly more sophisticated than parroting. It offers a brief summary of a small amount of content and helps to check the accuracy of what the interviewer has heard.

Summations are another form of responding to content and are usually somewhat lengthier and deal with a larger amount of information than paraphrases or parroting. Summations are used effectively throughout an interview to help the interviewer make sure that he has heard the story correctly. They also help patients stay focused on the problem as they are describing their situation.

Responses to feeling can take many forms. Such responses are particularly useful for demonstrating true understanding of the patient's plight and to communicate compassion. For example, a physician noting the angry scowl of a patient who has been waiting for over an hour to see her may respond, "You seem angry. Is it because you have been waiting so long to see me?"

Sympathetic responses communicate to the patient how the interviewer or physician feels about what has been said or what has happened. Sympathy demonstrates that the physician is in touch with the emotional aspects of a problem but does not always demonstrate that he is in tune with the patient's feelings or emotions. For example, a patient comes to the doctor because of trouble sleeping. During the course of the interview the doctor discovers that the insomnia started 6 weeks ago after the patient's father died in a nursing home. In response to this new piece of information, the doctor replies, "Oh, I'm very sorry to hear about your father; I know the two of you were very close." Although this expression of sympathy may be comforting to the patient, it does not fully demonstrate that the physician understands what the patient is feeling.

Empathetic responses demonstrate that the physician understands the feelings that the patient has experienced. For an empathetic response to be effective, the patient must perceive it as genuine and sincere. To illustrate this, reconsider the previous scenario. Instead of expressing only her sympathy, the doctor could lean forward to the patient, reach out, and touch her hand, establish good eye contact, and say, "I know how close the two of you were; I imagine you feel very much alone without him." This conveys to the patient a genuine level of understanding by the physician. In contrast, the same statement made while the physician is leaning back and leafing through the chart is less likely to be received as sincere.

Interchangeable responses are responses that link content with feelings. Interchangeable responses very clearly and effectively demonstrate to patients that they have been heard and understood. An interchangeable response to the previous example might be phrased as, "You're feeling some deep regret because you had to place your father in the nursing home." Interchangeable responses frequently encourage patients to be more open and more honest during the interview process.

Like leading questions, the denial type of response should be avoided. **Denial** responses negate the feelings expressed by the patient. For example, a patient may say, "I was absolutely terrified that this lump may be cancer!" A denial response would be, "Oh, I'm sure it wasn't that frightening for you," or, "That's ridiculous, it's just a simple bump." Clearly, denial responses detract from the interview process.

Sharing Skills

Sharing skills are a set of communication skills that enable the interviewer to communicate clearly his or her perspective to the patient. These skills are useful when information is shared with the patient. Sharing skills enable the patient to be aware of the physician's point of view and help the patient to acquire needed information. They also serve to help the patient focus on important issues and, when effectively applied, facilitate the acceptance of the physician's opinion by the patient. In response to sharing skills, patients will frequently be stimulated to explore and resolve discrepancies in their understanding of the problem when compared to the physician's perspective. Sharing skills include description, genuineness, self-disclosure, and constructive confrontation.

Description is a simple skill that allows the interviewer to state objectively what was seen, heard, or observed over the course of the interview. Description skills are frequently used to validate or explain why the physician has come to a given conclusion. For example, a patient presents to the office with an upper respiratory tract infection and, during the course of an interview, expresses particular concern about pneumonia. A descriptive statement such as, "You don't have any fever and I don't hear any abnormal sounds in your chest. I think pneumonia is extremely unlikely," provides explanation and reassurance to the patient.

Genuineness is a communication skill that enables the interviewer to express feelings about the patient or about some aspect of the patient's problem. Genuineness differs from empathic responses in that empathy identifies the feelings within the patient whereas genuineness identifies feelings within the interviewer. The interviewer must be careful that genuine statements be made in a nonthreatening, accurate, and specific context. Frequently, genuine statements can be used to acknowledge a patient's compliance to a medical treatment plan or ability to articulate a problem. For example, a patient who has recently been diagnosed as having diabetes mellitus and has been put on a weight reduction diet returns to the office for a follow-up visit having lost 5 lb. A genuine statement that recognizes this success might be, "I noticed you have lost 5 lb since your last visit. I'm very pleased with your progress."

Self-disclosure is a method by which the interviewer shares a personal experience and any related feelings with the patient. Self-disclosure statements are most effective when the interviewer perceives that the patient will benefit from hearing about his or her own personal experience. For example, a physician who recently coped with the death of her father from colon cancer may wish to share that experience with a patient who is having difficulty sleeping because her father is dying of cancer in order to model effective coping behavior.

Frequently during the course of a medical interview, occasions arise when the opinion or goals of the patient are in conflict with the opinion or goals of the interviewer. **Constructive confrontation** allows the physician to communicate those differences of opinion respectfully. In other words, constructive confrontation places the perspective of the patient and the perspective of the physician in juxtaposition. For example, a patient may present with an upper respiratory tract infection and sore throat and be convinced that he has streptococcal pharyngitis and needs an antibiotic. Based on the interview, physical exam, and laboratory data, the physician is able to rule out streptococcal pharyngitis. A constructive confrontation statement would be, "You seem convinced that an antibiotic would help, but your history, exam, and tests indicate that this is a virus; antibiotics are not effective against viruses."

Summary

The essential attitudes of unconditional positive regard, genuineness, and empathy are basic attributes of an effective medical interviewer. These interpersonal attitudes and skills establish doctor–patient rapport. Communication skills, both nonverbal and verbal, enable the physician to gather accurate information, communicate an understanding of the patient's perspective, and communicate to the patient clearly the doctor's opinion and perspective. Used skillfully throughout the medical interview, these skills promote effective clinical decision making and management.

Many authors have written about the medical interview process and have described it using a variety of terms and stages (Coulehan & Block, 1987). In its simplest form, the medical interview is a process that enables the patient and doctor to explore an issue or issues, to come to an understanding of the problem, and to develop goals and strategies to address the problem. For the purposes of this chapter, the interview process is described in four stages: joining, tracking, intervening, and closing.

Joining

Joining is usually the first phase of the medical interview. Joining is the process by which the physician and patient meet, develop initial rapport, and set the stage for an effective exchange of information. Creating a positive environment for the medical interview is an essential first step in effective interviewing. A positive environment allows time for the physician to suspend judgment, briefly review the medical record, and clear his or her mind of distractions. The physician should insure the patient's comfort, and environmental distractions should be minimized. For example, it is unlikely that a physician could effectively join with a patient in an un-air-conditioned office on a hot afternoon when the patient is an hour late for his appointment and the physician has just finished talking to a disgruntled patient who has not paid his bill.

Once a positive environment is established, the process of joining generally continues with a warm greeting from the physician. A warm greeting frequently includes a handshake or other gestures that minimize the social and cultural barriers inherent in the health care process. Appropriately, the interviewer should introduce himself clearly by name, identify his role in the health care team, and state the reason for the interview. For example, a medical student who is about to see a patient might say, "Good morning, Mrs. Jones. I am John Smith, a first-year medical student working with Dr. Brown. He asked me to talk with you this morning about why you came to see him today." When a patient is known to the physician, joining is enhanced by making a personalized comment. For example, the physician may ask about the patient's job or recent vacation. With a new patient, a sociable comment about the weather or a recent event will often help put the patient at ease. It is important that these types of social interactions be sincere, warm, and reflect congruence.

Attending skills are the most important skills used during joining. If the joining process has been successful, both the physician and patient should feel at ease in each other's presence. The patient should feel respected, and the physician should experience acceptance.

Case 3-2. Mrs. Jones, a 33-year-old woman, is a new patient to Dr. Smith's office.

Doctor: Good morning Mrs. Jones. I'm Dr. John Smith. (Dr. Smith extends his hand to greet the patient.)

Patient: Hello Doctor, it's nice to meet you.
Doctor: I see from your chart that you are from out of town. How was your trip in?
Patient: It was O.K.—traffic was a little heavy.
Doctor: It can be a little slow this time of day. Before we talk about why you are here today, please tell me a little about yourself.
Patient: Well, I'm married and have three lovely children.
Doctor: I see. Do you work outside the home?
Patient: No, I haven't worked since my children were born.
Doctor: Don't underestimate yourself. It's a lot of work to raise three children and keep a house.
Patient: That's true—but my husband helps a lot.
Doctor: Good. Now, tell me, what has brought you to the office today?

Case 3-2 illustrates the joining phrase of the interview process. Notice how the physician greets the patient and demonstrates that he has prepared for the interview. The social dialogue helps put the patient at ease and also gives the physician useful information about the patient. When the physician senses that the patient is comfortable and ready to proceed, the physician progresses to tracking.

Problems with joining occur if the physician lacks respect for the patient or is unable to create a positive environment. Other common problems in joining are related to distractions such as leafing through the chart while talking to the patient, interruptions from outside the room, or ignoring the physical comfort of the patient. Joining can also be undermined by the patient because of feelings of distrust for doctors or from other negative experiences with the health care system.

Tracking

Tracking involves following the patient's description of his or her problem. The transition from joining to tracking is usually achieved by establishing the chief complaint. The chief complaint is the principal reason the patient came to see the doctor. This is usually elicited by asking an open-ended question that encourages the patient to state clearly and specifically why he or she has sought medical attention. Phrases such as "What brings you here today?" or "Tell me what is bothering you," or "How can I help you?" are common ways to elicit the patient's chief complaint. Frequently, patients may give a fairly complex answer; therefore, it is important to use responding and questioning skills to clarify the chief complaint.

Once the chief complaint is established, the physician continues to explore the patient's history. Initially, tracking is usually open-ended. The physician encourages the patient to talk freely about his or her problem. Phrases such as "tell me more about that," or "can you describe that more fully," are open-ended phrases that encourage the patient to think about the problem and describe it more fully to the physician. The physician continues the tracking process by using questioning skills and responding skills to help the patient elaborate on the chief complaint. Responding skills enable the physician to clarify his or her understanding of the problem and demonstrate that the patient has been heard. During this time the physician is forming hypotheses and testing these hypotheses with other questions and responses. Simultaneously the patient is developing a better understanding of his or her problem and a greater understanding of the physician's opinion. Commonly, as the tracking process begins to focus, the physician uses more closed-ended questions to fill in specific details necessary for the clinical decision-making process. At the end of the tracking phase, there is usually a transition from the medical interview to the physical examination. But frequently during the physical examination the physician may continue tracking, filling in other details about the patient and his or her problem. While tracking with the patient, the physician must keep the patient focused on the problem and avoid ramblings and other distractions.

The tracking process requires the skillful use of questioning and responding skills. Throughout the process, the physician's communication skills facilitate the patient's ability to describe his or her problem, articulate his or her agenda, and enhance the physician's understanding of the patient's problem and needs. These skills allow the physician to address the cognitive and emotional aspects of the patient's problem.

Case 3-2 (continued). Dr. Smith's interview with Mrs. Jones continues and illustrates some of the principles involved in the tracking process.

Doctor: Good. Now, tell me, what has brought you to the office today?
Patient: Well, I'm not sure it's anything, but I've been having some pains in my stomach.
Doctor: Can you show me where?
Patient: Down here. (Patient rubs her hand across her lower abdomen.)
Doctor: O.K. So your main concern is this lower abdominal pain. (Confirming the chief complaint.)
Patient: Yes, but I'm not sure if it is anything I should be worried about.
Doctor: Why do you say that? (Noting two remarks of denial.)
Patient: Well, I'm pretty healthy, and I just don't think it could be anything serious.
Doctor: But you're unsure. (Tracking with patient's feelings.)
Patient: I suppose so. It's sort of silly, but my mother said this is how Daddy started out before the doctors discovered he had colon cancer.
Doctor: So you're worried you may have the same thing.
Patient: A little, I guess.
Doctor: Well, tell me more about your symptoms and then we'll see whether there is cause to worry. O.K.?
Patient: All right. The pain really started about 3 weeks ago and has sort of come and gone since then. But in the last week it has gotten worse, and I have been constipated.
Doctor: Mm-hm—anything else? (Encouraging patient to elaborate.)
Patient: It seems a little worse after I eat, and I feel a little sick.
Doctor: A little sick? (Requests clarification of a common term to avoid confusion.)

Patient: Yeah, like I might throw up if it gets worse. But I never have.

Doctor: So the pain has been gradually increasing for the last 3 weeks and is associated with constipation and some nausea after meals. (Patient nods.) How would you describe the way the pain feels?

Patient: It's a crampy, aching pain that can last off and on all day.

Doctor: Anything relieve it?

Patient: Well, I do feel better after a bowel movement, especially if I've been constipated.

Doctor: Any diarrhea? (Focusing the interview to obtain specific details.)

Patient: Occasionally, especially when it first started.

Doctor: Any mucus or blood in your stools?

Patient: Yes, there is some mucus with the diarrhea, but not blood.

Doctor: Any change in your appetite?

Patient: Well, I'm trying to lose weight and only eat one meal a day, but my appetite is still there, unfortunately.

Doctor: Do you think the symptoms and diet are related?

Patient: Come to think of it, they did start about 2 weeks after I started dieting.

Doctor: Did anything like this ever happen before?

Patient: When I was in college I used to get cramps and diarrhea before exams, but it never persisted after exams were over and was never this bad. I just thought I had a nervous stomach.

Doctor: Nervous about anything now?

Patient: Well, Daddy isn't doing very well, and my husband has lost some overtime work we counted on.

Doctor: Sounds stressful.

Patient: I feel a little stressed out right now plus not feeling well.

Doctor: Let me see if I have everything. The pain started 3 weeks ago after you started dieting and has slowly gotten worse. You had a change in bowel habits with diarrhea and constipation but no bleeding. And it sounds like you're under some new stress and a little scared that this could be serious. (Summation)

Patient: That about it. What do you think it is?

Doctor: Well, I want to examine you first, but I don't believe there is need for alarm.

Patient: That's good to hear.

In Case 3-2, notice how the physician used questioning skills to encourage the patient to talk without leading her. Responses were used to confirm information, clarify symptoms, and address strong feelings. Also, notice how questions or responses used words that the patient had just used, hence the term *tracking!* During the physical exam, other details of the history can be sought as the physician processes the information he has gained.

Problems with the tracking segment of the interview are usually created by introducing bias or confusion into the process. Bias can be introduced by asking leading questions. Leading questions usually occur because the interviewer is thinking too far ahead and coming to premature conclusions about the diagnosis or solution to the problem. In other words, he or she "second guesses" the patient. Similarly, bias can be introduced when responding to a patient by imposing the interviewer's opinion of what the patient is trying to say without confirming it. Confusion is created by a disorganized approach, an interviewing "flight of ideas." This usually results from asking too many questions and not doing enough listening and responding. Likewise, confusion is created by dwelling on a point for an excessive amount of time. This suggests to the patient that what in reality is a minor point is actually an area for major concern. Confusion also occurs when the physician asks compound questions or a sequence of questions. Excessive use of medical terminology should also be avoided.

Intervening

Intervening is the process by which the physician communicates his or her perspective or understanding of the problem to the patient. The transition from tracking to intervening usually occurs after completion of the physical exam, as the physician begins to discuss his findings. The physician may offer a diagnosis, recommendations for further testing, or suggestions for treatment. The physician should determine the patient's acceptance of the information, understanding of the information, and carry on the process until the physician and patient are comfortable with the final goals and strategies. During this stage of the interview, the physician needs to pay particular attention to nonverbal behaviors the patient may demonstrate and take advantage of the opportunity to clarify any confusion that may exist. It is important that the physician speak clearly, use terms that are familiar to the patient, and be concise.

Sharing and responding skills are most important during the intervening process. Description and genuineness are primarily used to convey content, whereas self-disclosure more often communicates emotional information. Constructive confrontation is used to resolve discrepancies between the doctor and the patient. Questioning skills also play a role in intervening by checking the patient's understanding and acceptance of the physician's perspective. All too often, physicians, in a patronizing or authoritative manner, tell the patient what to do or how to feel. Sharing skills insure that the patient is a participant in his or her own health care.

Case 3-2 (continued). In the following dialogue, demonstrating intervening, Dr. Smith shares his findings and recommendations with Mrs. Jones after he has completed the exam.

Patient: Well, Doctor. Do I have anything serious?
Doctor: I don't find any evidence of anything serious.
Patient: That's a relief!
Doctor: I believe that with your change in diet and recent stress you have experienced, that you are having symptoms of irritable bowel syndrome. Have you ever heard of that?
Patient: I think I read about it in a women's magazine. Is there anything you can do for it?

Doctor: Yes, A regular diet, high in fiber, plenty of water, exercise, and trying to establish regular bowel habits resolve symptoms in the majority of patients.
Patient: How can I eat a regular diet and still lose weight? I definitely want to lose weight.
Doctor: You're reluctant to change your diet because you're afraid you'll gain weight, but I'm sure your symptoms will improve if you eat more regularly.
Patient: That makes sense. Do you have a specific diet in mind?
Doctor: Would you be willing to see a dietician to discuss a weight reduction diet that will allow you to eat regularly and increase the fiber in your diet?
Patient: That would be great!
Doctor: Fine, let's make those arrangements.

In Case 3-2, the diagnosis was fairly straightforward, and the patient readily accepted the doctor's opinion. Description was used to substantiate his opinion. Notice how Dr. Smith used constructive confrontation to negotiate an important therapeutic point regarding diet.

Problems with intervening occur when the physician is too authoritative or fails to confirm the patient's acceptance and understanding of the physician's perspective. Excessive use of medical terminology and verbosity in explaining things to a patient are likely to undermine this important stage of the interview.

Closing

Closing marks the end of the interview process. Frequently, the transition from intervening to closing is initiated by agreeing on a time for follow-up, either in person or by phone. The physician should acknowledge the patient by name, express appropriate appreciation for the efforts directed at cooperation with the interview, and, when appropriate, personalize closing remarks.

Case 3-2 (continued). The following example of the interview between Dr. Smith and Mrs. Jones illustrates the stage of closing.

Doctor: Do you have other questions about your abdominal pain or treatment?
Patient: No, I think everything is clear, but what if the symptoms persist?
Doctor: I'm glad you asked. I want to see you back in 6 weeks to review your progress. If your symptoms haven't improved, there are some specific diagnostic tests that can be done to investigate other possibilities. How does that sound to you?
Patient: That sounds fine.
Doctor: Good. I'll see you in 6 weeks then. It was nice to meet you, Mrs. Jones, and I hope that you will be feeling better shortly.
Patient: Thank you, it was nice meeting you, too. I'll see you in 6 weeks.
Doctor: Good. Have a good day and a safe drive back.

In closing, the doctor confirms the patient's understanding and acceptance of the diagnosis and management plan. He also arranges for a follow-up visit and closes the interview with a caring statement.

Problems with closing occur when the interviewer is abrupt or unclear about follow-up. Much of the rapport and trust that have developed through an effective interview can be undermined by dismissing the patient in a manner incongruent with the rest of the interview.

Summary

The medical interview is at the heart of clinical decision making and management. An accurate, reliable, and reproducible medical interview requires effective communication between the patient and physician. The medical interview progresses in an orderly manner through four stages: joining, tracking, intervening, and closing. Interpersonal and communication skills are used during all stages of the interview process, but some are more important during specific stages (Table 3-1). Problems occurring during any of the phases of the interview process can result in an ineffective interview that benefits neither the patient nor the physician.

THE MEDICAL HISTORY

There are two types of medical histories: the comprehensive and the focused medical history. The **comprehensive** or systematic medical history is taken from a patient as part of the complete evaluation of a person newly admitted to the hospital or an ambulatory patient presenting to a physician for a complete evaluation, usually his or her first visit. By definition, a comprehensive history involves obtaining all information relating to the health of the patient. This generally includes:

1. The chief complaint.
2. The history of the present illness.
3. The past medical history.
4. The family history.
5. The social history.
6. A review of systems.

Table 3-1
Use of Important Interviewing Skills during the Interview Process[a]

	Joining	Tracking	Intervening	Closing
Attending skills	X			
Questioning skills		X		
Responding skills		X	X	
Sharing skills			X	X

[a] Important interviewing skills used during each phase of the interview process are marked with an "X" in that phase's cell.

The **chief complaint** (CC) is a brief statement, in the patient's own words, of his or her reason for consulting you. Listening carefully to the patient's reason for coming and recording it can elucidate the patient's perspective on the problem. For example, the patient may tell his or her physician, "I have a sinus infection," "I'm having trouble with chest pain," or "I need some medicine for my migraine headache." Obviously, the physician may not agree with the patient's conclusions about what is wrong with him or her. The patient's sinus infection may be a simple cold, her angina may be heartburn, and his migraine headaches a brain tumor. In fact, the patient's chief complaint may not reflect the real reason for the patient's visit at all. For example, a patient may want a "general check-up" or tell the nurse that he has "groin pain" when his real concern is about a penile discharge. A patient with marital or work stress may complain of "trouble sleeping." Thus, the chief complaint may not accurately reflect the patient's agenda, real diagnosis, or the most serious threat to his or her health.

The history of the present illness (HPI) is an elaboration of the patient's chief complaint and has several important dimensions. Depending on the nature of the chief complaint, there will be a need for more or less depth in each dimension.

What does the patient mean by the symptoms? What is the symptom like? For instance, when the patient complains of "dizziness," does the patient mean a rotatory sensation (vertigo) or lightheadedness? Is the patient's pain sharp, dull, crushing, burning, or achey? Determining the *what* of the symptoms can help establish a diagnosis. For example, in a patient with chest pain, sharp or stabbing pain is almost never caused by angina.

Where is the symptom located? Determining the where is especially important for patients presenting the pain, for example, headaches, back pain, abdominal pain, or leg pain. Where does it seem most severe? Does it radiate to other areas?

When did the problem start? What was the patient doing at the time when it started? How has the problem evolved over time? For instance, in a patient presenting with a sore throat, the diagnostic implications are different if the sore throat has been steadily worsening over 2 days versus if it has been worse in the morning but better later in the day. The diagnosis of headache provides another good example. Patients with tension headaches or headaches related to depression may complain of a constant headache of several weeks' duration. In contrast, the rare patient who has a brain tumor will complain of an insidious worsening of symptoms over time. The patient with cluster headaches will alternate between being headache-free and having periods of frequent severe headaches of short duration.

How severe are the symptoms? For example, in a patient presenting with shortness of breath, does he or she develop shortness of breath after climbing six stairs or after running a mile? In a patient presenting with fatigue, is the fatigue so severe that he or she is unable to get out of bed, or does the patient mean that he or she feels a little tired at the end of the day? This dimension of the history can give you insight into how severely affected the patient is (or feels he or she is) by his or her symptoms.

Most patients will be able to relate the above information reasonably well; other aspects of the history of present illness may be more difficult. The patient may not think to volunteer certain important information; therefore, it is important for the physician to ask about the following: exacerbating and alleviating factors, environmental and social factors contributing to the patient's problem, and associated symptoms.

Exacerbating and alleviating factors are those things that make the patient's symptoms worse or better. For example, with epigastric (upper abdomen) pain, it is important to ask whether eating certain types of food affects the symptoms. Classically, gallbladder symptoms worsen with fried and greasy foods. Peptic ulcer disease may be relieved by food or antacids. Lower abdominal pain associated with irritable bowel syndrome will often times be aggravated by food and relieved after a bowel movement. It is also important to ask what remedies the patient has tried and how those remedies have affected the problem. The fact that a rash has not responded to a topical antifungal cream may have diagnostic importance. In a patient presenting with symptoms of nasal drainage, it would be important to know that the patient has not responded to previous treatment with a particular decongestant.

Environmental and social factors are those events that seem linked chronologically with the start of the patient's symptoms and thus might be causally related. A good example of this is insomnia beginning at the time of a marital separation. A particularly stressful event at work may be associated with an increase in the frequency and severity of the patient's headaches.

Associated symptoms are other symptoms that have (or haven't) occurred with the patient's current problem. For example, has the patient noted heartburn or regurgitation with his or her chest pain (a clue for reflux esophagitis)? Has the patient noted dark urine or clay-colored stools in association with nausea (a clue for hepatitis)? Has the patient noted cough or nasal drainage with a sore throat (both of these would decrease the chance that the sore throat is caused by bacterial infection)?

Without much detailed knowledge of disease pathophysiology, it may seem impossible to know about what associated symptoms to ask. A helpful guideline is to ask questions pertaining to the organ system in question. For example, with chest pain, the cardiovascular, gastrointestinal, pulmonary, and musculoskeletal systems could be involved. Therefore, it would be worth asking about upper gastrointestinal, cardiac, pulmonary, and musculoskeletal symptoms. In some circumstances, however, the search for associated symptoms should include organ systems besides the obvious ones. For example, elderly patients may develop loss of urinary control, falls, or confusion as a result of a pulmonary infection.

Case 3-3. Dr. Smith obtains a history of the present illness from another patient.

Doctor: I'm Doctor Smith. You look like you're in quite a bit of pain. Can you tell me a little bit about what sort of problem you've been having?
Patient: You're right about the pain. It's my back.
Doctor: Can you tell me about it?
Patient: It started about 3 days ago.
Doctor: Do you remember what you were doing when it started?

Patient: I was lifting a big tub at work when I felt this sharp pain in my back.
Doctor: Can you show me where the pain is located?
Patient: It's down low, right here (points at her low back area).
Doctor: And the pain has been bothering you a lot since then?
Patient: Oh yes; I have trouble trying to get up after I've been sitting down, and I have trouble if I bend at all.
Doctor: Does the pain stay in your back, or does it go anywhere?
Patient: No, it stays right there. I don't know what I'd do if it went anywhere else!
Doctor: Have you had any numbness or tingling or weakness in your legs?
Patient: No.
Doctor: Have you had any trouble controlling your water or your bowels?
Patient: No, thank goodness.
Doctor: What have you done to make the pain better over the last few days?
Patient: Well, I've had to miss work, and I've tried to rest in bed, but that can be difficult because I have two young children.
Doctor: Have you tried anything else, like any pills, or heat, or anything else?
Patient: All I have at home is some aspirin, and I've tried using a heating pad sometimes.
Doctor: Is this the first time you've had trouble with this problem, or has this occurred in the past?
Patient: Oh, I've had problems like this before, but usually it gets better after a couple of days of resting.
Doctor: When was the last time?
Patient: Oh, about 6 or 8 months ago.
Doctor: Does the pain usually go away completely? Are you usually fine in between the times when your back hurts?
Patient: Yeah, I usually don't have too much trouble.
Doctor: Do you do any special things to take care of your back in between the times when you're having trouble?
Patient: No, nobody's ever talked to me about anything special.
Doctor: What kind of work do you do?
Patient: I work as a nurse in a nursing home.
Doctor: I suppose that means you have to do quite a bit of lifting.
Patient: Oh, yes, you know a lot of those patients can't get around too well.

The past medical history (PMH) often contains important clues regarding the cause of the patient's difficulties. For example, in a patient with right lower abdominal pain, the list of likely diagnoses is different for a patient who has already had an appendectomy. Likewise, the tests ordered in patients with right upper abdominal pain will be affected by the knowledge that the patient has had a cholecystectomy (gallbladder removal). Knowing that an individual presenting with cough had been hospitalized this time last year with pneumonia can provide new insight into the patient's apparent anxiety regarding his or her current problem. Important elements of the past medical history are childhood and adult serious illnesses, including traumatic events, immunizations, operations, including dates and diagnosis, medications, and medication allergies. In a pediatric patient, the past medical history will be somewhat different depending on the patient's age. For example, if the child is young it may be important to inquire about the mother's prenatal and perinatal course, childhood growth, and developmental milestones.

The family history (FH) contains information about inherited illnesses for which the patient is at risk and information about the family structure and milieu in which the patient grew up and is currently living. Family support can have an important influence on health. Thus, the family history provides a bridge to the next element of the history.

The most effective method for obtaining the family history involves constructing a genogram. The **genogram** is a pictorial representation of the patient's family, including one to two generations above and below the patient when possible, indicating the sex, age, occupations, illnesses, and deaths in family members (cause and year of death). After the genogram is constructed, an inquiry should be made into other illnesses that run in the family. The physician should inquire specifically about a history of the following problems in the patient's immediate family (parents and siblings): allergies, alcoholism, arthritis, blood pressure problems, bleeding tendency, cancer, diabetes mellitus, epilepsy, gout, glaucoma, kidney disease, mental problems, migraine headaches, muscle disease, and early myocardial infarctions. All these illnesses are reasonably common problems with strong hereditary patterns. More information on genogram construction is contained in Chapter 9.

The social history (SH) is extremely important. According to Osler, "It is more important to know what kind of patient has the disease than what kind of disease the patient has." The social history provides insight into an individual's values, attitudes, habits, and support systems. The elements of a social history can be organized into the mnemonic SCREEEM: **S**ocial, **C**ultural, **R**eligious, **E**conomic, **E**ducation, **E**nvironmental, and **M**edical Resources (Smilkstein, 1980).

The purpose of the *social* element is to explore the patient's family and other close relationships. Aspects include with whom the patient lives, the patient's relationship with his or her biological family, emotional and geographic closeness to members of her biological family, and to whom the patient feels closest (biological family members or others). Other important aspects of this component of the social history are contained in Chapter 9.

One should find out about the patient's *cultural* background, including ethnic and geographic origins and how well the patient feels he or she fits into his or her current cultural milieu. Generally, the patient's culture also has an effect on what the patient believes about his or her illness and what will be most effective in curing the illness. Such beliefs should be explored. Other important aspects of this component of the social history are contained in Chapter 10.

The *religious* element of the social history should explore the importance of religious beliefs to the patient, whether the patient considers him- or herself a religious person, as well as the patient's degree of involvement in a religious community. Some patient's religious beliefs have profound implications for medical care, for example, Jehovah's Witnesses or Christian Scientists.

Important information to obtain in an *economic* history include (1) the patient's current employment, (2) adequacy of his or her current employment to meet his or her lifestyle needs, and (3) availability of medical insurance.

The *educational* element should clarify the patient's level of education, whether it is high school, college, or postgraduate level. It is also helpful to find out about the educational attainment of the patient's significant other.

The *environmental* component should contain information about the patient's environmental and personal habits, including (1) job site, (2) home, and (3) participation in such habits as smoking, drinking, illicit drug use, and exercise.

Finally, it is important to find out about the patient's current and past involvement with and perceptions of the medical community, *medical resources*. This can be accomplished by asking about current and past physicians and their specialities. It is also helpful to find out about who else the patient relies on for medical advice.

Case 3-3 (continued). The following is an example of a social history.

Doctor: Next, Ms. Brown, I'd like to ask you a little more about your family and day-to-day life. Are you happy with your marriage and family life?

Patient: We've had our ups and downs, but, yes, I'd say things are going pretty well now.

Doctor: So you'd consider your marriage pretty stable?

Patient: Yes, I would.

Doctor: You mentioned earlier that you are a nurse. Are you a registered nurse (RN), or a licensed practical nurse (LPN)?

Patient: I'm an RN. I graduated from the University of Oklahoma School of Nursing longer ago than I'd like to remember!

Doctor: Where do you work?

Patient: I've worked as a nurse at the Happy Rest Nursing Home for the past 5 years.

Doctor: What kinds of things do you do there?

Patient: I'm kind of a jack of all trades, since we're sort of short staffed. I'm the charge nurse for one wing; I also distribute medications, and sometimes I help the aides with lifting and moving the patients.

Doctor: It sounds like there is a lot of variety in your work. Do you still enjoy it?

Patient: Oh yes, by and large, I do. No two days are the same, and I get a lot of satisfaction from helping those poor old people!

Doctor: What's a typical day in your life like?

Patient: Well, I get up about six in the morning, usually have a cup of coffee, some juice or cereal, and head off to work so I can be there by about 7 a.m. I usually get home by about four in the afternoon, fix supper for my husband and children, spend the evening with them watching a little TV or do some reading, and then go to bed.

Doctor: You mentioned drinking coffee. Do you drink much coffee?

Patient: Usually only one cup a day.

Doctor: Do you drink much alcohol?

Patient: I don't drink at all.
Doctor: Cigarettes?
Patient: No, I don't smoke.
Doctor: Do you usually eat just two meals a day?
Patient: Usually I'll have a salad or hot dish in the cafeteria at work at noon, but sometimes if things are busy, I'll miss lunch.
Doctor: What about dinner?
Patient: We usually have meat and potatoes and a salad.
Doctor: It sounds like your days are pretty busy. Do you get any chance to exercise?
Patient: Well, I get some exercise at work, and my husband, kids, and I try to get out for a two-mile walk two to three times a week.
Doctor: That's good. How about hobbies or other interests?
Patient: I enjoy reading and needlepoint, and we're pretty active in a local Baptist church.
Doctor: What kinds of things are you involved in there?
Patient: Oh, choir and one of the woman's groups.
Doctor: Would you say you have a pretty good network of friends.
Patient: Oh yes, I'm very fortunate in that regard, what with friends at church and neighbors, and of course we've lived around here quite a while.
Doctor: How long?
Patient: Both my husband and I were born here, and my grandparents moved here from Missouri.
Doctor: You mentioned earlier that you and your husband both work outside the home. Has your financial situation been okay, or has it been a little bit difficult?
Patient: No, we're living pretty comfortably now, but we're trying to save a little here and there for the kids, hoping they'll go to college.
Doctor: Do you have health insurance?
Patient: Yes, Blue Cross from work.

The **review of systems** (ROS), as the name implies, involves a systematic review of possible symptoms or problems in the major organ systems of the human body. Parts of the review of systems that were covered while obtaining a history of present illness do not need to be repeated. Initially, it is helpful to use a checklist to obtain the review of systems; later physicians develop their own approach, tailoring the questions to the individual patient. For example, asking about urinary incontinence in 20-year-old men is unlikely to yield many positive responses, but it is crucial to ask about incontinence in an elderly woman, where it is a highly prevalent problem. Items commonly included in the review of systems, by organ system, include:

- *General.* Fevers, chills, weight loss, appetite changes, general statement of the patient's health.
- *Psychological.* "Nervousness," depression, insomnia, anxiety, sexual disturbances, psychosis, deviant or criminal behavior.

- *Skin.* Itching, bruising, petechiae, moles, infections, rashes.
- *Hematopoietic system.* Anemia, unusual bleeding after tooth extraction or other minor trauma, enlarged or tender lymph nodes.
- *HEENT.*
  Head: headache, facial pain.
  Ears: discharge, tinnitus, hearing loss.
  Eyes: vision change, blurry vision, pain.
  Nose and sinuses: epistaxis (nosebleeds), nasal drainage or blockage.
  Mouth and throat: sores in the mouth that haven't healed, bleeding from the gums, date of last dental exam, persistent hoarseness or sore throat.
- *Breasts.* Lumps, discharge, or pain.
- *Respiratory tract.* Cough or change in chronic cough, sputum production, hemoptysis, pain associated with respirations.
- *Cardiovascular.* Exertional chest pain or dyspnea, nocturnal dyspnea, orthopnea (shortness of breath when lying flat but not when upright), palpitations, history of high blood pressure or heart murmur, exertional calf pain.
- *Gastrointestinal.* Nausea, vomiting, hematemesis (vomiting up blood), gas, sour eructations, difficulty swallowing, heartburn, abdominal pain, jaundice, change in bowel movements (frequency, blood in stool, black stools, change in the shape of the stool, bowel habits), hemorrhoids.
- *Urinary tract.* Dysuria (pain on urination), frequency, urgency, pyuria, hematuria, history of gravel or stones, weak stream, incontinence, enuresis.
- *Male genital tract.* Penile discharge, masses of the testicles, pain.
- *Female genital tract.* Menstrual history, menarche, frequency, regularity, duration of periods, pads/day, date of last menstrual period, use of contraception, vaginal itching, vaginal discharge, dyspareunia (pain on intercourse), pelvic pain, history of venereal disease, age at menopause, postmenopausal vaginal bleeding.
- *Musculoskeletal system.* Pain, stiffness, limitation of motion in any joint, swelling of joints, sprains, redness of any joint.
- *Nervous system.* Seizures, fainting spells, dizziness, difficulty with speaking, difficulty with gait, balance, weakness, numbness or tingling.
- *Endocrine.* Tremor, heat or cold intolerance, voice change, change in hair distribution, polyuria, polydipsia, polyphagia, change in glove or shoe size, fertility.

Example review-of-systems questions include:

- I am going to ask you a series of questions to be sure that you haven't forgotten to tell me something that may be important. Have you recently experienced any fevers or chills?
- Have you had any problem with unusual or unexpected weight loss or changes in your appetite?

- How would you describe your health in general?
- Would you describe yourself as a tense or nervous individual?
- Do you have problems with frequently crying, feeling blue, or depressed?
- Do you have trouble sleeping at night?
- Are you satisfied with your sexual life?
- Have you ever been in trouble with the law?
- Have you noticed any unusual rashes, bumps, or sores on your skin, or do you bruise more easily than usual?
- Have you had any trouble with anemia or low blood or bled an unusual amount after having a tooth pulled or getting cut?
- Have you noticed any enlarged or sore lymph glands?
- Have you had any unusual headaches, any unusual pain in your ears, discharge from your ears, or trouble with hearing?
- Have you had any trouble with your vision, pain in your eyes?
- Do you wear glasses, and when was the last time you had your vision checked?
- Do you have any problem with nosebleeds, unusual blockage or drainage from your nose?
- Have you noticed any sores in your mouth that haven't healed? When was the last time you were checked by a dentist?
- Have you noticed that you have a sore throat that doesn't seem to go away or that you've had any change in your voice, particularly hoarseness?

If a positive response is elicited, further questioning may be needed. For example, if the patient indicates that he or she has chest pain, additional questions might include: "Can you show me where the pain is? How long has this pain bothered you? How severe is the pain? Can you describe the pain to me? What have you noticed tends to bring the pain on? Have you noticed anything that tends to relieve the pain?"

Although obtaining a review of systems completes the comprehensive medical history, data gathering continues with the physical examination, which corroborates findings suggested by the history and may uncover new diagnostic possibilities (see Chapter 4). Laboratory tests, such as blood tests, urinalysis, or radiological studies, are indicated in some patients to confirm or rule out a diagnosis suggested by the history and physical examination or to monitor a patient's clinical status.

After data gathering is complete, an assessment is made, which is an interpretation of the information gathered during the medical encounter, by synthesizing this information into a single diagnosis or a list of possible diagnoses (see Chapter 5). A well-thought-out assessment helps make sense of the clinical data gathered and provides a springboard to the management plan.

Finally, a plan is formulated. The plan is the management strategy for the case. This may involve further diagnostic testing to help arrive at a diagnosis or determine the severity of a known diagnosis, medication to relieve the condition, patient education to help the patient understand and take steps to prevent worsening or recurrence of the condition, and provision for follow-up visits.

Effective clinical management involves weighing issues such as the risk versus the benefit of interventions and their cost effectiveness (see Chapter 6).

THE FOCUSED MEDICAL HISTORY

The second type of medical history is the **focused history.** It is useful for gathering information during a limited period of time, during a 10- to 15-min office visit, for example, and thus is much more limited in scope. The objective of a focused history is to obtain only that information needed to arrive at the heart of the patient's problem as quickly as possible. The basic components of a focused history include the reason for the visit (chief complaint) and a history of the current problem, including, to a varying degree depending on the problem, amplification of the chief complaint, elements of the past history, family history, social history, and review of systems if they pertain to the current problem.

The information obtained from a focused medical history is usually recorded in a *SOAP note.* The SOAP format is the standard way of recording progress notes in hospitalized patients as well. "S" stands for *subjective* information. This information includes the patient's chief complaint, history of present illness, and relevant information from the past history, family history, social history, and review of systems. Physical findings, laboratory data, old records, x-ray reports, and other information not colored by the patient's interpretation comprise *objective* information, the "O" in SOAP. The "A" in SOAP means *assessment,* that is, the physician's diagnosis. "P" is the plan or strategy to be used to diagnose and solve the patient's problem.

THE MEDICAL RECORD

Once the physician has obtained the history and done a physical exam, the important task of recording the information still remains. The written record is the documentation of these carefully obtained findings and will be what the physician or others will consult for questions about the patient's status. Therefore, it is important that the findings be clearly and concisely recorded. Findings can either be recorded as a complete medical history or as a progress note utilizing the SOAP format, depending on the extent of the evaluation. Figure 3-1 is an example of how Ms. Brown's complete medical history would appear in the written record. Figure 3-2 illustrates that same history written in a SOAP format.

Gathering a medical history is an essential first step in helping patients improve their health. The comprehensive history includes chief complaint, history of present illness, past medical history, social history, family history, and review of systems. The focused history includes a chief complaint and history of the current problem, usually organized into a SOAP format. It is important for the student to develop skills in obtaining both types of history, since a carefully taken history will reveal important clues to the patient's problem, will often help focus the student's attention on certain aspects of the physical examination, and will often direct the student toward a particular diagnosis.

CC: Ms. Brown is a 38-year-old woman who presents with a 3-day history of low back pain.

HPI: Ms. Brown states that she noticed the sudden onset of lower back discomfort while reaching over to pick something up at work. The pain does not radiate. She hasn't noted paresthesias or weakness in her legs but has noticed that the pain hasn't improved much in spite of using a heating pad, aspirin, and resting when she can. The discomfort has bothered her enough that she has had to miss work as a nurse at a local nursing home. She mentions that she had similar episodes of pain in the past (the last bout was 6–8 months ago), but past episodes seemed to improve more quickly that this current episode.

PMH:
1. Illnesses: Hospitalized 3 years ago at Oklahoma Memorial Hospital (OMH) for deep vein thrombosis of the leg.
   Injured left knee skiing 1976, no surgery or sequelae.
2. Surgeries: appendectomy, 1956, OMH,
   bilateral tubal ligation, 1977, OMH,
   cholecystectomy, 1984, OMH.
3. OB: 3201 [Three pregnancies, two pregnancies to term, no premature deliveries, one miscarriage (pregnancy terminated prior to 20 weeks' gestation)].
4. Immunizations: last dT more than 10 years ago.
5. Medications: Aspirin, two tablets four times a day; for headaches and back pain.
6. Allergies: None.

Genogram:

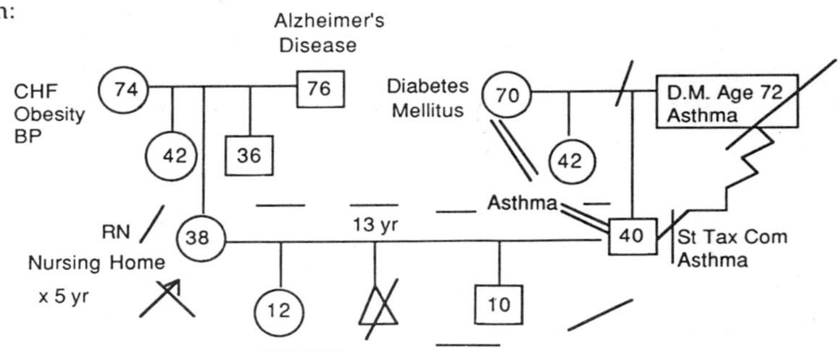

SH: Works for the past 5 years as a charge nurse at the Happy Rest Nursing Home. She enjoys her work there. She is happy with her marital and financial situation. She says she has a good social support network through church (Baptist Church) and family. She denies use of cigarettes, ethanol, but drinks one cup of coffee per day. She usually eats three meals per day, salad or casserole at lunch, salad with meat, potatoes with family at suppertime. She walks two to three times a week, 2 miles at a time, with her family.

ROS:

General health: Approximately 10 lb weight loss over past 4 months, but this has been intentional (overweight). Denies fevers, chills, appetite changes.

Psychological: Occasionally (no more than once per month) can't get to sleep because she worries about things at work, but even then gets to sleep by midnight at the latest. Denies any trouble falling or staying asleep, feeling blue or depressed, or feeling more tense or anxious than most other people are.

Skin: Mentions a couple of "moles" on her neck × 2 years. They tend to get caught in her necklace. She wonders if they can be removed. Otherwise denies, itching, bruising, petechiae, infections, or rashes.

Figure 3-1. Ms. Brown's complete medical history.

Hematopoietic system: Denies anemia, unusual bleeding after tooth extraction or trauma, or enlarged or tender lymph glands.

HEENT:

Head: She complains of "migraine headaches" × 10 years, occurring each month or so, associated with menses. The headaches are throbbing, sometimes on the left side, sometimes on the right, associated with nausea and some photophobia, and improve with rest. They usually respond to aspirin or other over-the-counter medications.

Ears: Denies discharge, tinnitus, or hearing loss.

Eyes: "Nearsighted" since teen years, wears glasses, last correction about 1 year ago. She says that they still seem to be okay. Denies blurry vision or pain.

Nose and sinuses: Gets stuffy nose, scratchy throat, and sneezing, usually during April of each year. She treats this with over-the-counter antihistamines. She denies nasal drainage, epistaxis, or blockage.

Mouth and throat: She denies sores in the mouth, bleeding from the gums, or hoarseness. Her last dental exam was about 6 months ago. She was told her teeth were fine.

Breasts: She does breast self-exam. She has not noticed any lumps or discharge but was wondering if she needs a mammogram.

Respiratory: She denies cough or change in chronic cough, sputum production, hemoptysis, and pain associated with respirations.

Cardiovascular: She denies exertional chest pain or dyspnea, nocturnal dyspnea, orthopnea, palpitations, history of high blood pressure or heart murmur, and exertional calf pain.

Gastrointestinal: She had a 10-year history of intermittent lower abdominal cramping, sometimes associated with loose brown stools, and relieved by defecation. She says her symptoms seem to be worse when she is feeling "uptight." She denies any weight loss, blood in her stool, black stools, nausea, vomiting, hemetemesis, sour eructations, or difficulty swallowing.

Urinary tract: She denies dysuria, frequency, urgency, pyuria, hematuria, history of gravel or stones, weak stream, incontinence, or enuresis.

Female genital tract: Menstrual history: She became menarche at age 12. Her periods now occur every 28 days, and last 4 or 5 days. Her last menstrual period began on August 2, previous menstrual period about July 4. She denies vaginal itching or discharge or history of venereal disease.

Skeletal: See History of Present Illness. She denies pain, stiffness, or swelling in any of her joints.

Nervous system: She denies seizures, fainting spells, dizziness, difficulty with speaking, gait, balance, weakness, numbness, or tingling.

Endocrine: She denies tremor, heat or cold intolerance, voice changes, changes in hair distribution, polyuria, polydipsia, polyphagia, change in glove or shoe size, or fertility problems.

PE: A record of a complete physical exam is omitted here [see Chapter 4]

Lab: Lumbar-sacral spine films: within normal limits.

A: Mid- and low back muscle and ligamentous strain, which seems to be gradually improving.

P: Discussed with patient:

1. Continue taking current meds if helpful.
2. Gave written low back exercises and information regarding proper bending and lifting.
3. Follow-up visit scheduled for 7–10 days.

Figure 3–1. Continued

S: Last Wednesday, 10/7/87, at work, the patient was lifting 45- to 50-lb tubs on her own. During the lifting and following it she developed pain in her mid- and lower back. She states that it is confined to her lower back and does not spread into her legs. She denies numbness, tingling, or weakness in her legs or feet or any problem with control of her bowels or bladder. The pain gets worse when she moves around and is somewhat better when she rests. She denies any past history of back injuries but has had occasional milder episodes of low back pain, occurring about once a year.

O: Pleasant black female in no distress. Range of motion of the trunk is full. There is some paravertebral muscle spasm but no pain over the lumbar or sacral spine. Neurological exam is normal. Straight-leg raising was negative.

A: Mid- and low back muscle and ligamentous strain, which seems to be gradually improving.

P: Discussed with patient:

1. Continue taking current meds if helpful.
2. Gave written low back exercises and information regarding proper bending and lifting.
3. Follow-up visit scheduled for 7–10 days.

Figure 3-2. Ms. Brown's focused medical history.

CONCLUSIONS

The medical interview is a scientific method used to "measure" the patient's signs and symptoms and should reflect the desirable characteristics of any scientific test, including objectivity, precision, accuracy, sensitivity, specificity, and reproducibility. The physician is the instrument, quantifying the patient's signs and symptoms through his or her interviewing skills. The scientific basis of the process is influenced by both physician and patient. The physician serves as both test instrument and analysis instrument, and his or her clinical knowledge, skills, and beliefs influence the process and may also serve as a source of bias undermining the scientific basis of the process. Like the physician, the patient's account of the situation will be influenced by his or her knowledge, values, and beliefs as well as past experiences with the health care system.

These biases can be minimized through knowledge and application of several interviewing attitudes and skills. These include attitudes such as unconditional positive regard and congruence. Nonverbal skills also facilitate effective communication, and these include attending skills and facilitative cues. Finally, verbal skills include questioning skills (open-ended, focused, circular, and leading questions), responding skills (paraphrasing, summation, and sympathetic and empathetic responses), and sharing skills. Proper use of these skills during the appropriate phase of the interview process facilitates accurate data gathering.

The content of the medical interview depends on whether a focused or comprehensive evaluation is needed. Traditionally, a comprehensive history includes chief complaint, elaboration of the chief complaint (history of the present illness), past history, family history (including genogram), personal social history, and a review of systems. The focused history incorporates chief complaint and history of present illness with elements of past history and other parts of the comprehensive history relevant to the problem at hand. Both approaches conclude with an assessment and plan.

The medical interview and history form the foundation for the clinician's assessment and management decisions. A well-taken history, using the interviewing skills described, will produce accurate information, leading to accurate assessments and appropriate management plans; poorly taken information may lead to erroneous assessments and ineffective or even dangerous management steps. Therefore, it is vitally important for the student aspiring to be an effective clinician to develop and continue to fine-tune the interviewing skills described in this chapter.

CASES FOR DISCUSSION

Case 1

A 23-year-old male comes in to his physician because of a "sore throat." He describes his throat as scratchy, and he has had some nasal drainage. The physician determines it is a viral sore throat and prescribes a decongestant and symptomatic treatment. To the physician's surprise, instead of seeming relieved at the news, the patient seems upset.

1. How might you have handled the interview to prevent this "end of visit" surprise?
2. Assume he tells you he's always needed antibiotics in the past for sore throats. How would you respond to him?

Case 2

A 40-year-old male comes in to see his physician with an itchy rash on his hands. The physician looks at the chart, says to the patient, "It says here you have a rash on your hands. Let's take a look at it." He examines the rash briefly, then writes out a prescription and says, "Here, use this cream."

1. Indicate which phases in the interview process (i.e., joining, tracking, etc.) this physician performed.
2. Which phases in the process did he not perform or perform incompletely?
3. What additional information might have been helpful?

Case 3

A 28-year-old female comes in to see her physician with complaints of "neck pain." The physician asks her if she has any numbness or tingling in her arms, and she says she hasn't. The physician then writes her a prescription for a pain reliever and muscle relaxer and leaves the room.

1. Indicate which phases of the interview process were performed.
2. How might you have handled the encounter differently?
3. How would you feel if you'd been the patient in this encounter? Why?
4. What additional information, which the physician did not obtain, could have a bearing on the management of this case?

Case 4

A 25-year-old Caucasian male comes in for a general check-up. He has no particular problems today but just felt it was time to have a check-up. His insurance pays for an annual examination. He had asthma as a child and also had his tonsils and adenoids removed. His last tetanus booster immunization was 10 years ago. His siblings and parents are all "alive and well." He's been married for a little over 2 years and says the marriage is "happy." They have no children. He has worked in the state auditor's office for the past 3 months and says he enjoys his work. He has had a college education.

1. Indicate in which part of the history the items above belong.
2. Would you obtain additional family history? Why or why not? What would you obtain?
3. What personal social history was not obtained? Why would this be important?

Case 5

Arrange the information below into SOAP format: Problem of depression. Patient's affect appears brighter today than 1 month ago. Her depression seems to be responding to the antidepressant medication. She has generally been feeling more "upbeat" lately. Depression improving on medication. Is job hunting and plans to interview soon in South Carolina. Says she is much more in control of her work situation and is coping well there. She should continue taking the medication and come back to see me in 1 month.

EXERCISES FOR PRACTICE

The best way to learn interviewing and history-taking techniques described in this chapter is to practice them on either real or simulated patients. If real or simulated patients are not available, then role-playing a medical encounter can be equally effective.

During the role play, one student should play the patient, one the physician, and one should observe the interview. The "patient" should "make up" a plausible scenario, perhaps from his or her own experience, or a short clinical vignette can be supplied by the instructor. The "physician" then interviews the "patient," obtaining either a comprehensive or a focused medical history. After the interview, both the "observer" and the "patient" provide feedback to the "physician" on his or her interview style. The roles among the group of three students then change, and the process repeats itself as time allows.

RECOMMENDED READINGS

Reiser, D. B., & Rosen, D. H. (1985). *Medicine as human experience.* Rockville, MD: Aspen.

Chapter 5 of this book provided a nice discussion of the science of observation, following the patient's affect, the concept of process, and the "A.R.T." of medical interviewing. Later chapters discuss the distinction between disease and illness and between curing and healing, using examples from their patients and the author's own illnesses.

Enelow, A. J., & Swisher, S. N. (Eds.). (1986). *Interviewing and patient care,* 3rd ed. New York: Oxford University Press.

This text provides an in-depth examination of the interview process including dealing with difficult patients, recognizing the patient's emotional and behavior response to illness and the provider, and describing techniques to interview children, older adults, and the entire family.

Coulehan, J. L., & Block, M. (1987). *The medical interview: A primer for students of the art.* Philadelphia: F. A. Davis.

This text provides an in-depth examination of the interview process but also discussed difficult clinical management issues such as noncompliance.

CHAPTER 4

The Physical Examination

William M. Chop, Jr. and Stephen J. Spann

Case 4-1. A 14-year-old single black female presents to the emergency room at 11 p.m. complaining of severe bilateral lower abdominal pain of 24 h duration. The physician finds the patient to be crying hysterically and writhing in pain. Unable to elicit a history from the patient, the physician approaches the bedside to begin a physical examination.

The physician begins by gently and systematically feeling the patient's abdomen while talking with her in a soothing, reassuring voice. The examination reveals her to be quite tender in both lower abdominal quadrants, with mild to moderate direct and rebound tenderness (pain both with deep probing of the abdomen and with suddenly releasing the probing fingers). As the patient begins to calm down, the physician is able to obtain a history.

The patient admits to being sexually active without the use of contraception. Her last menstrual period started on schedule 2 days ago. Her past medical history and review of systems are otherwise unremarkable.

The physician suspects a diagnosis of acute pelvic inflammatory disease (a bacterial infection of the uterus, fallopian tubes, and surrounding tissues) secondary to *Neisseria gonorrhoeae* or *Chlamydia trachomatis*. The physician explains to the patient that a pelvic examination is needed to confirm or disprove the diagnosis. The young woman is initially very resistant to this idea. Therefore, the physician carefully explains the physical examination maneuver and the importance of the information that it yields. The patient then gives her consent.

The physician proceeds to perform a gentle vaginal speculum and bimanual pelvic examination, all the while explaining each step. The examination reveals a mucopurulent cervical discharge, with marked tenderness of the uterine cervix and both fallopian tubes. The physician explains to the patient the need for a urine pregnancy test to rule out a tubal pregnancy. The patient consents, and the test proves negative. The physician feels that the previous suspicion of acute pelvic inflammatory disease is the most likely diagnosis and treats the patient with an intramuscular injection of ceftriaxone followed by oral doxycycline. A culture of the uterine cervix taken at the time of the pelvic examination subsequently grows *Neisseria gonorrhoeae.*

INTRODUCTION

The physical examination is a very special and important part of any patient–physician encounter, as illustrated by case 4-1. It serves mainly a diagnostic role that tends to be overrated by most patients (and by many physicians), but it also has an often underrated therapeutic role in patient care.

The first part of this chapter describes physical examination principles. The second part consists of a series of figures comprising a detailed framework for a "core physical examination" useful for the new student of medicine to learn and practice during patient encounters.

GATHERING OBJECTIVE INFORMATION

An observation that a patient makes about himself or herself is classified conventionally as "subjective" information. An observation made by a physician about a patient is classified conventionally as "objective" information. Objective information also comes from laboratory tests, x rays, and other machine-related measurements, but in most cases the majority of objective information comes from the physical examination.

Physicians gather objective information by four methods: inspection, percussion, auscultation, and palpation. **Inspection** uses the sense of sight to gather global and specific information about the appearance of the patient, such as noting that a patient's skin appears yellow (jaundice). **Percussion** uses the senses of hearing and feeling to gather specific information about the relative density of body areas. It involves a technique of tapping on body parts, usually with the middle finger of one hand, while listening and feeling for the degree of resonance elicited. For example, tapping on the chest can be used to determine the level of the diaphragm. **Auscultation** uses the sense of hearing in listening with a stethoscope to draw inferences about the physiological functioning of specific body areas. For example, listening to heart valves may assist in determining if the valves are leaking. **Palpation** uses the sense of feeling to define textures, masses, and thickenings and to determine the degree of tenderness of specific body areas. For example, feeling an abdomen helps to determine if the liver is enlarged and if it is abnormally tender. **Smell** occasionally serves as a fifth information-gathering method.

POSSIBLE ERRORS IN THE INFORMATION OBTAINED BY THE PHYSICAL EXAM

The quality of information obtained during the physical examination may vary because of several factors even when correct indicated observations are made. Even though the information gathered during the exam is considered objective, it may unavoidably include subjective components. For example, during abdominal palpation a patient might cry out because of psychological problems. The physician is likely to interpret such a reaction erroneously as objective evidence of physical pain.

Likewise, there is a subjective component to the physician's interpretation of physical findings (degree of retinal vasoconstriction, amount of abdominal tenderness, presence or absence of an enlarged spleen, degree of enlargement of the liver, degree of loss of touch sensation). Subjective interpretation of physical findings is minimized by defining criteria for abnormal findings and, when possible, using a measurement standard (percentage reduction in the diameter of the retinal arteries, measured span of the liver, etc.).

There may also be significant intraobserver and interobserver disagreement. The same examiner may obtain conflicting physical findings on the same patient during different examinations. Different examiners may differ in their physical findings on the same patient. Even when consistency between observations and among observers is present, the observations or test results may not accurately reflect the true clinical state. Bias, a systematic deviation of an observation from the true clinical state, can occur even in the presence of consistent observations. Inconsistencies and biases in information gathering are attributable to the examiner, to the patient, and to the examination process.

Examiner-Related Causes of Inconsistency and Bias

Biological variation in the senses used during the physical examination may arise both between observers and within the same observer. One clinician may hear a subtle heart murmur that another clinician does not appreciate because of a hearing impairment. An intern who has been awake for 36 h may not appreciate a subtle joint effusion, yet may recognize it the next day following an appropriate period of rest.

There is also a *tendency to record inference rather than evidence*. Physicians often interpret clinical findings instead of describing them. For example, "mitral regurgitation murmur" may be recorded rather than the more descriptive "grade II/IV holosystolic apical murmur radiating into the left axilla."

Physicians may also fall prey to *entrapment by prior expectation*, based by what they hope or expect to find in a patient. They may consequently be interpreting diagnostic information in light of this expectation.

Ignorance (as a lack of knowledge on the part of the physician) is also a possible source of misinterpretation of diagnostic findings.

Patient-Related Causes of Inconsistency and Bias

Biological variation in the system being examined may occur. For example, it is normal for a patient's blood pressure to vary from hour to hour and day to day.

The effects of illness and medication may alter the patient's ability to provide a cogent history, as could be caused by dementia, delirium, or tranquilizers. Illness and medication effects may also alter the clinical manifestations of disease, as when blood pressure becomes normal after a heart attack in a patient who previously had high blood pressure.

Memory problems may cause a patient to ruminate over past events, searching for explanations for his or her problems. Serial histories may change as the patient reinterprets past events.

Examination-Related Causes of Inconsistency and Bias

A *disruptive examination environment* may adversely affect the examination results. For example, a subtle heart murmur may not be heard in a noisy room, or jaundice may not be appreciated in dim light.

Improper operation of diagnostic tools may produce biased test results. For example, the use of an incorrectly sized blood pressure cuff yields inaccurate blood pressure readings. An uncalibrated manometer could produce equally biased results.

Minimizing Inconsistency and Bias

It is important to take steps to minimize bias in the information-gathering process. Sackett, Haynes, and Tugwell, in their book on clinical epidemiology, recommended that examiners minimize bias by the following methods: (1) corroborate key findings by repeating key elements of the examination, by checking important findings with other available information sources, by confirming key findings with appropriate lab studies, and by asking colleagues "blinded" to the clinical history to examine the patient; (2) report evidence as well as inference; (3) use appropriate diagnostic instruments; and (4) arrange for independent interpretations of diagnostic laboratory studies that involve subjective observer interpretation (Sackett, Haynes, & Tugwell, 1985).

PSYCHOLOGICAL RISKS INHERENT IN THE EXAMINATION PROCESS

The information-gathering process is fraught with potentially difficult psychological issues for both the patient and the physician. The physical examination may constitute a threat to the patient's self-image of health and wholeness. To have this self-image threatened is to be reminded that one is mortal. To be examined is to risk the finding of disease. To undergo certain physical examination maneuvers is to have one's body invaded. The physical examination often violates sexual taboos (breast exams, pelvic exams, male genital exams, rectal exams) and can be very frightening to patients. Furthermore, despite the fact that society permits the physician to ask psychologically invasive questions and perform physically invasive examinations, the physician (especially during the early stages of training) may feel anxious and apprehensive about exercising such invasive prerogatives.

These issues are best dealt with when the physician is aware of both the patient's and his or her own anxieties and apprehensions and makes every effort to address the patient's fears with empathy and respect. Careful attention should be given to the patient's physical comfort. The ambient temperature should be comfortable. The examining room should offer privacy. If physically able, the patient should be allowed to undress and dress in private. The patient should be carefully gowned or draped, and anatomic areas such as the female breasts and the anogenital region should be kept covered except when being specifically examined. A female attendant should accompany a male physician examining a female patient. It may be desirable for a male attendant to accompany a female physician examining a male patient. Painful physical examination maneuvers such as otoscopy, deep abdominal palpation, pelvic examination, and rectal examination should be carried out gently. All maneuvers and procedures should be explained to the patient as they are being performed, since this will usually reduce the patient's apprehension. Abnormal findings should be explained to the patient. When the physician spends an unusual amount of time examining a specific body area, the reasons and findings should be communicated to the patient.

THERAPEUTIC ASPECTS OF THE PHYSICAL EXAMINATION

In addition to gathering information, the process of the physical examination involves touching and the "laying on of hands" and thereby has an independent therapeutic effect on the patient. In many cultures the importance of the physician's touch in the healing process has been recognized for centuries. Historically, healing power was attributed to the touch of a great person. The Bible gives many examples of Christ touching persons and healing various illnesses. A touch and the sign of the cross were used in England and France to heal scrofula. Priests were seen as possessing sacred healing powers. The touch did not always cure. Those who complained of not being healed were said to lack faith.

In our own culture, the physical examination is part of the therapeutic context of medicine. Laying on of the hands in some manner is expected by most patients. Touch is experienced affectively. Touching implies communication and is a significant statement of intimacy. Touching means taking part, taking matters in hand. Touching and being touched is an expression of caring. Touching, to many patients, is part of the process of getting well (Bruhn, 1978). Experienced clinicians recognize the contribution that touching makes to healing and deliberately use their touch as a therapeutic tool.

THE FLOW OF THE PHYSICAL EXAM

Physicians tend to develop their own patterns for proceeding through a physical exam. Generally, the exam proceeds from general observations to vital signs and then from the head toward the toes. However, the best physicians often begin the physical examination even before meeting the patient. For example, if the patient has filled out some paperwork, inspection of the patient's handwriting can be a clue to level of education, attentiveness, tremor, anger, etc.

Certainly during the joining process of the interview, the physician is beginning to make objective observations about the patient's handshake, voice, appearance, and general mental status. As the more formal aspects of the physical examination begin, physical contact begins. The initial touching during the exam is especially important in communicating to the patient an attitude of respect and caring.

By the time the formal examination begins, the physician may already have decided which of its aspects will be most important and as such are diagnostically necessary. Other aspects of the physical may be performed automatically and routinely, even when they are not diagnostically necessary, because several other useful purposes may be served. These routine maneuvers serve to provide some thinking time for the physician. They also serve as neurosensory feedback for the physician in that the physical act of performing the maneuver prompts the physician to the next act in the sequence and serves as a focal point for subsequent recall of the exam findings. Routine maneuvers also establish the patient's base-line responses, which may be useful for comparison to the responses elicited by other more important aspects of the exam. Finally, certain routine maneuvers may be expected by the patient, so that their performance enhances the patient–physician bond.

A CORE MODEL OF THE PHYSICAL EXAMINATION FOR USE BY NEW STUDENTS OF MEDICINE

Performing a physical examination should feel like driving a car, where the driver thinks about where he or she is going rather than about how to steer and brake. When a physical exam is performed naturally, with each part flowing smoothly into the next, it requires less conscious effort and frees one to focus on the clinical problem at hand rather than on the mechanics of the exam. Figures 4-1 through 4-20 comprise a "mental tape" to help the first-year medical stu-

Table 4-1
Sample "Write-up" of the Core Physical Examination

General	Pleasant, cooperative, mildly anxious 32-year-old white female appearing her stated age.
Vital signs	Temp 98.6°; HR 72; BP 130/70; Resp 16.
Eyes	Normal fundal exam.
Ears	Tympanic membranes and ear canals appear normal.
Mouth/throat	Good dentition and no lesions noted.
Lungs	No dullness noted on percussion. Clear lungs in all areas, with no wheezes or rhonchi or rales.
Heart	Regular rate and rhythm with S1 and S2 heard but no extra sounds noted.
Abdomen	Bowel sounds normal. Soft and nontender without any masses. Liver edge normal. Liver span 10 cm by percussion.
Neuro	Patellar reflexes 2+/4+ on both right and left. Achilles reflexes 2+/4+ on both right and left.

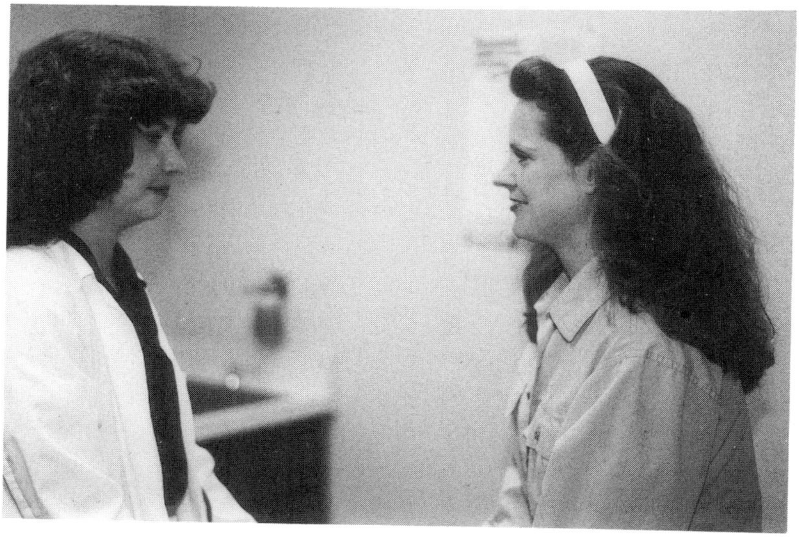

Figure 4-1. General inspection. After the interview, a brief screening examination begins. A general inspection of this patient reveals both obvious physical attributes and an initial psychosocial impression. This patient may be described as a "pleasant and cooperative but mildly anxious 32-year-old white female appearing her stated age."

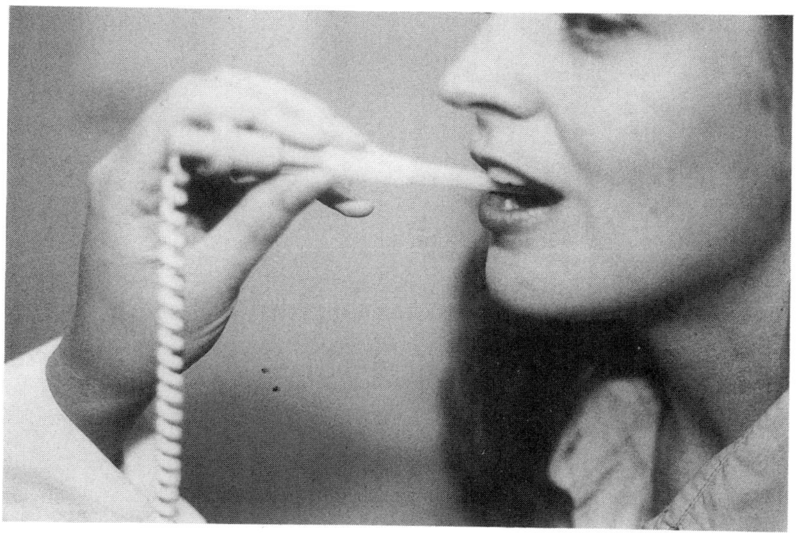

Figure 4-2. Vital signs: Temperature. First take the vital signs, starting with her temperature. Seat the patient comfortably on the end of the examination table and place a thermometer under her tongue. Record her temperature in 2 or 3 min. In the meantime, take the other vital signs.

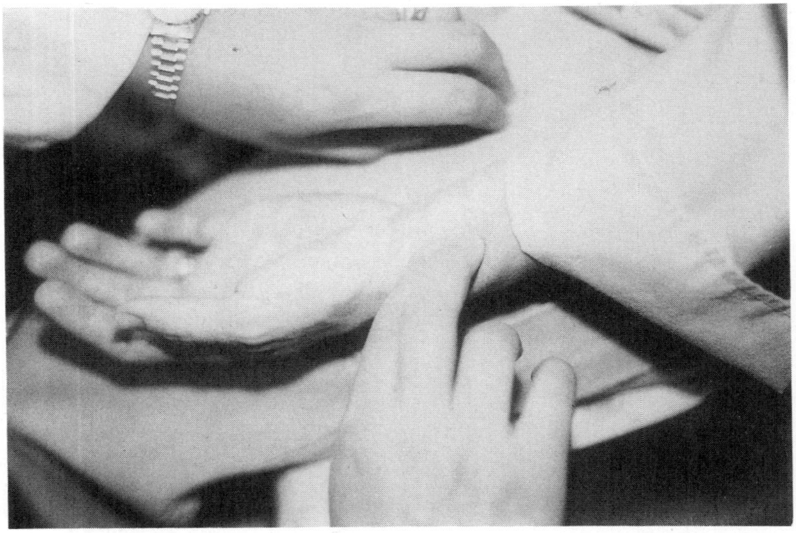

Figure 4-3. Pulse rate. Next take the radial pulse rate. Gently take hold of the patient's left hand and palpate her radial pulse on the flexor surface of the thumb side of her wrist. Count her pulse rate for 30 s timed with a watch. Her count is 36. Multiply it by 2 and make a mental note of her pulse rate, which is 72 beats per minute.

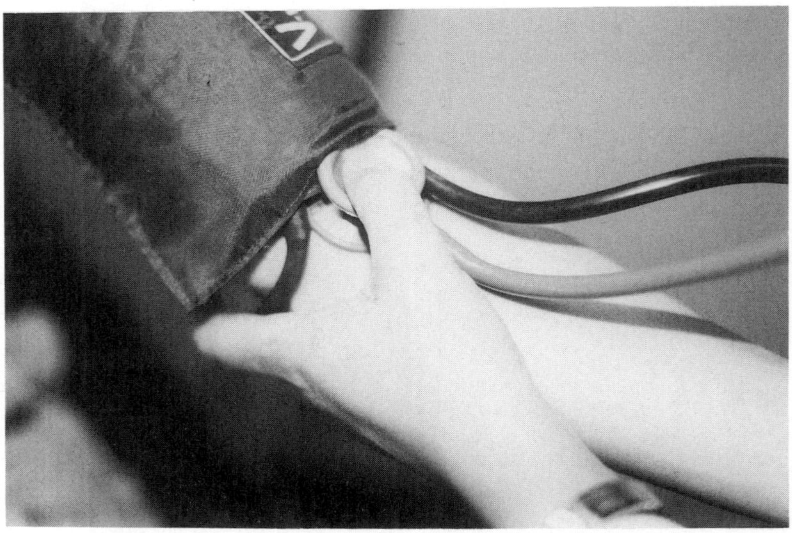

Figure 4-4. Blood pressure. Hold her left arm up and support it. Wrap the blood pressure cuff around her upper arm. Check to be sure it fits properly by looking at the sizing marks. Prepare to listen through the stethoscope, then palpate her brachial pulse on the medial flexor surface of her arm just below the cuff. Place the stethoscope diaphragm directly over the pulse and quickly inflate the cuff by pumping the bulb until the gauge rises to at least 180 mm Hg.

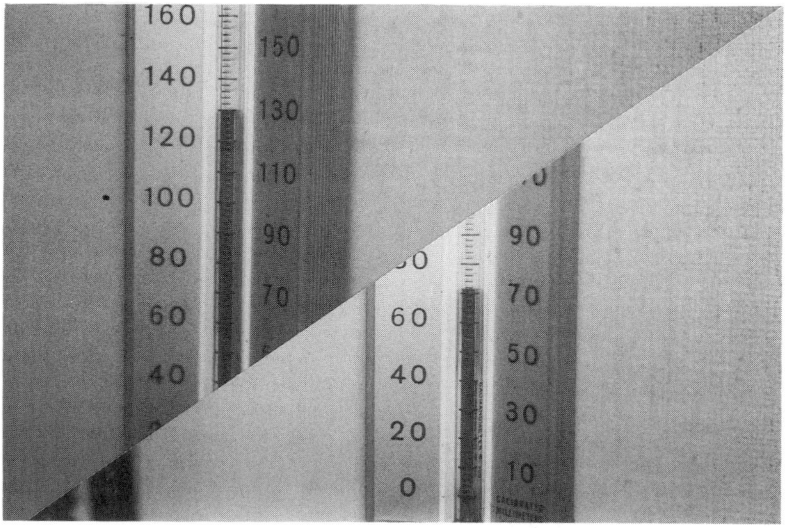

Figure 4-5. Systolic and diastolic blood pressures. After the cuff is adequately inflated, open the valve on the bulb slightly and allow the gauge to fall at about 3 mm Hg per second. As the column falls, auscultate (listen) closely for the systolic pressure, which is the gauge reading at which the pulse first becomes heard (the point at which it pushes past the cuff). Her systolic pressure is 130 mm Hg. As the column continues to fall, the sounds disappear at the patient's diastolic pressure, 70 mm Hg. Her blood pressure is therefore recorded as 130/70. Allow the cuff to deflate completely; then remove it and place it back in its rack.

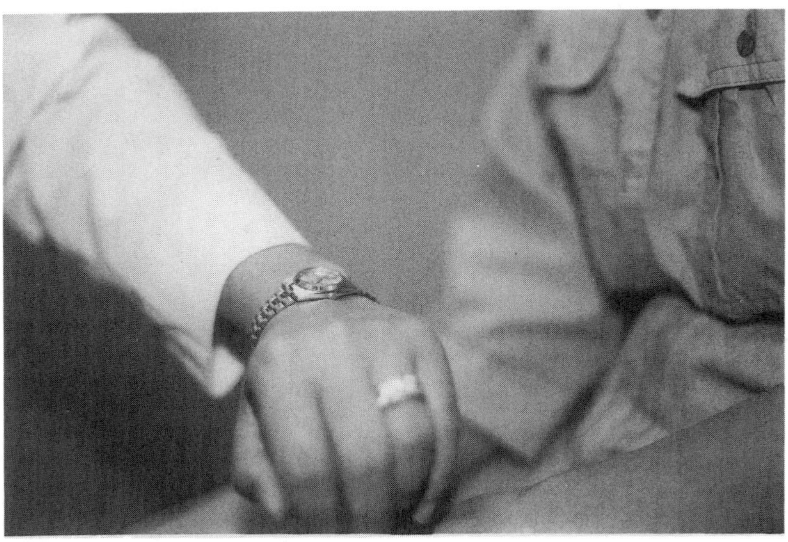

Figure 4-6. Respiratory rate. Count breaths for 30 s and multiply by 2 to get the respiratory rate per minute.

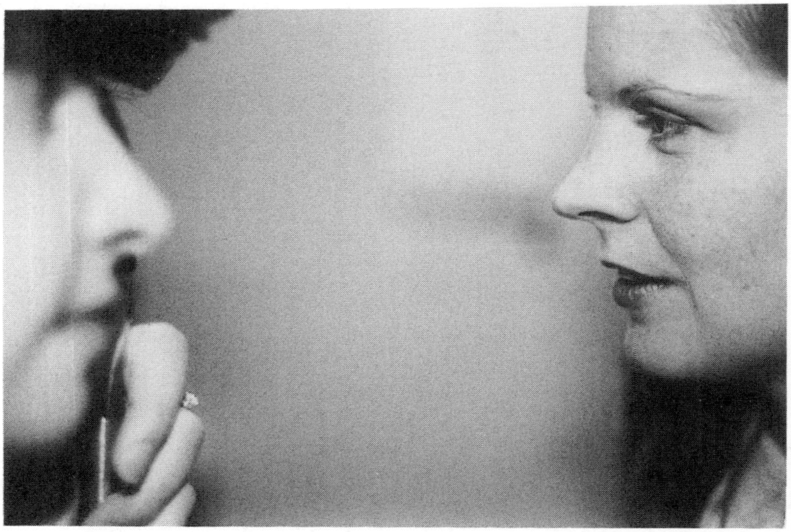

Figure 4-7. Eyes. Pick up the ophthalmoscope and turn it on. Flip off the room lights and direct the patient's gaze toward the opposite wall. Turn the lens on the scope to zero and set the light aperture to a large circle. The scope is held in the left hand and looked through with the left eye while the right hand stabilizes the patient's head and left eyelid. Once in position, swing the circle of light onto the patient's left pupil.

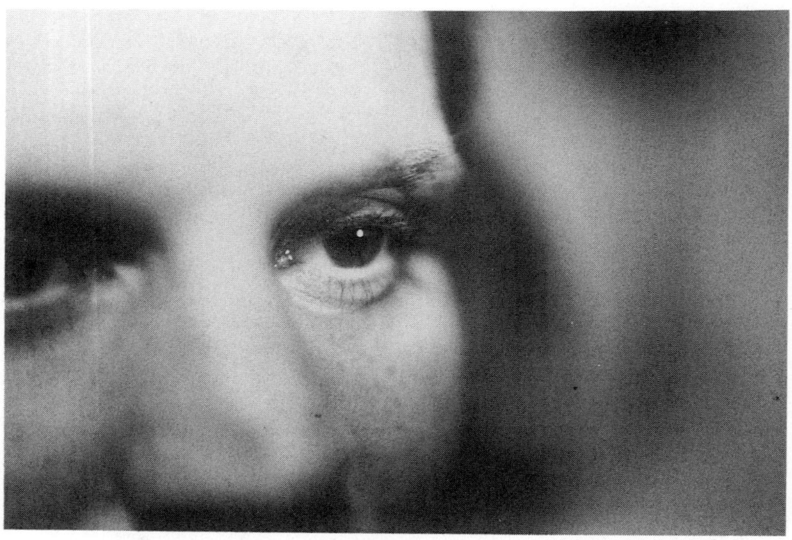

Figure 4-8. Red reflex. Note the usual "red reflex" appearance of the fundus. Then, begin moving slowly closer to the patient's eye, keeping the edge of the light barely over her pupil.

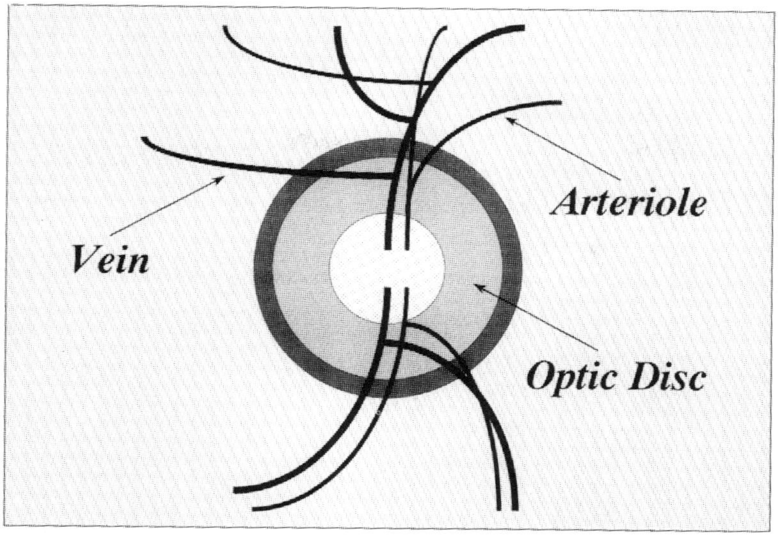

Figure 4-9. Fundus. As the fundus comes into view, adjust the scope's lenses to get the retinal vessels into focus. Follow the vessels along until the optic disk is located, then sweep outward, inspecting the patient's normal-appearing fundus. Then move to the patient's right side, switching the scope to the right hand and right eye to examine the patient's right eye.

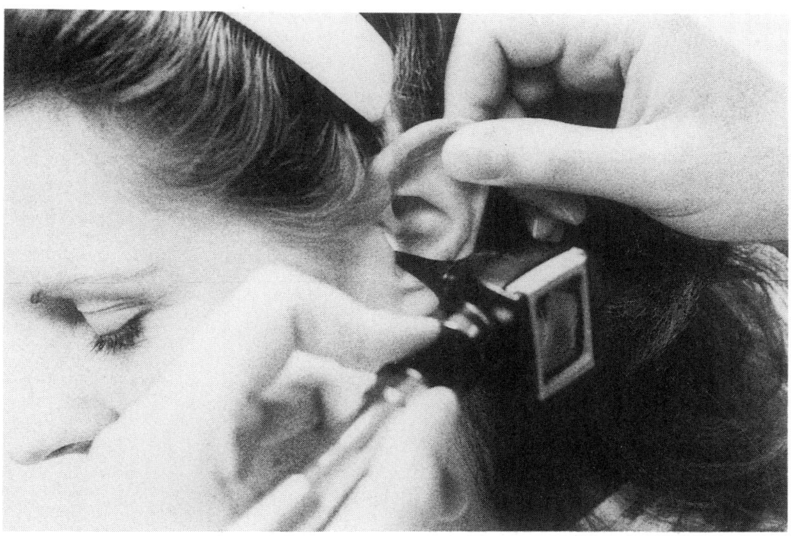

Figure 4-10. Ears. Hang up the ophthalmoscope and pick up the otoscope. Attach a speculum; then hold the otoscope horizontally in the left hand and examine the left ear, after first pulling the ear upward and backward with the right hand to straighten the ear canal.

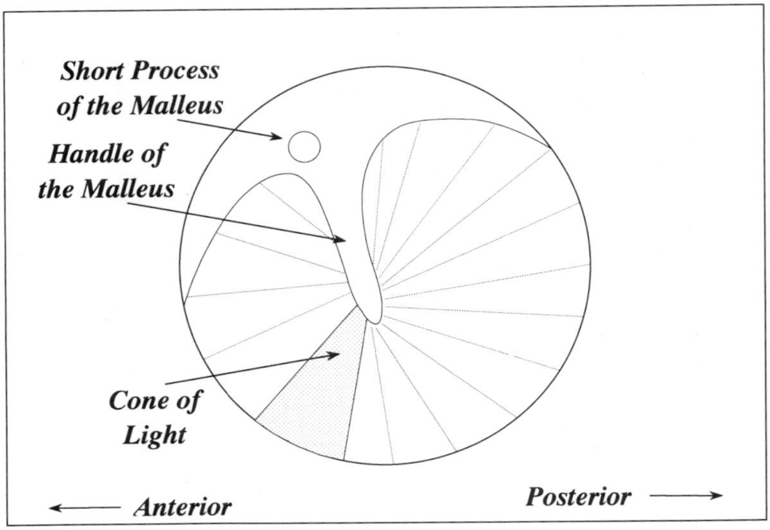

Figure 4-11. Ear canal and tympanic membrane. Gently insert the speculum tip into the ear canal. Allow the small and ring fingers of the left hand (holding the scope) to touch the patient's face just in front of and below the ear, so that if the patient moves the scope will move with the patient. Then look through the scope and inspect the ear canal and the tympanic membrane. Switch the otoscope to the right hand to examine the right ear; then remove and dispose of the otoscope speculum. Don't hang up the scope just yet.

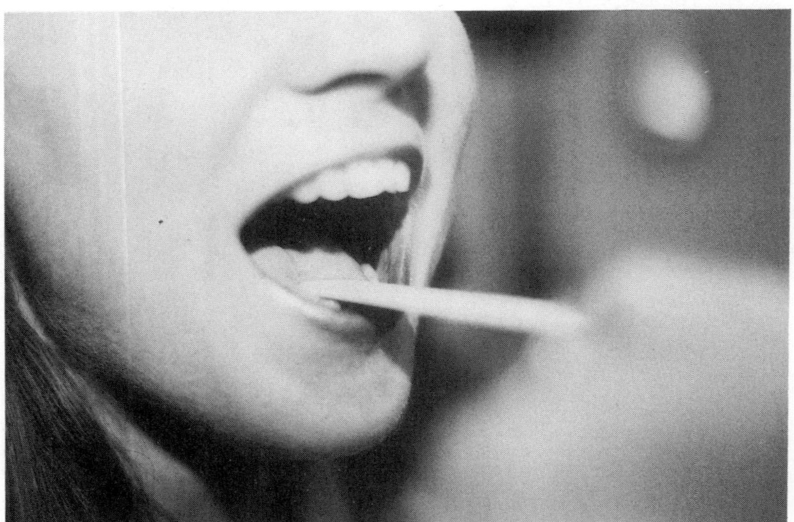

Figure 4-12. Mouth. Pick up a tongue blade and use it and the otoscope light to inspect the patient's mouth and throat. Hang up the otoscope and dispose of the tongue blade.

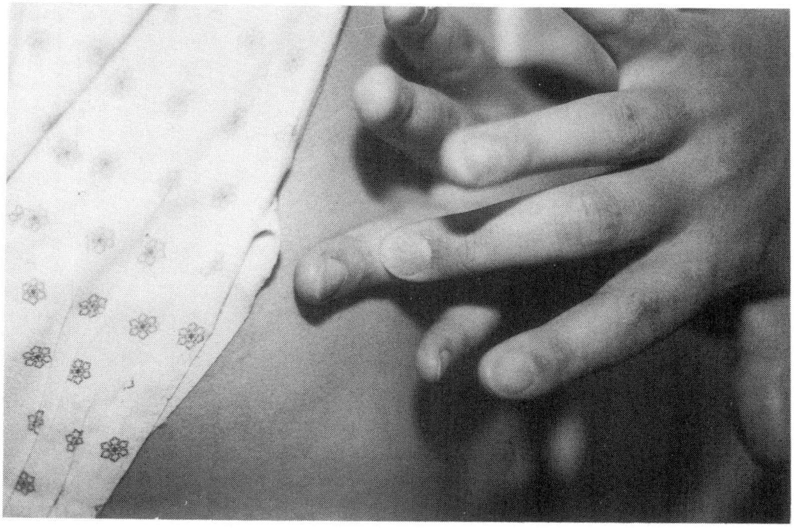

Figure 4-13. Lungs. Step to the side and back of the patient and percuss the posterior lung fields for asymmetric resonance and to identify the level of her diaphragm. The examiner's left middle finger is placed flat on each area of the chest and then smartly "thumped," using the tip of the examiner's right middle finger. Listen and feel for the degree of resonance. Compare the right and left sides of the chest.

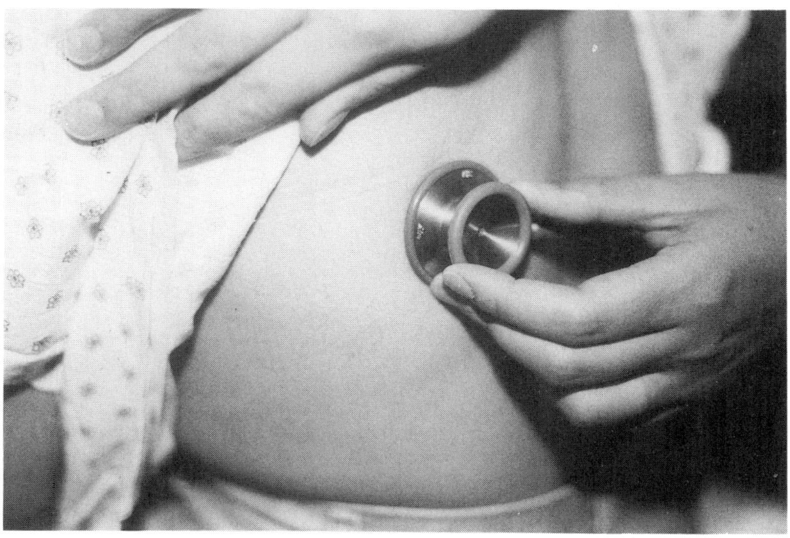

Figure 4-14. Wheezes, rhonchi, and rales. Ask the patient to breathe through her mouth and auscultate for wheezes, rhonchi, and rales. (Rhonchi are coarse crackles caused by fluid in airways, and rales are fine crackles caused by fluid in the alveoli.) Press firmly using the diaphragm of the stethoscope, which is best for hearing the higher-frequency lung sounds. Check upper and lower posterior lung fields, each axillary lung field (to hear the middle lobe and lingula), and the anterior lung fields.

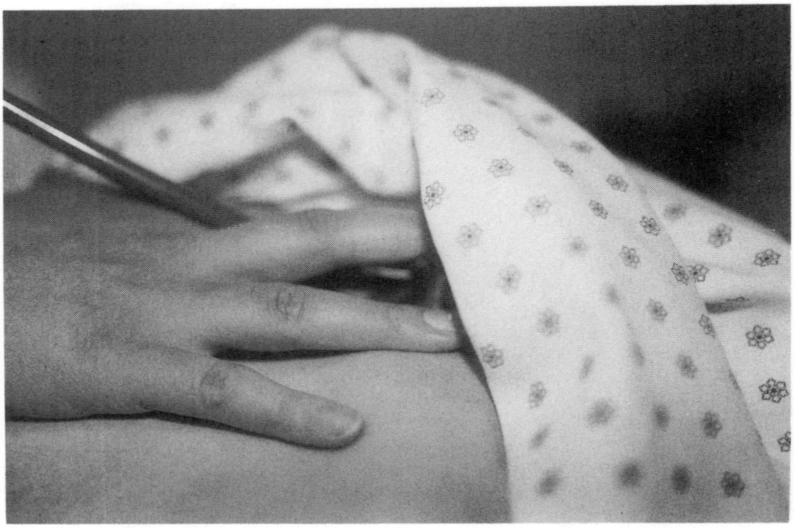

Figure 4-15. Heart. Ask the patient to lie back on the exam table. Pull out the shelf to support her feet. Gently lift the gown up to her rib cage, exposing her abdomen. Prepare to auscultate the heart in order to observe its rate and rhythm (regular or irregular), its first and second sounds, and any extra sounds such as murmurs or rubs.

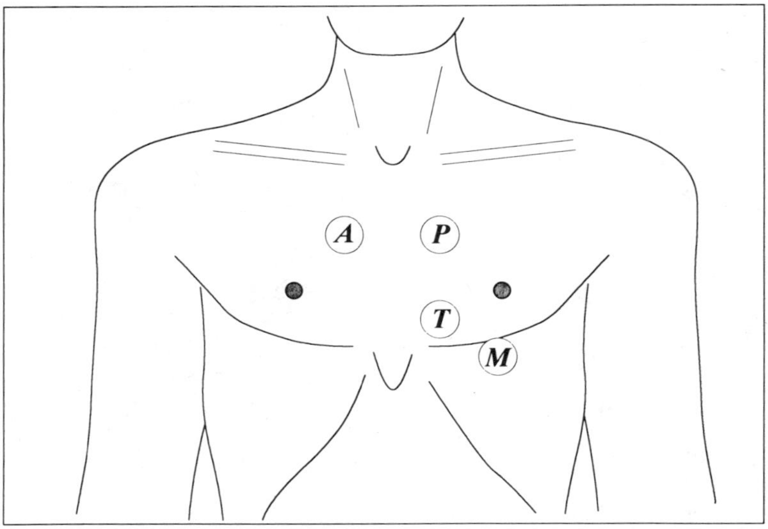

Figure 4-16. Heart valves. Using the stethoscope (diaphragm portion), auscultate in each of the four main valvular areas. Start at the left lower sternal border (T, tricuspid area) and proceed successively to the apex (M, mitral area), the left upper sternal border (P, pulmonic area), and the right upper sternal border (A, aortic area). Then use the stethoscope's bell to listen again at the apex, pressing only very lightly in order to make the skin act as a very loose diaphragm and thereby enhance low-pitched sounds.

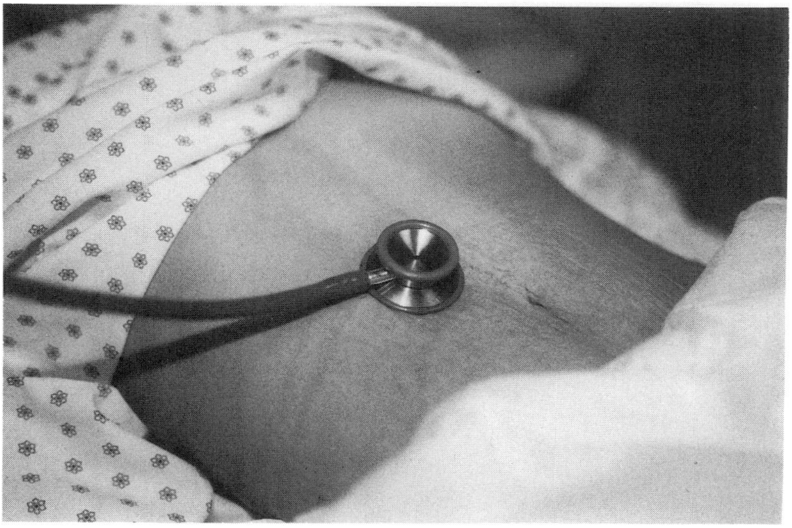

Figure 4-17. Abdomen. The abdominal examination is next. Inspect the abdomen for shape, scars, and skin lesions. Auscultate for bowel sounds. Note whether the bowel sounds are absent, hypoactive, normal, or hyperactive.

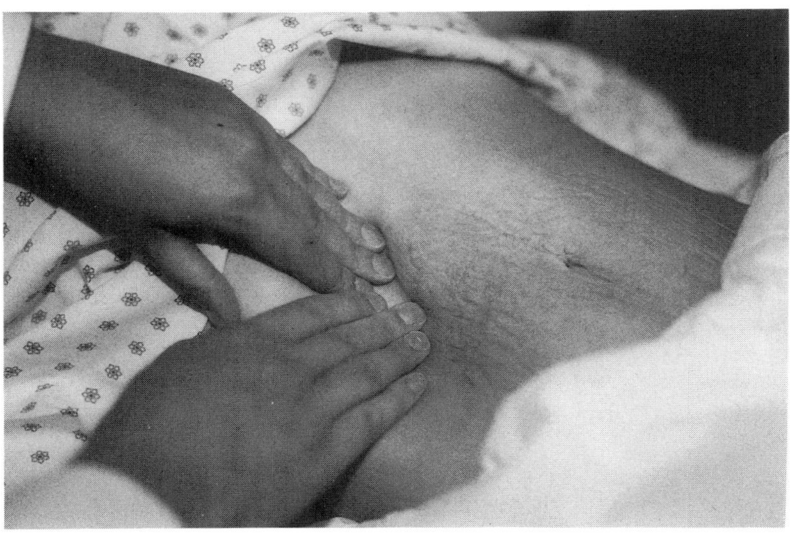

Figure 4-18. Liver palpation. Continue the abdominal exam by palpating gently in each quadrant. Note any abnormal mass or tenderness. Palpate the liver by pressing gently into the right upper quadrant and asking the patient to take in a deep breath. Feel the liver tap the examining fingers as the diaphragm pushes the liver down, a maneuver that is normally slightly tender to the patient.

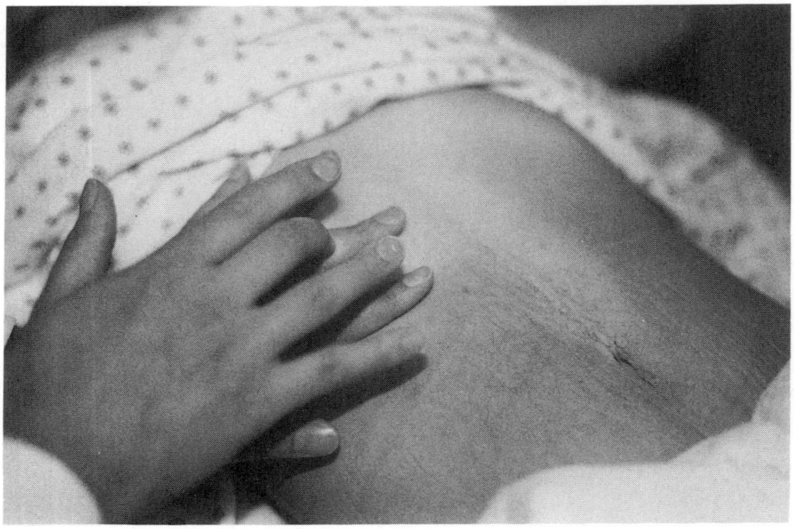

Figure 4-19. Liver percussion. Finally, examine the liver by percussion. Note the liver's size by measuring the area of dullness between the resonance of the right lung superiorly and the slightly tympanitic abdomen inferiorly.

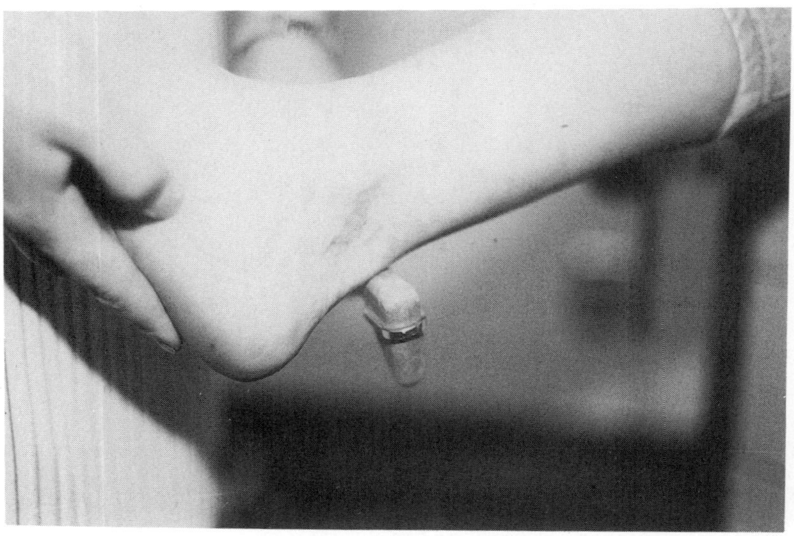

Figure 4-20. Deep tendon reflexes. Pick up the reflex hammer and percuss the patellar and Achilles tendons. Palpate the strength of the reflexes and record it on a 0 to 4+ scale. The core examination is now complete and ready to be recorded in the medical record as shown in Table 4-1.

dent's efforts to flow smoothly and naturally when learning to perform the parts of a simplified, "core" physical examination. The core exam will be greatly expanded in the years to come, but a smooth flow will always be important. A sample "write-up" of the findings of the exam is presented in Table 4-1.

CONCLUSIONS

The physical examination is a very special and important part of any patient–physician encounter. It serves diagnostic and therapeutic roles in patient care. In its diagnostic role it is used to gather objective information by the methods of inspection, percussion, auscultation, and palpation. In the basic examination these methods are applied in an orderly regional manner that progresses from general observations to vital signs and then from the head toward the feet. The physical examination unavoidably includes subjective components and is subject to biases attributable to the examiner, the patient, and the environment. It may also cause some psychological discomfort to the patient and the performing physician. However, because of the therapeutic significance of the physician's touch, the physical examination may contribute greatly to the patient's healing.

CASES FOR DISCUSSION

Case 1: A Modestly Uncomfortable Situation

As you prepare to see your first patient of the afternoon you pull the chart from the rack on the examination room door and note that you will be seeing Mrs. Jones, a new patient who is here for evaluation of a problem your nurse has recorded as "chest pain."

As you enter the room, you note your patient to be an attractive, anxious-appearing, 21-year-old, married, white female dressed in a business suit and seated in the examination room chair. During the joining process of the interview, the patient provides you with her chief complaint: "I'm worried about a pain I've had in my right breast for the last 2 days." The pain is in her right upper lateral chest. She first noticed it the morning before yesterday, and it has become progressively more severe. It becomes more intense when she takes a deep breath and lessens when she is still but never completely relents. She is unaware of any recent trauma to her chest. She had a cough and upper respiratory symptoms 10 days ago but considers herself to be nearly recovered at this point. She performs breast self-examination, has never had a breast problem in the past, and has noted no skin changes, retraction, dimpling, or nipple discharge. She takes oral contraceptives and has no significant symptoms of pregnancy. No one in her family has had breast disease. She is a nonsmoker. She relates no other health problems and says that she moved to this state 3 months ago and therefore until now has not needed to establish a personal physician.

Your nurse has already recorded the patient's vital signs: all normal. You are therefore ready to proceed with additional examination maneuvers.

1. What specific examination maneuvers should be performed?
2. How will you initiate the examination?
3. Will you have the patient change into a gown? Will you use any additional drapes or precautions to protect the patient's modesty?
4. Will you have a female chaperone present for any portion of the examination?

Case 2: For Crying out Loud

As you approach the second examination room door, you hear the loud cries of a small child from behind the door. As you enter the room, Michael, your 3-year-old patient, screams even louder and clings to his mother, who continues to try to calm him. She says that he has had an earache and a fever since the previous evening. Additional history is remarkable only for a mild runny nose and cough. Whenever you begin to approach Michael, he cries more loudly and clings more tightly to his mother.

1. What portions of the physical examination should be performed? In what order?
2. What additional questions might you ask Michael's mother before beginning the physical examination?
3. What are some of the advantages and disadvantages of attempting to calm Michael prior to examining him? What are the advantages and disadvantages of restraining him?
4. If Michael were an equally upset and uncooperative 8-year-old, would you handle the situation any differently? Why? What if he were 13 years old?

Case 3: With a Jaundiced Eye

Your next patient is Mr. Smith, a 48-year-old gentleman who was discharged from the hospital 1 week previously after a prolonged stay for treatment of decompensated alcoholic cirrhosis. During his hospitalization you had noted many of the typical problems of his underlying disease: (1) reduced hepatic clearance of bilirubin from the blood, resulting in a yellowing of his skin and sclera (clinical jaundice); (2) reduced protein in the blood with concurrent elevated portal pressure, resulting in enlargement of the abdomen with fluid (ascites); (3) portal system hypertension putting back-pressure on the portal tributaries, resulting in dilation of the abdominal wall veins and of the anal canal veins ("caput medusa" and hemorrhoids); (4) scarring of the liver, resulting in shrinkage and hardening of the liver (cirrhosis); (5) reduced hepatic clearance of endogenous estrogen, resulting in vascular changes of the skin and testicular changes ("spider angiomata" and testicular atrophy).

1. If you wanted to recheck all of the above classical findings, in what order would you make observation of the body regions or organ systems involved?
2. What examination modalities (inspection, percussion, palpation, auscultation) would you use for each finding?
3. How would you "write up" the findings?

Case 4: Home Sweet Home

For your last patient of the day, your nurse has arranged a home visit for Alice Brown, a 16-year-old white female with severe cerebral palsy and mental retardation. She lives at home, where her mother provides most of her care. The family is poor and does not have a car. It is difficult for them to arrange transportation to your office for Alice. You are equipped with your "little black bag."

1. What equipment will you need in your "little black bag" in order to examine Alice properly?

On arrival at Alice's small home you note that the windows are open. It is quite hot, and you can hear the traffic on the expressway and street. A window fan drones. Mrs. Brown takes you into Alice's room, where Alice is lying in a small single bed. The radio is on, the shades are drawn, and a small bare-bulb light glows dimly. The room is cooler because of a window unit air conditioner. You greet Alice, sit down, hold her hand, check her pulse, take an interval history from Mrs. Brown, and prepare to perform a physical.

2. What observations about Alice's status are likely to be more accurate in the setting of her home?
3. What observations about Alice's status are likely to be less accurate in the setting of her home?
4. What could be done to optimize physical examination accuracy in this setting? Clue: What factors would interfere with inspection, percussion, palpation, and auscultation?

Case 5: Little Men and Maids All in a Row

Last fall you and your partner performed all of the "preparticipation sports physicals" for the football team at the local high school. There were 65 athletes. You had the parents of each athlete complete an athletic history form and then conducted the examination in three stations in the locker room, with the boys lined up in gym shorts. At the first station your nurse took heart rate and blood pressure. At the second station your partner examined head, eyes, ears, neck, and back. At the third station you examined lungs, heart, abdomen, and scrotum (for inguinal hernia).

The coaches at the school now consider your practice to be their "team doctors," and this fall you have also consented to perform physicals on all of the female athletes.

1. Will you conduct the examinations the same way as the year before? Why or why not?
2. What are the advantages and disadvantages to such an "assembly line" approach to performing physicals?

EXERCISES FOR PRACTICE

The best way to learn the elements of the core physical examination and to develop a "mental tape" of the physical examination process is to practice these elements on patients. If patients are not available, then it is certainly acceptable to practice on classmates in groups of two. The classmates should alternate performing each exam maneuver on each other, with an instructor who demonstrates each maneuver and provides feedback to the students as they practice each maneuver. New students of medicine should realize that many of these maneuvers, for example, visualizing the optic fundus using an ophthalmoscope, are very difficult to master. The student should not expect mastery after one practice session. However, practicing these few physical exam maneuvers early in the student's career will allow early familiarity with physical examination instruments, familiarity with the vocabulary of the physical exam, and the formation of a conceptual framework on which subsequent learning can occur. The student also will begin to build self-confidence.

RECOMMENDED READINGS

Bates, B. (1987). *A guide to physical examination*, 4th ed. Philadelphia: Lippincott.

This is a classic text used by many medical students in learning to understand, perform, and refine their skills at physical examination. The text nicely combines attention to detail with an overall head-to-toe "flow" of the exam.

DeGowin, E. L. (1987). *DeGowin and DeGowin's bedside diagnostic examination*, 5th ed. New York: Macmillan.

This text is an excellent thick but pocket-sized source of great detail and insight into the many subtleties of the physical examination. It is a timeless classic, useful to physicians at all levels.

Swartz, M. H. (1989). *Textbook of physical diagnosis: History and examination.* Philadelphia: W. B. Saunders.

Although there are brief sections on taking a history and clinical decision making, most of this book is an in-depth description of the physical exam, including clinicopathological correlates, with an emphasis on how findings relate to different diseases.

CHAPTER 5

Clinical Decision Making

Daniel S. Marley and Mark B. Mengel

Case 5-1. Dr. W., while on evening call, was awakened from a brief 15-min nap by her pager. She phones the emergency room to find that they have a 60-year-old white female complaining of headache. Dr. W. reluctantly pulls herself together and trudges off to the emergency room (ER).

While walking through the halls, she finds herself thinking of the possibilities: (1) tension headache, (2) migraine, (3) cerebrovascular accident, (4) accelerated or malignant hypertension, or (5) sinus infection. She reminds herself that she needs to keep temporal arteritis and brain tumors in mind, even though those conditions are fairly rare.

She gets to the emergency room and looks at the chart. The patient's blood pressure is 130/82 mm Hg. Her temperature is 99.0°F. Her heart rate is 80 beats per minute. Dr. W. goes to the patient and introduces herself, thinking, "Well, if her pressure is really 130/82, I can forget about hypertension causing this headache." She asks the patient a few questions about the headache and finds out that it is not very severe and that the patient does not have a history of migraine or other vascular-type headaches.

Dr. W.'s differential diagnosis is now (with probabilities):

1. Tension headache—60%
2. Sinusitis headache—35%
3. Cerebrovascular accident—3%
4. Temporal arteritis—1%
5. Brain tumor—1%

Dr. W. asks a few more questions while she performs an examination of the patient's head, eyes, ears, nose, throat, and cranial nerves. The patient describes the pain as behind her eyes and in her forehead and face. It is a pressure-type pain that is especially worse when she bends over. The patient has had a mild cold for about 2 weeks. Dr. W. finds retracted ear drums, swollen nasal turbinates with yellowish drainage, and a slightly raw throat.

Given this new information, Dr. W.'s differential diagnosis changes to:

1. Acute sinusitis—90%
2. Tension headache—9%
3. All other causes—1%

A brief neurological exam is totally normal. Now Dr. W. is faced with another differential diagnosis dilemma. Does this patient have a significant infection of her frontal or sphenoidal sinuses, which may require hospitalization? Sinus percussion reveals only tenderness over the maxillary sinuses with no frontal sinus tenderness. The patient is afebrile, and the headache is not severe. Dr. W. wonders whether she should obtain sinus x rays but feels that she is already 95% sure that the patient has no dangerous forms of sinusitis. Therefore, she gives the patient a prescription for oral antibiotics and a decongestant, recommends acetaminophen and hot compresses for pain, and asks the patient to see her family doctor in 3 days for a follow-up visit.

INTRODUCTION

One of the primary functions of a physician is to diagnose a patient's illness. How a physician does this is a question that has been asked as long as there have been students of medicine, but the answers are still elusive. Furthermore, although some decision-making patterns used by physicians have been identified, they do not necessarily follow the "classical" methods taught in medical school. Many of the traditional methods of approaching difficult medical decisions, such as formulating an exhaustive differential diagnosis, have been found to be fraught with "traps" that may lead an unsuspecting doctor to make a decision that is seriously flawed.

This chapter introduces the four basic patterns of clinical decision making, emphasizing the one most frequently observed in experienced physicians. A discussion of how to formulate a differential diagnosis and clinical decision-making thresholds occurs next. Finally, a discussion of test characteristics, an understanding of which is essential to rational decision making, concludes this chapter.

METHODS OF CLINICAL DECISION MAKING

Because treatment is usually diagnosis-specific (antibiotics will usually cure acute sinusitis but not malignant hypertension), the health and well-being of the patient depend on an accurate "labeling" of the problem. Many investigators have tried to determine how physicians proceed through the diagnostic process. In a recent textbook on clinical epidemiology, Sackett and colleagues, having reviewed the literature in this field, described four basic ways that clinicians make a diagnosis: (1) pattern recognition, (2) arborization, (3) the process of exhaustion, and (4) the hypotheticodeductive approach (Sackett *et al.*, 1985).

Case 5-2. A 36-year-old female comes into a physician's office feeling very anxious with heart palpitations, difficulty sleeping, and being constantly hot and flushed. When the physician first stepped into the room and looked at the patient, she noted that the patient was a fairly thin woman whose eyes were bulging. The patient also had a broad-based neck. The physician further noted that she was sweating a great deal despite the cool temperature of the office. A diagnosis of hyperthyroidism instantly leaped to the physician's mind. This diagnosis was confirmed by laboratory testing a few days later.

Pattern recognition is the "instantaneous realization that the patient's presentation conforms to a previously learned picture or pattern of disease" (Sackett *et al.*, 1985). By this method, a single diagnosis quickly comes to mind once the patient is observed. The most important components of the pattern are usually visual, as in Case 5-2, but they can also be auditory, for example, the mashed-potato voice of a patient with tonsillitis, or olfactory, for example, the fruity breath odor of diabetic ketoacidosis. Pattern recognition is often very helpful to physicians, but only with certain "pathognomonic" presentations. "Pathognomonic" means that a finding is seen with only one specific diagnosis.

One danger of relying on this method is that often a physician bases his estimate of the probability of the patient having the disease on the number of "textbook" characteristics the patient has instead of the true "disease prevalence" in that patient (Sox, Blatt, Higgins, & Marton, 1988). Another danger is that once a doctor makes a "pattern recognition" diagnosis, it is often hard for him or her to consider other diagnostic alternatives.

Arborization

Case 5-3. A 56-year-old female with hypertension and non-insulin-dependent diabetes mellitus (NIDDM) presented to a physician's office with a 2-h history of acute substernal chest pain. She described the pain as dull and achy in quality. It took her breath away. The pain did not radiate, nor was it accompanied by nausea, vomiting, hemoptysis, or fever. She did give a history of occasionally getting a sour taste in her mouth at night. She had not taken anything for the pain. The pain was not made worse by inspiration or change of position. Food helped the pain somewhat. She denied ingestion of aspirin, alcohol, or other antiinflammatory medications.

She has smoked one pack of cigarettes per day for 30 years. Her high blood pressure was well controlled on captopril, 12.5 mg twice daily. Unfortunately, her NIDDM was poorly controlled on glyburide, 5 mg once daily. She had no past history of heart disease, peptic ulcer disease, or gallbladder problems. She had no family history of heart disease.

Physical examination revealed a pulse of 80 beats per minute, blood pressure 150/90 mm Hg, respiration 16 per minute and unlabored, and temperature of 98.6°F. Her skin was warm and dry. Examination of the neck showed no jugular venous distension. The carotid pulses were 2+ bilaterally without bruits. The lungs were clear to auscultation and percussion. The chest exam revealed no costochondral joint tenderness. Heart exam revealed no murmurs, clicks, rubs, or gallops. Abdominal exam was normal by palpation. Bowel sounds were normal. Murphy's sign (a sign of gallbladder tenderness) was negative. Rectal exam found no masses, and a test of the patient's stool was negative for blood. Extremities were without clubbing or edema.

At this point, a diagnosis of reflux esophagitis was made. The patient was given a slurry of antacids, viscous xylocaine (a local anesthetic), and a smooth muscle relaxant as a therapeutic trial. Five minutes after ingestion of this slurry, the patient's pain resolved.

Arborization is "the progression of a diagnostic process along but one of a large number of potential preset paths by a method in which the response to each diagnostic inquiry automatically determines the next inquiry to be carried out and ultimately the correct diagnosis" (Sackett *et al.*, 1985). Proceeding through a clinical algorithm in a logical fashion is one of the best examples of arborization. For example, using the information given in Case 5-3 and the clinical algorithm shown in Fig. 5-1, one begins in the upper left corner and moves through the algorithm depending on the response at each point. In this way the correct clinical diagnosis of reflux esophagitis can be reached very quickly.

Because the arborization strategy is so logical and tedious, it is rarely used by physicians except when they are confronted with rare symptoms or signs. It is used most often by physician-extenders and by medical students who are learning the diagnostic process. After medical school, because it is so time consuming and does not really correspond to the way physicians think, it is soon discarded.

Method of Exhaustion

The method of exhaustion is a diagnostic process in which clinicians perform a very complete history and physical exam, undertaking a "painstaking, invariant search for (but paying no immediate attention to) all medical facts about the patient, followed by sifting through the data for the diagnosis" (Sackett *et al.*, 1985).

The strategy of exhaustion depicts the diagnostic process as a two-stage event. First, all the data that might possibly be pertinent to the case are collected. When that stage is finished, the second stage begins as the clinician searches through the data to make a diagnosis. Even though many clinicians are taught in medical school that this is the preferred method for making a diagnosis, it is not. Not only is this method highly inefficient, it may be detrimental to the patient, as many studies have documented the hazards of collecting excessive amounts of information when solving clinical problems (Koran, 1975; Sisson, Schoomaker & Ross, 1976; Stein & Mold, 1988). Most importantly, this method does not correspond with the way clinicians really think. Thus, the strategy of exhaustion is the method of a novice soon abandoned with experience. Many studies have confirmed this fact (Barrows, Norman, Neufeld, & Feightner, 1982; Elstein, Shulman & Sprafka, 1978).

Barrows *et al.* videotaped a random sample of family physicians and inter-

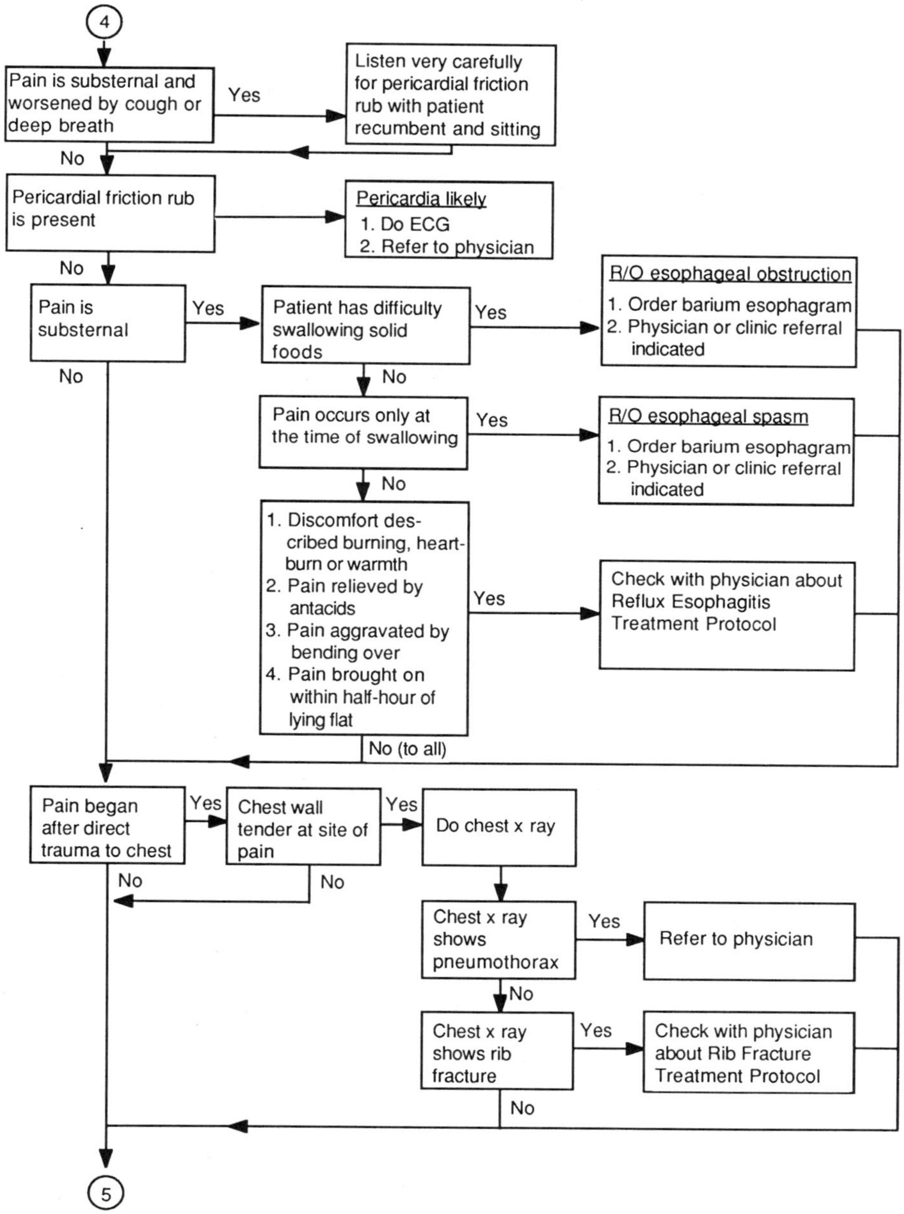

Figure 5-1. Part of a chest pain algorithm, courtesy of Harold C. Sox, Jr., M.D. Reprinted with permission from Sackett *et al.* (1985)

nists as they worked through a series of programmed patients. Even though these seasoned clinicians used the method of exhaustion at times, primarily to keep their patients occupied while they thought of something else to ask, it was not their primary diagnostic method. Interestingly, despite the accurate and efficient diagnoses most clinicians made during the study, many apologized to the investigators for not using the method of exhaustion (Barrows *et al.*, 1982). What was their diagnostic method of choice?

The Hypotheticodeductive Approach

This approach involves "the formulation, from the earliest clues about the patient, of a short list of potential diagnoses or actions, followed by the performance of those clinical and laboratory maneuvers that would best reduce the list" (Sackett *et al.*, 1985). This method was the preferred clinical decision making strategy used by physicians in the Barrows *et al.* study. In that study, family physicians and internists examined simulated patients with pericarditis, duodenal ulcer, peripheral neuropathy, and multiple sclerosis. They documented that the first hypothesis was generated on average 28 s after hearing the chief complaint. The correct hypotheses (these clinicians were right 75% of the time) were generated an average of 6 min into these half-hour workups, with an average of 5.5 hypotheses generated for each case. At the same time the clinicians were generating their lists of hypotheses, they were simultaneously performing those bits of history making and physical examination that would best help them shorten their lists.

In case 5-1, the physician's current hypotheses were described during their development from initial presentation to final management. Each new piece of data acquired through history or physical exam caused a change in the ranking, the elimination of some possibilities, or the addition of other conditions. Finally, Dr. W. was "comfortable" with a given hypothesis, such that she acted on that hypothesis by treating the patient.

Further studies of the hypotheticodeductive approach have revealed that this process can be further divided into four subprocesses: (1) cue acquisition, (2) hypothesis generation, (3) cue interpretation, and (4) hypothesis evaluation (Elstein, Shulman, & Sprafka, 1978).

During the **cue acquisition** phase, data are collected. An important event here, since the amount of data that could be collected is vast, is bounding of the problem space. This is accomplished by generating the first hypotheses from the initial bits of information obtained from the patient.

Hypothesis generation is the subprocess during which all potential hypotheses are generated. This process is of fundamental importance since these hypotheses will dictate the amount and quality of further information to be obtained from the patient. The usual number of hypotheses physicians generate is limited by short-term memory to an average of three to five, with a maximum of seven. Further hypotheses may be generated by nesting them hierarchically, for example, nesting myocardial infarction, pericarditis, and angina under "heart disease" as a single category.

Cue interpretation is a poorly understood process during which the physician confirms or "rules out" hypotheses generated during the previous phase. Physicians appear to go through a process of organizing the data and then comparing the organized data to a list of classical disease presentations contained in their memory. Experts in a particular field, who are often confronted with similar problems again and again, utilize "strong" methods of cue interpretation in which a few readily selected cues that have been found in that clinician's experience to be very useful in guiding decision making are sought. If present, these cues enable physicians to confirm or "rule out" hypotheses quite quickly (Mancuso & Rose, 1987).

The last subprocess, **hypothesis evaluation,** follows naturally from the cue interpretation phase. During this phase the clinician picks the most likely hypothesis. It is important to point out that the process of developing hypotheses does not require one to step through each of these subprocesses in order. Many physicians will jump to hypothesis generation after a short cue acquisition phase but then go back to cue acquisition to collect more data prior to moving onto cue interpretation.

At what stage do medical students start to adopt the hypotheticodeductive approach? A similar study to the one done on family physicians and internists was performed on medical students (Elstein *et al.*, 1978). Surprisingly, medical students used the hypotheticodeductive approach immediately on arrival to medical school. The difference between beginning and graduating medical school students, and for that matter between students and seasoned clinicians, is primarily quantitative, not qualitative. With additional education and experiences, clinicians become more likely to generate the correct hypothesis, to generate it earlier, and to obtain more pertinent historical and physical exam data about their working hypotheses in less time.

Is there anything clinicians can do to improve their diagnostic abilities? Elstein and colleagues also examined that issue using a large number of seasoned clinicians (Elstein *et al.*, 1978). The first finding of this study was that the ability of these clinicians to make an accurate diagnosis from simulated patients was very variable, problem specific, and not related to the physician's ability to gather data or to his or her familiarity with the diagnostic process but was primarily a result of their past experiences. Like chess masters who are actually not better at planning a large number of moves in advance than a novice, the ability of these clinicians to diagnose correctly was dependent on the amount of disease-specific knowledge that they had stored in long-term memory (just as chess masters have more chess board patterns stored in long-term memory) and on their ability to access that stored information quickly and compare it to the organized information from the case. From research on memory, diseases that were organized under diagnostic cues, such as symptoms and signs, were accessed much faster than when cues were organized under specific diseases.

Second, and unfortunately, physicians would often distort cues to support their favorite hypothesis during the cue interpretation phase, would not think probabilistically, and would often not attend to or even collect information that refuted or ruled out other hypotheses. In other words, physicians were often biased in favor of their "favorite" hypotheses. For example, a cardiologist might be biased toward heart disease as a cause of chest pain, to the detriment of the diagnostic process.

Third, it appears that knowledge of the diagnostic process did not improve these clinicians' ability to make a diagnosis. Fortunately, and for reasons that are not well understood, teaching medical students the diagnostic process and asking them to work through cases does appear to improve their ability to make a diagnosis. Additionally, clinicians who are able to think "probabilistically" and selectively order lab tests based on the likelihood of that test either "ruling in" or "ruling out" tentative diagnoses are probably more cost-effective than physicians who use the method of exhaustion (Cherkin, Rosenblatt, Hart, Schneeweiss, & LoGerto, 1987).

Finally, because diagnostic ability does depend on level of knowledge and how that knowledge is organized in a clinician's brain, it is clear that learning vast amounts of disease-specific information should not be done haphazardly but by an organized process in which medical information is arranged by symptoms and signs of disease, nested hierarchically, so that the information can be rapidly accessed during the diagnostic process. Unfortunately, the organization of information in medical school, usually by disease state rather than by diagnostic cues, will not help the student with this formidable task. All of the above reasons do, however, combine to underscore the benefit of learning the diagnostic process while a novice and practicing it throughout medical school.

DIFFERENTIAL DIAGNOSIS

Assuming the use of the hypotheticodeductive approach, we can analyze what goes into establishing a rational differential diagnosis. Dr. W., in Case 5-1, began formulating a list of possible diagnoses the moment she heard the patient's chief complaint. That initial list served to form a "boundary" around the problem, so she could concentrate on what to ask or examine next. She then chose her questions and exams to "test" her hypotheses.

There is no short cut for knowing or learning what the most likely hypotheses are in a given case. Experience and training are necessary to recognize the patterns in patient's symptoms and signs and then generate a list of likely causes. The list of *all possible* causes may be immense and of little value. For example, the patient's headache in Case 5-1 may have been caused by cysticercosis, but the *probability* of that hypothesis is so low that it is not even worth entertaining. Thus, it is essential that the clinician have a good idea of what is *probable*.

Probability

Probability is the chance that a particular event will occur. In medicine, usually an event has already occurred (the disease), and the physician must determine the probability that a particular disease is responsible for the patient's illness. Probability is expressed as a percentage or as a decimal fraction of 1. A probability of 1.0 means that the event *will* occur (or that a diagnosis is certain). Likewise, a probability of 0 means it will *not* occur. Of course, the probabilities of all possible outcomes (or disease possibilities) must add up to 1.0.

When a doctor sees a patient, an initial hypothesis list is formed. Usually at the subconscious level, the physician attaches to each hypothesis a probability of that hypothesis being the cause of the patient's problem. As cues are acquired, those probabilities change in a very dynamic way. For example, Dr. Y. sees a 65-year-old woman in his office.

She says:	Doctor, this cough is driving me crazy!
He thinks:	Cold = 80%, chronic bronchitis = 15%, lung cancer = 5%
She says:	I've been coughing up some phlegm and even streaks of blood. I've smoked two packs of cigarettes a day since I was 15.
Dr. Y. thinks:	Cold = 20%, chronic bronchitis = 70%, lung cancer = 10%
She says:	The cough has been getting worse over the past 3 months, and I have lost about 30 lb over that time also.
Dr. Y. thinks:	Cold < 1%, chronic bronchitis = 19%, lung cancer = 80%

Dr. Y is probably not even aware of his thoughts or the change in his probabilities as he learned new information. However, when he is finished with the interview, he will be able to list those hypotheses with the highest likelihood as his working differential diagnosis. Each physician has his or her own cut-off for when to include a hypothesis in the differential. Some may choose to ignore a hypothesis with a probability that has slipped below 20%, but others may not be comfortable ignoring a hypothesis with even a small 5% probability of being a possible cause of a patient's illness. The smaller the probability required to push a hypothesis onto the "back shelf," the closer to an "exhaustion" model of decision making that clinician is using.

What does the physician use as a starting point when initially assigning probabilities to the differential diagnosis? The basis for this is prevalence. **Prevalence** is defined as the number of persons with a specific disease at any one time per given number of "parent" population.

For example, the prevalence of breast cancer in all women in the United States (the parent population) is 100 per 100,000, or 0.1%. If a physician were to see a new female patient, he or she would immediately assign a probability of at least 0.1% to that patient for breast cancer. As more information is gathered (breast cancer in a first-degree relative, for example), that probability may change (increase, in this case).

Most physicians do not actively memorize prevalence data. Their initial assignment of probability is more often based on experience in their own practice. Although this has the advantage of "custom fitting" the prevalence of certain diseases to the particular type of population seen by the physician, it also has the disadvantage of causing some physicians to significantly over- or underestimate the true prevalence of certain diseases in their practice.

An important point to remember about prevalence is particularly applicable to medical students. The prevalence of a disease in a primary care clinician's office may be markedly different from the prevalence of that same disease in a specialist's office or on a teaching hospital ward. For example, the prevalence of brain tumors in the general population is less than 1%. Assume for the sake of argument, that of 1000 patients with headaches who are seen in a primary care physician's practice, one will have a brain tumor. That primary care doctor may send 10 of those 1000 patients (including the one with a brain tumor) to a specialist because of unusual characteristics or findings. Therefore, the specialist will see one brain tumor out of 10 patients. The prevalence for the primary care doctor is $^1/_{1000}$ or 0.1%, but the prevalence for the specialist is $^1/_{10}$ or 10%. Specialists and tertiary care hospitals receive patients screened through a primary care filter, with prevalences of diseases much higher than "the real world." Because medical students learn clinical medicine largely in tertiary care hospitals, they tend to inflate estimates of the prevalence of unusual diseases.

Importance

Certain diagnostic possibilities may be of fairly low probability (like brain tumors) but be of such grave importance that they are kept in the differential diagnoses. Therefore, *importance* is another characteristic of a hypothesis that may lead to its inclusion in the differential diagnoses. Other examples of important conditions would be myocardial infarction in anyone over 40 years of age with chest pain, ectopic pregnancy in a woman with pelvic pain or nonmenstrual vaginal bleeding, meningitis in infants, and pulmonary embolism in adults with acute shortness of breath.

Treatability

One other consideration that may lead to a hypothesis being kept on the "active" list even though it may be of low probability is *treatability.* For example, in a middle-aged woman with vague complaints of fatigue, intermittent fevers, and diffuse joint pains who lives on a farm, Lyme disease might be kept in the differential diagnosis because it is relatively easy to treat, especially when compared to other connective tissue disorders that would also be included in this woman's differential diagnosis, even though its probability would still be quite low.

CLINICAL DECISION-MAKING THRESHOLDS

Case 5-4. A patient presents to the ER with chest pain. He is a 48-year-old male nonsmoker, nonhypertensive, with no previous history of heart disease. His pain is substernal, not "crushing," does not radiate, but is associated with some diaphoresis. His pain is also not positional or pleuritic but has been going on for about 2 h without abatement. His physician's biggest question is, "Is this a myocardial infarction (MI) or not?"

The probability that this particular patient with this particular set of symptoms is having a true MI is estimated by the physician to be 70%. Suppose an ECG is done and is negative for any acute changes suggestive of a MI, is it safe then to say that this patient has *not* had a heart attack? How sure does the physician need to be? How sure would the patient want the physician to be? What are the ramifications if he is wrong and sends the patient home if in fact the patient has had an MI?

How sure does the clinician need to be that the patient in the ER has had a myocardial infarction before admitting him to the intensive care unit (ICU)? The doctor must consider the costs (not just in dollars but also in terms of health) of sending him to the ICU if in fact he has not had an MI. The patient could easily be billed $5000 for a 2- or 3-day ICU stay. However, if the clinician needs to know beyond a "shadow of a doubt" that the patient has had an MI before admitting him, several expensive, invasive tests may need to be done before the physician is sure enough to either admit or discharge the patient.

The physician performs an electrocardiogram (ECG) on the patient. It is totally normal and shows no evidence of any changes suggestive of ischemic heart disease. Are these data helpful to the physician?

Pauker and Kassirer (1980) have developed a way of utilizing the probability of disease in decision making to help make decisions about further testing, called the *threshold approach*. If the physician in Case 5-4 would like to be 75% sure that the patient has had an MI before admitting him to the ICU, then this physician's "test/treatment threshold" is 75%. In other words, 75% is the probability of MI *above* which the doctor will no longer test and will consider the patient to have the disease, for all practical purposes (Fig. 5-2).

On the other end of the spectrum, at what probability will the clinician be comfortable that the patient has *not* had an MI so that he can be sent home? Where a physician sets the no-test/test threshold depends on several factors. Certainly, the natural history and prognosis of the diseases in the differential diagnosis influence the threshold. If a disease is not very serious (viral upper respiratory infection, for example), then the no-test/test threshold may be quite high. A very serious and life-threatening disease, however, for which there is

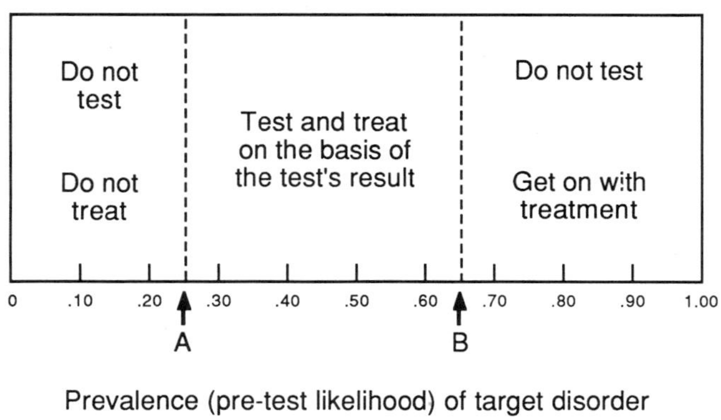

Figure 5-2. Clinical decision-making thresholds based on the probability of disease. A is the no-test/test threshold. B is the test/treatment threshold. Reprinted with permission from Sackett *et al.* (1985).

excellent treatment (syphilis, for example) should probably have a very low no-test/test threshold associated with it since the consequences of missing the diagnosis would be severe. Costs and risks of testing procedures may influence the positioning of the no-test/test threshold also. For example, if the only way to rule out a small suspicion of coronary artery disease in a certain patient is by cardiac catheterization, a physician may raise the no-test/test threshold somewhat to avoid the unnecessary procedure.

Other important influences on the no-test/test threshold include the availability of testing resources and the patient's or patient's family's wishes. If the only test available is a magnetic resonance imaging (MRI) scan and the scanner is located 400 miles away, it is quite likely that this will influence the physician's no-test/test threshold as well as possibly affecting the patient's desire to proceed. Patient wishes obviously must be considered when setting thresholds. For example, when a surgical procedure is the only test available, and the patient, even though well informed, wishes to avoid surgery if at all possible, the no-test/test threshold might be moved higher, or the test/treat threshold might be moved lower.

For the sake of argument, the physician in Case 5-4 would be comfortable sending the patient home if he knew the patient's probability for MI was less than 5%. This is the physician's no-test/test threshold. In other words, this is the level of probability of disease below which the doctor is comfortable that the patient does not have the disease and, thus, no further tests are needed (Fig. 5-2).

When the physician performed an ECG on the patient, it showed no acute changes suggestive of an acute MI. It was totally "normal." Does that mean that the probability of MI is now below the physician's 5% no-test/test threshold? How does he know if the ECG is "accurate" enough in helping him decide what to do with this patient?

These are the steps the physician in Case 5-4 used in his decision making:

1. He made an initial estimate of this patient's probability of disease using the patient's history and physical exam findings, his own practice experience, and published data on the prevalence of MI in patients similar to this one. This was his pretest probability or prior probability of disease, before any testing was done.
2. He then made his best estimate of the probability of disease he would need to commit this patient to treatment versus continuing to test for the presence of disease. This was his test/treatment threshold.
3. He then made another "best estimate" of the probability of disease below which he would feel comfortable considering the patient "not diseased," at least from the standpoint of further evaluation and testing. This was his no-test/test threshold.
4. He then ordered a test on the patient that he hoped would raise or lower his estimate of probability of disease either above the test/treat threshold or below the no-test/test threshold. To determine if this actually occurred, the physician would need to know the operating characteristics of the ECG he ordered.

Most clinicians realize that tests aren't 100% accurate. Sometimes a test result might indicate that a person has a disease when in fact he or she does not. This is called a **false positive** result. Conversely, a test may indicate that someone does not have a disease when in fact he or she does. When a test "misses" a true case of disease, it is called a **false negative** result. Why do these inaccuracies occur?

Tests very often have a range of possible values. For example, serum amylase (a pancreatic enzyme) is a test used to determine if someone has pancreatitis. When the test was initially developed, it was applied to a large population of "normal" people without pancreatitis. As would be expected, some "normal" people had high amylase values and some had very low amylase values. Therefore a *range* of values distributed about a mean characterized "normal" people.

A group of patients *with* pancreatitis was then tested, and it was found that they tended to have higher serum amylase values than the "normal" group; i.e., they have a higher mean. However, there were a small number of pancreatitis patients who had lower amylase values than normal persons, and some normal persons who had levels higher than pancreatitis patients (Fig. 5-3).

Thus, there are some "normal" people whose values fall above the normal limit (false positive) and some "diseased" people whose values falls inside the "normal" range (false negatives). This phenomenon is inherent in virtually every test known. It is also not limited to tests. One can think of a question on history or a physical examination finding as a "test" for a disease. Symptoms and signs also have "false positive" and "false negative" results.

If we set up a "truth" table of two by two divisions with "true disease" and "no disease" across the top and "positive test" and "negative test" along the left side, then we can place *all* tested patients in any one of the four resulting cells (Fig. 5-4).

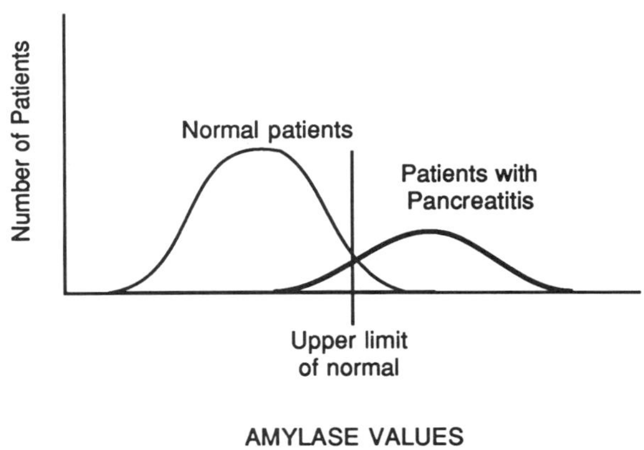

Figure 5-3. Distribution of serum amylase values in a group of patients with pancreatitis and a group without pancreatitis (normals).

Tests are evaluated using these 2 × 2 truth tables. For example, in evaluating the usefulness of the "wet prep" test for *Trichomonas vaginalis* infections as a cause of vaginitis, 600 women who came into a sexually transmitted disease (STD) clinic were tested with the "new" test as well as the "gold standard" test, *T. vaginalis* culture. Patients were defined as having "true disease" if they had a positive *T. vaginalis* culture. The new test, which involves looking at a saline suspension of vaginal secretions under the microscope for motile *T. vaginalis* organisms, was then evaluated by seeing how often it was positive in truly diseased patients and how often it was negative in those without infection.

Assume 100 women had positive cultures for *T. vaginalis,* a prevalence of 100/600 or 17%, at the STD clinic. Of those 100, 78 had "positive" wet prep tests and 22 had "negative" wet prep tests. One woman who did not have a positive culture had a positive wet prep test. With just this information, it is possible to calculate the **operating characteristics** of this new wet prep test and to help determine how good it is in "ruling in" or "ruling out" suspected *T. vaginalis* vaginitis, using a 2 × 2 truth table (Fig. 5-5).

The **sensitivity** of the test is defined as the percentage of those with a positive test among those who have true disease. In order to derive sensitivity from the 2 × 2 table, the formula below is used:

$$\text{Sensitivity} = \text{True positive}/(\text{True positive} + \text{False negatives})$$

In other words, sensitivity is how often a test is positive when a disease is truly there. In the *T. vaginalis* example, it would be 78/(78 + 22) = 0.78. This means that the test can be expected to be positive 78% of the time it is performed in someone with *T. vaginalis* vaginitis.

The **specificity** of the test is defined as the percentage of those who have a

	True Disease	No Disease
Test Positive	True Positives	False Positives
Test Negative	False Negatives	True Negatives

Figure 5-4. A 2 × 2 "truth" table of disease status by test results.

	True Trichomonas	No Trichomonas	
Wet Prep Positive	78	1	79
Wet Prep Negative	22	499	521
	100	500	600

Figure 5-5. A 2 × 2 "truth" table comparing wet prep results with *T. vaginalis* disease status as determined by culture in 600 women presenting to a STD clinic.

negative test among those have no disease. The formula for deriving specificity from the 2 × 2 table is:

Specificity = True negative/(True negatives + False positives)

In other words, specificity characterizes how well a test accurately identifies those people who do not have disease. In the *T. vaginalis* example, the specificity is 499/(499 + 1) = 0.998. This means that a physician can be >99% sure that if she performs this test in someone without disease, the test will be negative.

PREDICTIVE VALUE

Unfortunately, the definitions of sensitivity and specificity require that the clinician know whether the person has disease before testing is performed. Obviously, what the physician really wants to know in a clinical setting is if the person has disease given a positive test. The clinician also wishes to know the converse: that a person does not have disease given a negative test. It is important to realize that these statements are not the same as sensitivity and specificity, and similarly, the probabilities associated with them are much different. However, sensitivity and specificity can be used to help determine if the person has disease given a positive test or does not have disease given a negative test.

The **positive predictive value** is defined as the probability that a person truly has disease given a positive test. Positive predictive value can be derived from a 2 × 2 table using the following formula:

Positive predictive value = True Positives/(True positive + False positives)

In other words, positive predictive value is the ability of the test to predict that a person truly has disease if she has a positive test. In the *T. vaginalis* example, the positive predictive value is 78/(78 + 1) = 0.987. Therefore, if a person has a positive test, she has a 99% probability of actually having the disease.

Negative predictive value is defined as the probability that a person truly does not have disease given a negative test:

Negative predictive value = True negatives/(True negatives + False negatives)

In other words, negative predictive value is how well the test predicts who does not actually have disease if she has a negative test. In the *T. vaginalis* example, the negative predictive value is 499/(499 + 22) = 0.96. Therefore, if a patient has a negative wet prep test, the physician can be 96% sure that she does not have the disease.

An important difference that separates sensitivity and specificity from positive and negative predictive value is that predictive values vary with the prevalence of the disease. The vertical line down the middle of the 2 × 2 table is a prevalence boundary; that is, if a calculation is done that uses data from both sides of that line, prevalence influences those calculations. Specificity and sensitivity calculations do not cross that line and are therefore independent of prevalence. However, calculating positive and negative predictive value does require input from both sides of the line; therefore, prevalence, or the pretest probability of disease, is a major determinant influencing the predictive value of a test.

As an example of how prevalence affects predictive values, consider testing for the presence of acquired immunodeficiency syndrome (AIDS) using the human immunodeficiency virus (HIV, the AIDS virus) antibody test, assuming the HIV antibody test is 99% sensitive and 99% specific. In a relatively low-risk population of 100,000 college students, where the prevalence of AIDS is 0.1%, the 2 × 2 table is shown in Fig. 5-6.

	AIDS+	AIDS-	
HIV+	99	999	1098
HIV-	1	98901	98902
	100	99900	100,000

Figure 5-6. A 2 × 2 "truth" table comparing HIV-testing results with AIDS status in a population of 100,000 college students.

The positive predictive value (probability of AIDS given a positive test) is: 99/(99 + 999) = 0.09. A student with a positive test would, no doubt, want to be more than 9% sure he had AIDS virus before being labeled "AIDS positive." (In reality, a second different test is always performed on any positive initial HIV test for just this reason.)

The negative predictive value is 98,901/(98,091 + 1) = 0.999, which means that a student might rest assured that she does not have disease if her test is negative, as she could be >99.9% sure.

Therefore, it's clear that in screening large populations for diseases of low prevalence, the best one can hope for is to identify those who do *not* have the disease, as it is very difficult to prove who truly *does* have the disease.

Next, consider a relatively high-risk population, such as 100,000 drug addicts, where the prevalence of true AIDS is 25%. The same sensitivity and specificity values are used to form the 2 × 2 shown in Fig. 5-7.

The new positive predictive value is now 24,750/(24,750 + 750) = 0.97, which means that a person with a positive test is much more likely to truly have AIDS (97% versus 9%). The new negative predictive value is 74,250/(74,250 + 250) = 0.996. The test is still very good at "ruling out" AIDS if the test is negative.

This example shows how it is easier to "confirm" a disease with a positive test when testing a group with a fairly high initial likelihood of disease. Note that the number of false positive tests went from 999 in the low-prevalence group to 750 in the high-prevalence group. This shows the value of trying to screen the population being given the test to include only relatively high-risk persons. This raises the pretest probability or prevalence so that there will not be 249 additional new labels of "AIDS positive" in persons who are in fact absolutely normal. In fact, the greatest gains in posttest probability are made when pretest probability is between 40% and 60% (Fig. 5-8).

In actual clinical practice, predictive values are usually not available. All that

	AIDS+	AIDS-	
HIV+	24,750	750	25,500
HIV-	250	74,250	74,500
	25,000	75,000	100,000

Figure 5-7. A 2 × 2 "truth" table comparing HIV-testing results with AIDS status in a population of 100,000 drug addicts.

is usually available is either a prevalence estimate or a pretest probability estimate and the sensitivity and specificity of the test in question. Therefore, one cannot use the method above to calculate positive and negative predictive value. Instead, a mathematical derivation, Bayes' theorem, which uses sensitivity, specificity, and pretest probability or prevalence can be used to generate positive and negative predictive value:

$$\text{Positive predictive value} = \text{Sensitivity} \times \text{prevalence}/\{(\text{Sensitivity} \times \text{Prevalence}) + [(1 - \text{Specificity}) \times (1 - \text{Prevalence})]\}$$

$$\text{Negative predictive value} = \text{Specificity} \times (1 - \text{Prevalence})/\{[\text{Specificity} \times (1 - \text{Prevalence})] + [(1 - \text{Sensitivity}) \times \text{Prevalence}]\}$$

In Case 5-4, the physician is faced with a patient whom he suspects of having an MI with a 70% probability. An ECG is obtained that is absolutely negative for any changes associated with myocardial infarction. The sensitivity of initial ECG for myocardial infarction is 0.57, and the specificity is 0.98 (Behar, Schor, Kariv, Barell, & Mondan, 1977). Plugging these values into the above equation for negative predictive value yields a result of 0.49, meaning that given

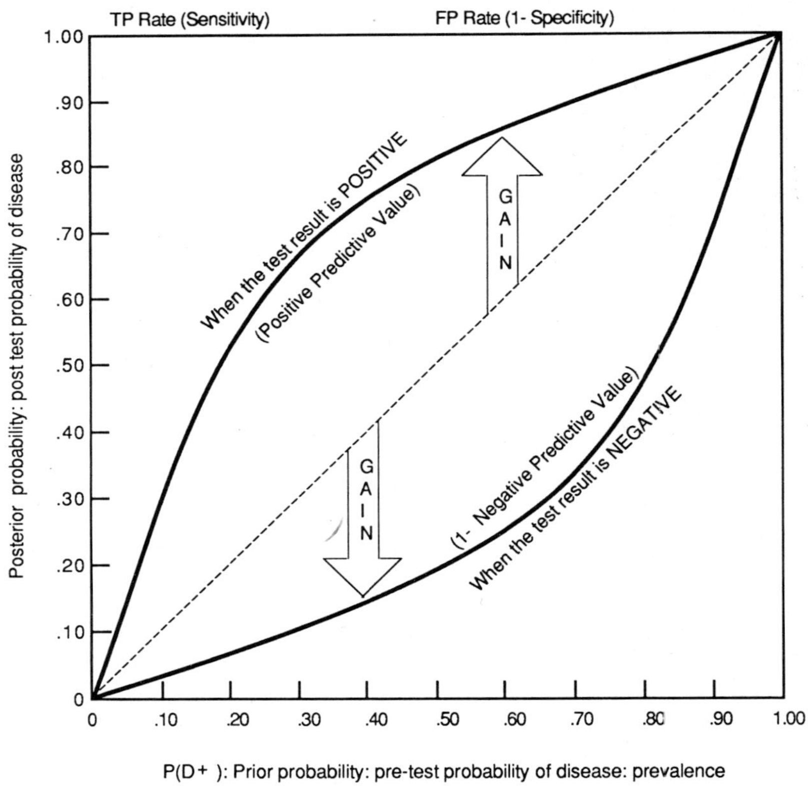

Figure 5-8. Gains in posttest probability, measured from the diagonal, given various pretest probabilities, with greatest gains realized at a pretest probability of between 40% and 60%. Reprinted with permission from Sackett et al. (1985).

a negative ECG the patient has a 49% probability of not having had an MI. The complement of this, the probability that he has had an MI given a negative ECG, is equal to one minus the negative predictive value, 1 − 0.49, or 51%. Therefore, his "posttest" probability for having had an MI given a negative ECG is 51%. The negative ECG has not helped to get below the 5% no-test/test threshold, so further evaluation is necessary.

According to Bayes' theorem, diseases that have a very low prevalence or pretest probability are very difficult to confirm; that is, it is difficult to obtain a high positive predictive value. Low-prevalence diseases are, however, relatively easy to "rule out." A test does not need much sensitivity or specificity if the prevalence is sufficiently low to obtain a very strong negative predictive value. Conversely, diseases with high prevalence are more difficult to "rule out" but are more easily confirmed.

Inspection of the formula of Bayes' theorem reveals that sensitivity "drives" the equation for negative predictive value to a greater extent than specificity. The clinical implication is that if one wants to choose a single test to rule out a given condition, one should choose the test with the greatest sensitivity, sacrificing some specificity. Similarly, in the equation for positive predictive value, the specificity term has a greater effect on the result than does sensitivity. Therefore, one should choose a test with the highest specificity to rule in or confirm the presence of disease.

Case 5-5. A 35-year-old female presents to her family physician with complaints of epigastric (upper midabdominal) pain. The physician suspects the possibility of duodenal ulcer disease. The prevalence of duodenal ulcer disease in 35-year-old women presenting to family physicians with epigastric pain has been reported to be 11% (Mollmann, Bonnevie, Gudbrand, & Wulff, 1975). There are several tests the physician could perform to increase his level of certainty regarding the presence or absence of duodenal ulcer disease. Some of these tests are listed in Table 5-1, along with their operating characteristics obtained from the medical literature (courtesy of S. Spann, M.D.).

Suppose that the physician asks if her pain is relieved by eating. What is the probability that she has duodenal ulcer disease given a positive or negative answer? Using the sensitivity and specificity values in Table 5-1 and the preva-

Table 5-1
Tests for Duodenal Ulcer Disease

Test	Sensitivity	Specificity	Reference
Interview Question:			
Is pain relieved by food?	76%	45%	Mollman *et al.* (1975)
Physical examination:			
Is there epigastric tenderness to deep palpation?	27%	75%	Priebe, Laurington, & Beck (1982)
Laboratory study:			
Does the upper GI x ray show duodenal ulcer disease?	58%	79%	Montagne, Moss, & Margulis (1978)

lence (pretest probability) for duodenal ulcer of 11%, a calculation using Bayes' theorem yields the results shown in Fig. 5-9.

If the patient answers "yes," the probability that she has duodenal ulcer disease increases from 11% to 15%. If she answers "no," the probability that she has duodenal ulcer disease (100% − PV) decreases from 11% to 6%. Assuming that the patient answers "yes" to the above question and that the physician decides to perform deep epigastric palpation on physical examination to obtain more information. Using the sensitivities and specificities in Table 5-1 and the new prevalence (pretest probability) of duodenal ulcer disease of 15% (because of the history of pain relief with food), a calculation using Bayes' theorem yields results shown in Fig. 5-10.

If the patient is tender, the probability that she has duodenal ulcer only increases from 15% to 16%. If she is not tender, the probability of duodenal ulcer still increases from 15% to 16% (because of the test's dismal sensitivity). Clearly, deep abdominal palpation has a very low information content.

Assume that the physician, in total frustration, decides to perform an upper GI x ray to see if the probability estimates for duodenal ulcer disease can be improved. Again, using the sensitivity and specificity values in Table 5-1 and the new prevalence (pre-test probability) of 16% (given the history of relief with food

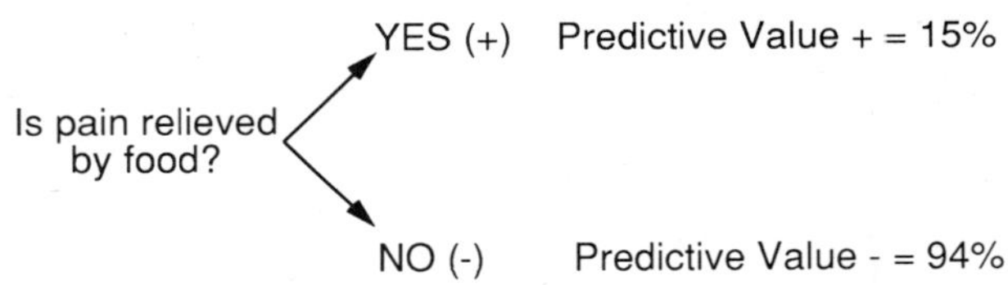

Figure 5-9. Effect of information gained from the question "Is pain relieved by food?" on the probability of duodenal ulcer disease.

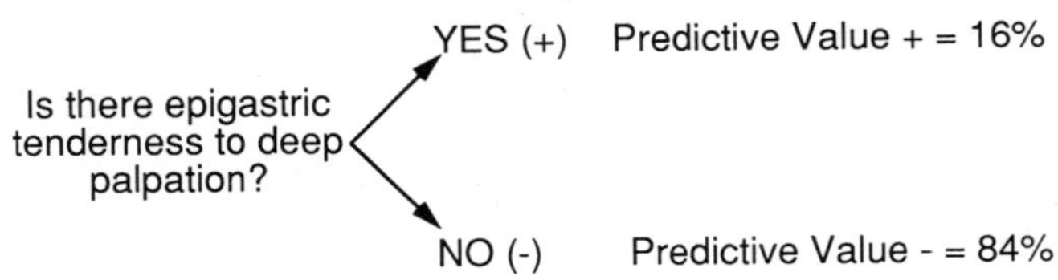

Figure 5-10. Effect of information gained from epigastric palpation on the probability of duodenal ulcer disease.

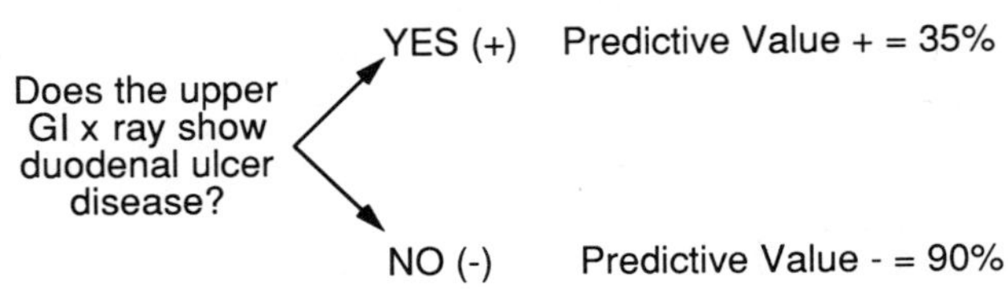

Figure 5-11. Effect of information obtained from upper GI x ray on the probability of duodenal ulcer.

and the physical finding of epigastic tenderness on deep palpation), a calculation using Bayes' theorem yields results shown in Fig. 5-11.

If the x-ray study is positive, then the probability that the patient has an ulcer increases from 16% to 35%. If the x ray is negative, the probability of ulcer decreases from 16% to 10%. Even the x-ray study doesn't offer very much in the way of information content.

This case illustrates several points: (1) interview questions, physical examination observations, and laboratory studies can all be considered as discreet tests; (2) when test sensitivity and specificity data are available from the literature and one has an estimate of the prevalence of the disease in the population to which the patient belongs, one can calculate the probability of disease after a given test result; (3) by performing predictive value calculations one can determine the information content of the test and decide whether the test is worth performing; and (4) laboratory studies, unfortunately, often add little to the information content of symptoms and signs obtained from the interview and physical examination.

CONCLUSIONS

Physicians must make many important, even life-and-death, decisions, often with very limited data. Using data appropriately and knowing the limitations of data on clinical decision making have been the focus of this chapter.

Four patterns of clinical decision making have been discussed: pattern recognition, arborization, the method of exhaustion, and the hypotheticodeductive approach. There are occasions when all of these may be appropriate. However, pattern recognition requires the presence of several "textbook" illness characteristics as well as the physician being able to recognize them as a pattern. Arborization requires a specific diagnostic protocol (or decision algorithm) to be available as well as proper interpretation of each decision step. When arborization strategies work, they usually work well, but they are not frequently used by experienced physicians. The method of exhaustion is often time consuming and inefficient and as such is often abandoned by more experienced physicians.

The hypotheticodeductive approach to decision making is the method most often used by experienced clinicians. Using it, a physician gathers initial data during the cue acquisition phase, develops a preliminary differential diagnosis during the hypothesis generation phase, and then reorders these hypotheses during the cue interpretation phase from most likely to least likely. Cue interpretation involves determining which cues (symptoms, signs, or test results) support or refute the various hypotheses generated, so that the hypotheses may be ranked accordingly. Hypothesis evaluation is the final step where the physician decides which hypothesis is most likely and initiates treatment.

Studies have shown that the hypotheticodeductive approach is the most efficient and intuitive method. The primary determinant of its accuracy in making the final correct diagnosis is the experience of the physician. The greater the physician's catalogue of diagnostic cues and their associations with specific disease states, the better the physician will be able to assimilate the patient's findings into an appropriate differential diagnosis.

A rational differential diagnosis, or hypothesis list, is formulated based on these criteria: (1) probability, (2) importance, and (3) treatability. Probability is determined from prevalence of the disease in a population of patients with risk factors similar to the patient being seen. Often, this is not known and must be a "best guess" based on the physician's experience. Prevalence may change significantly depending on the setting. For example, the prevalence of renal cancer in a primary care physician's office will be much lower than that in a university medical center urologist's office. Importance concerns the harm that might be done if a particular hypothesis is not considered, even though it may be unlikely, such as occult malignancy. Treatability implies that easily treatable conditions may be included within a differential diagnosis even if they are of low probability.

Once the hypothesis list is formed, the clinician must know how additional information changes the probability that the patient actually has a particular disease. The physician must also know at what probability level he or she will be comfortable considering the patient to have that disease and at what level the physician will be comfortable considering the patient to be without that disease.

The physician must first make a "best educated guess" that the patient has a given disease from the prevalence of that disease and from his clinical judgment and experience. This becomes the pretest probability that the patient has the disease in question. Next, the clinician must decide on the test/treatment threshold he or she will use with this patient, based on the seriousness of overdiagnosing or underdiagnosing the disease. If a test yields a posttest probability that is above the test/treat threshold, the physician considers the diagnosis "confirmed" and begins treating.

The physician must also set a no-test/test threshold to be used to rule out disease, such that if the posttest probability of disease is below the no-test/test threshold, the physician considers the patient to be disease-free.

To know just how far to adjust the probability of disease for a patient who has had a test with either a positive or negative result, the operating characteristics of that test must be known, as well as the pretest probability of disease (or prevalence) for that patient. Those operating characteristics can be defined using a 2 × 2 truth table obtained when the test in question is compared to a "gold standard" test. That gold standard defines the "true" presence or absence of disease.

Sensitivity is the ability of a test to be positive in patients who truly have disease. Specificity is the ability of a negative test to identify those who do not have disease. Sensitivity and specificity alone cannot be used to adjust the probability that the patient has a specific disease. However, by utilizing Bayes' theorem, positive and negative predictive values can be generated, which can be used to adjust the probability of disease.

These quantitative decision-making concepts are not immediately intuitive, but they do represent a more detailed analysis of how physicians think during everyday interactions with patients. With the advent of microcomputers and other easily accessible data-retrieval and -processing devices, a physician can have immediate access to the key elements necessary to quickly get an answer to a testing strategy or differential diagnosis dilemma (Pauker & Kassirer, 1981). A more rational clinical decision-making approach is the likely result.

Case 1

Mr. Bates is a 58-year-old black married executive in an insurance agency. He came to your office today with complaints of the sudden onset 1 h earlier of sharp left-sided chest pain associated with shortness of breath. He had had no previous history of serious illnesses, but his father did die of a myocardial infarction at age 67.

1. What disease hypotheses are you considering in Mr. Bates's case at this time?
2. Are there any other historical pieces of information that you would like to ask Mr. Bates before performing a physical exam?
3. What physical exam findings would you look for in this case?
4. Would you order either an ECG or a chest x ray on Mr. Bates?

Case 2

Mrs. Phillips is a 43-year-old white female with a 2-week history of pelvic discomfort, pain on intercourse, and two episodes of postcoital vaginal spotting. She is married and sexually active with one partner. She does not use any form of contraception at this time. Her last menstrual period was 6 weeks ago and was somewhat shorter than her usual periods.

1. What hypotheses would you consider at this time?
2. What additional historical and physical exam information would you collect?
3. If the physical exam revealed a slightly enlarged uterus and a urine pregnancy test was positive, what hypotheses would be more likely?
4. If the physical exam revealed a mucopurulent cervical discharge with a normal-size uterus that was slightly tender and no adnexal masses, which hypothesis would be most likely?

Case 3

A 14-year-old boy is brought to your clinic because of a rash and a fever of 2 days' duration. He does not feel very well but is not "toxic" or in severe distress. He says that about a week ago he had been camping in a grassy field for 2 days but denies any tick bites. He also has a mild headache and sore throat. He has had no congestion, nausea, vomiting, or diarrhea. The rash started on his thighs and then spread all over his body. It itches a little. He is on no medicines and has no known allergies.

1. What are the disease hypotheses that you are considering?
2. What do you feel is the pretest probability that this patient has Rocky Mountain spotted fever?
3. The treatment for Rocky Mountain spotted fever is oral tetracycline in patients over 8 years of age. If you know that Rocky Mountain spotted fever has a mortality if left untreated of 80%, what is your test/treatment threshold for this patient? (What is the probability in this patient to consider him to have the disease so that you would go ahead and treat him?)

4. If this patient were 5 years old instead of 14 years old and the only treatment available is oral chloramphenicol with its 1 in 40,000 risk of irreversible fetal bone marrow suppression, would this change your test/treatment threshold?

Case 4

Acute cerebral overload (ACO) is a hypothetical disease of junior medical students. It is characterized by inability to read, excessive desire to sleep or watch TV, and red, irritated eyes. The disease is definitively diagnosed by brain biopsy. In a first-year medical school class of 150 students, all allowed their brains to be biopsied. Twenty-six had evidence of ACO on biopsy. A new blood test for ACO has been developed, called the ACO-screen. In evaluating the effectiveness of the test, it was found that 23 of the students with ACO by biopsy were positive on the ACO-screen test. Of those with negative biopsies, 120 had negative ACO-screen tests; the other four were positive.

1. What is the "gold standard" for the diagnosis of acute cerebral overload?
2. What is the prevalence of ACO in first-year students at the school in question?
3. What are the sensitivity, specificity, positive predictive value, and negative predictive value of the ACO-screen test?

Case 5

There is another medical school 20 miles away from the medical school in Case 4. The first-year class at this school (call it school B) has 165 students. The two first-year classes are statistically the same in terms of age, sex, race, socioeconomic status, religion, general health status, and alcohol intake. The only thing different is that school B is notoriously "laid back," with the students learning the curriculum at their own pace. The prevalence of acute cerebral overload school B is only 3%.

1. What would be the sensitivity and specificity of the ACO-screen blood test at school B?
2. At which medical school would it be harder to confirm that a student has ACO if he or she has a positive ACO-screen test?

RECOMMENDED READINGS

Weinstein, M. C., & Fineberg, H. V. (1980). *Clinical decision analysis.* Philadelphia: W. B. Saunders.

The authors of the text have drawn from many disciplines to present formal decision-analytic concepts and how they apply to medical decision making. It is still considered the "bible" of medical decision making by many, and many portions are suitable only for the experienced reader.

Sackett, D. L., Haynes, R. B., & Tugwell, P. (1985). *Clinical epidemiology: A basic science for clinical medicine.* Boston: Little, Brown.

The authors of this test have been remarkably successful in bringing together two worlds, the world of epidemiology and the world of the decision, in order to describe the science behind the art of medicine. The section on diagnosis provides a lucid and entertaining discussion of clinical decision making for the novice and the experienced clinician alike.

Sox, H. C., Blatt, M. A., Higgins, M. C., & Marton, K. I. (1988). *Medical decision making*. Boston: Butterworths.

Sox *et al.* present both basic and advanced concepts of medical decision making in a very readable text suitable for the novice. The text is filled with excellent clinical examples that illustrate main points.

CHAPTER 6

Clinical Management

Mark B. Mengel

Case 6-1. A 39-year-old white male with hypertension and non-insulin-dependent diabetes mellitus (NIDDM) presented to his physician's office for the third time in 6 months complaining of fatigue and polyuria. When this patient presented 6 months earlier, the diagnoses of both NIDDM and essential hypertension were made, and the patient was placed on glyburide, 5 mg po qd (once a day), and captopril, 25 mg po bid (twice a day). A check of the patient's blood sugar and blood pressure 2 weeks later revealed that it was well controlled on the regimen.

However, 2 months later the patient returned with symptoms of fatigue and polyuria. At that time his blood sugar was 220 mg/dl (normal < 110 mg/dl), and his blood pressure was 160/105 mm Hg (normal < 140/90 mm Hg). He firmly stated that he was taking his medicine at that time. An increase in his glyburide to 10 mg po qd resulted in an attack of hypoglycemia 1 week later, necessitating a decrease in his glyburide therapy to 7.5 mg po qd.

At this current visit the patient's symptoms again suggest that his NIDDM is "out of control." When confronted, the patient again states that he is taking all of his medicines faithfully. Despite this reassurance, the physician is still concerned that the patient is not taking his medication. The physician stresses to the patient that he should continue his current regimen, emphasizing the importance of diet and exercise in the control of his blood sugar and blood pressure, and schedules more frequent follow-ups for the patient, asking him to return in 2 weeks.

INTRODUCTION

After an adequate diagnostic process has been completed, the clinician and the patient face what is probably the most challenging phase of the medical care process: clinical management. During the clinical management process, clinicians and patients attempt to restore the patient to health. If the patient has a transient, self-limited, or readily curable acute condition, health may be restored quite quickly, for example, by prescribing appropriate antibiotics for a child with an ear infection. On the other hand, if at the end of an appropriate diagnostic process the clinician determines that the patient has a chronic illness, designing an appropriate treatment plan is much more difficult, and the patient may not be quickly restored to health. Because the clinical management process is best illustrated in patients with a chronic illness, this chapter centers on those illnesses.

The science of how clinicians can best manage patients with chronic illnesses is still in its infancy. In fact, of all the processes used by physicians when encountering a patient, the process of clinical management is probably the one most closely tied with the notion of the "art of medicine." Medical students are frequently amazed that patients with very similar chronic conditions may receive very divergent treatments. For example, a mildly hypertensive patient in one physician's office may receive a once-a-day diuretic medication while a similar patient in another physician's office may be prescribed a low-salt diet and increased exercise. Another divergent management approach often occurs in the area of patient follow-up. For example, one physician may see diabetic patients every month, even when their blood sugars are in good control, whereas another physician seeing patients with the same severity of diabetes mellitus may schedule follow-up visits every 3 months. Because of this widespread variability and the general lack of well-designed studies in the area of clinical management, physicians are often as confused as patients as to what is the most appropriate course of action in managing a particular chronic illness. Fortunately, investigators are now beginning to study the clinical management process in an attempt to understand how physicians can help their patients to optimize their health.

Unfortunately, patients do not always follow their doctors' advice. Physicians, probably for want of a better term, have labeled such patients as noncompliant. Although many other physicians and scholars of the medical care process are not comfortable with this term, as it implies that the physician has ultimate overall authority in the clinical management process and ignores the confusion among physicians themselves on how best to manage patients, the term noncompliance has nonetheless stuck as a label for this problem. Unfortunately, noncompliant patients are not readily identifiable and, as in Case 6-1, often do not admit their noncompliance.

The goals of this chapter are to (1) develop an understanding of chronic illness and the burden of chronic illness on the patient's life, (2) develop an understanding of one clinical management process model, and (3) develop an understanding of noncompliance and several clinical strategies to help improve patient compliance.

CHRONIC ILLNESS

Case 6-2. A 13-year-old male was one of 50 patients a physician was seeing that afternoon for routine sports physicals. Previous to the physical exam, the patient had submitted a urine sample for analysis and given blood for a hematocrit determination. As the physician was about to enter the patient's room, he picked up the patient's chart and was shocked to find that the patient was spilling 3+ glucose in his urine. The patient also had 2+ ketones and 1+ protein in his urine.

The physician entered the room and noted that the patient was breathing fast. The patient complained of fatigue of 2 weeks' duration, always being thirsty, and despite eating his normal diet having lost 3 lb in the past 2 weeks. The physician simply could not believe that he had uncovered a case of insulin-dependent diabetes mellitus (IDDM) and so repeated the urinalysis, which verified the previous findings. He then verified the diagnosis by obtaining a random blood glucose value of 327 mg/dl from the patient. Overcoming his disbelief, the physician asked the patient's mother to come into the room and began to explain the abnormal laboratory findings.

As the physician began to explain, the patient and his mother gradually began to assume a look of shock and disbelief. With the mention of the diagnosis, IDDM, both the patient and his mother burst into tears. The physician did not expect such an emotional response even though he himself was shocked initially. After crying for 5 min, the patient and his mother revealed that they suspected something serious but had delayed coming to the doctor, hoping that the illness would resolve on its own. The physician then began to outline treatment options to the patient and ended with the statement that, as so much needed to be learned by the patient and his mother about IDDM, he felt the best place to begin treatment was in the hospital. Although initially resistant to this suggestion, both the patient and his mother eventually agreed to an immediate admission to the hospital for initiation of insulin therapy.

Although the prevalence of chronic disease clearly increases as people age (U.S. Department of Commerce, 1980), chronic disease also affects the young, as illustrated in Case 6-2. Certain types of renal failure, cystic fibrosis, Crohn's disease, asthma, and anorexia nervosa are all fairly common chronic diseases that usually present during childhood or in the teen-age years. Certain chronic illnesses can run in families, such as heart disease, NIDDM, and breast cancer. Others have environmental factors that increase their prevalence such as cigarette smoking, which increases the prevalence of chronic obstructive pulmonary disease, arteriosclerotic heart disease, and peptic ulcer disease. Additionally, as medical science has been successful in bringing what were once chronic infectious diseases under control and curing them, such as tuberculosis and osteomyelitis, other chronic infectious illnesses have inexplicably arisen to take their place, such as acquired immunodeficiency syndrome (AIDS).

It is difficult even to determine in some cases whether a disease is truly chronic. For example, in the case of a bricklayer who injured his back by falling from a scaffold and developed back pain that did not fully resolve until he had completed 3 months of physical therapy; would his illness be considered acute, since it did eventually resolve, or was it chronic, as it lasted more than a few days? Although the distinction is artificial, if an illness lasts for longer than 6 months it is generally considered chronic. A condition is considered acute if it lasts for less than 2 months and if, after it has been cured or resolves on its own, the patient sustains no ill effects. Many clinicians will often use the principles and techniques of chronic illness management to manage acute illnesses if they appear to exert a significant burden on the patient or if they fall within the gray area between an acute and chronic condition.

The Nature of Chronic Illness

There is great variability in the ways chronic diseases present and how much they affect the patient's health and life style. In attempting to categorize these highly variable illnesses in terms of their natural history and presentation, Rolland has developed a typology for chronic and life-threatening illnesses based on four characteristics: onset, course, outcome, and incapacitation (Rolland, 1984).

With regard to *onset,* chronic illnesses can develop either acutely or gradually. For example, strokes often have acute clinical presentation manifested by the sudden onset of neurological deficits, whereas rheumatoid arthritis develops gradually and slowly, at some point reaching a state where the patient is motivated to see a physician. Obviously an acute-onset illness will require much more readjustment on the part of the patient and his or her family, whereas more gradual illnesses don't require such an adjustment or rapid mobilization of resources.

With regard to *course* or *natural history,* chronic illnesses can be divided into three categories: progressive, constant, or relapsing. A progressive illness is one in which the course is generally symptomatic and progresses in severity, for example, widely metastatic cancer, rheumatoid arthritis, or NIDDM. A constant clinical course is one in which biological stabilization usually occurs after an initial event, such as a stroke or spinal cord injury. Relapsing illnesses are characterized by a course in which multiple exacerbations frequently occur, such as asthma, peptic ulcer, sclerosis, or migraine headaches. In between flare-ups of illness, a patient can often carry on a near-normal life style.

With regard to *outcome,* chronic illnesses can be divided into those that are obviously fatal, possibly fatal with a shortened lifespan, and nonfatal conditions. Examples of fatal illnesses include metastatic cancer, AIDS, and cystic fibrosis. Possibly fatal conditions that shorten lifespan include arteriosclerotic heart disease, NIDDM, and chronic obstructive pulmonary disease. Nonfatal conditions include spinal cord injuries, migraine headaches, and epilepsy.

With regard to *incapacitation,* a chronic illness can be divided into those conditions that are obviously incapacitating, in that they cause a severe impairment of functioning, and those that are nonincapacitating. Examples of incapacitating conditions include Alzheimer's disease (cognitive incapacitation), strokes (paralysis), chronic obstructive pulmonary disease (decreased respiratory function), and spinal cord injuries (paraplegia). Examples of nonincapacitating illness include a mild myocardial infarction, kidney stones, migraine headaches, psoriasis, and pernicious anemia.

Although somewhat artificial, these categories do serve as guides to clinicians in estimating the chronic illness burden on the individual and determining the adjustment that the individual and his or her family must make.

Phases of Chronic Illness

Patients with chronic illnesses typically progress through three phases: the crisis phase, the chronic phase, and the terminal phase (Rolland, 1984). During the *crisis phase,* which can be divided into prediagnosis with symptoms and the initial adjustment period, patients usually sense that something is amiss. Often, as in Case 6-2, they and their family become scared and do not immediately see a physician in the hope that the symptoms will eventually resolve. At some point during this phase patients are able to overcome their fear and eventually present to their doctor to find out what's wrong.

After a diagnosis has been made, then an initial adjustment period is necessary as patients grieve the loss of preillness identity and functional status and come to some acceptance of the permanent change in their life required by the demands of their chronic illness. For example, in Case 6-2, the adolescent who was just diagnosed with IDDM will have to integrate insulin injections and self-blood glucose monitoring into what is an already stressful period of individual development. Adhering to a diabetic diet will require significant changes in the timing and the amount of foods eaten. Because food consumption is associated with social activities and is in and of itself pleasurable, such changes will require much self-discipline and sacrifice. Physical activity and exercise must be approached by the teen-ager with more caution, as exercise might cause life-threatening attacks of hypoglycemia. In addition, because the management of IDDM does not occur in a vacuum, individual stresses may take from the time and energy required to actively manage the illness.

Because of the grief associated with the diagnosis of a chronic illness and the demands the chronic illness places on the individual to adapt, many authorities have compared the feelings individual patients experience to the well-researched grief response that terminal patients experience (Citrin, Kleiman, & Skyler, 1986). Although many diabetic patients do not go through the strict temporal sequence of feelings described by Kubler-Ross (1969), her model does provide a useful framework (Table 6-1).

Clearly the patient's family and other support systems are important as the patient attempts to adjust to the diagnosis of a chronic illness during the crisis phase. As with the individual patient, other family members and important

Table 6-1
Phases of Psychological Adjustment to a Chronic Illness

Denial
Anger
Bargaining
Depression
Acceptance

significant others may go through a psychological adaptation similar to the grief response. Denial, feelings of anger, and depression are common as family members realize that the patient may be unable to fulfill critical family roles, particularly during the initial adjustment period. For example, the elderly spouse of a patient who just received the diagnosis of Alzheimer's dementia may, after recovering from the initial shock, go into a depression herself as she begins to realize that she does not have the resources to cope with her demented spouse and must plan a nursing home admission for him.

Additionally, the diagnosis of a chronic illness may engender feelings of vulnerability and mortality in other family members. Thus, it is important for family members during the adjustment phase to be able to express their feelings in a supportive manner to the ill family member and renegotiate new family roles. This initial support is *crucial* to the family member who must begin a new life as an individual with a chronic illness.

Given the initial impact of a chronic illness on the patient's life, it is remarkable that so many chronically ill patients make a successful adjustment. Fortunately, most do. A recent study compared scores on the RAND mental health index in five groups of chronically ill patients (patients with arthritis, diabetes mellitus, cancer, renal disease, or dermatologic disorders) and a group of depressed patients (Cassileth, Lusk, Strouse, Miller, Brown, & Cross, 1984). Scores in patients with chronic illness did not differ significantly from each other or from the general public, and all patients with chronic illness had significantly better scores than the depressed patients under treatment. In addition, scores improved with age. This study also confirmed the existence of an initial adjustment process. Patients with a chronic illness who recently received that diagnosis had poorer mental health scores than those whose illness had been diagnosed more than 4 months previously.

The next phase of illness, *the chronic phase,* can be long or short depending on the course of the illness. The chronic phase is the time period after the patient and the family come to grips psychologically with the illness, institute appropriate adjustments, and devise an ongoing plan to manage the demands of the chronic illness. Unfortunately, during this "long haul," numerous problems can arise. If an illness is highly debilitating or incapacitating, the family can become exhausted with problems that seemingly have no end. In such circumstances, the primary caretakers in the family may become depressed or sick themselves from the large "burden of care." Sometimes, the demands of a chronic illness are so great that individuals and families seem developmentally frozen in time, halting the normal developmental stages individuals and families must proceed through in order to establish and maintain individual autonomy and family stability. Likewise, some individuals and their families, particularly those who do not progress successfully through the initial adjustment period, may not be able to face, either emotionally or physically, the traumas of chronic illness and become so disengaged that family dissolution occurs.

Finally, after successfully coping with the initial demands of the chronic illness, some patients and their families may forget that they even have an illness that demands continued management and forget to continue to take their medicines on schedule and perform those activities necessary to insure continued control over their disease. This is particularly true of hypertensive patients and patients with NIDDM, in which compliance with the treatment regimen seems to decrease the farther the patient is from the time of diagnosis.

The last phase of illness is the *terminal phase* in which the patient either succumbs to his or her chronic illness, succumbs to a complication of his or her chronic illness, or succumbs to another disease state. Often this phase begins with a preterminal stage in which the patient and his or her family begin to realize that life is at an end. This stage will often be marked by a great deal of patient and family anxiety as they attempt to cope with the fatal disease process. Physicians will often be asked by patients in this state to do anything possible to prolong their lives, and families will often bring the patient to the physician repeatedly, even if the patient is not in a state of crisis, in the hope of finding some way to prolong the patient's life. Gradually a period of grief and mourning begins in which the patient begins to proceed through the stages of grief. The physician, if closely involved with the patient, also often proceeds through such a grief response and can be very instrumental in helping the patient and the family by educating them about the stages of grief and even sharing some of his or her own feelings and vulnerability about the patient's imminent demise. On the other hand, physicians need to be cognizant that such a sharing of their own feelings and vulnerability may make a patient and his or her family even more anxious.

After the patient's death, the family must proceed through a period of grief in which the loss of the patient is mourned. The death of a loved one also demands another adjustment by the family as they must resume family life without the patient. Typically this stage takes 2 to 6 months. As in other phases of adjustment, families can become stuck. If family members take longer than 6 months to adjust to the loss of a loved one, then further intervention and help are warranted, perhaps even psychological counseling to help the family members readjust to the new situation.

Case 6-2 illustrates the *initial adjustment phase*. The patient in this case, like many patients with a chronic illness, tried to deemphasize his symptoms and did not present to a health care provider immediately in the hope that his symptoms would resolve. Despite the fact that both he and his mother knew something was amiss, when the physician finally made the diagnosis and presented that information to them, both the patient and his mother were shocked, an indication of the strength of their denial, and began an immediate grief response. The physician was also shocked and empathized with the patient, as he himself knew the burdens and potential complications of IDDM from taking care of other diabetic patients.

The physician in Case 6-2 recommended a period of hospitalization because the number of tasks to master and readjustments necessary was so great that the physician felt the patient needed access to the resources of the hospital in learning initially how to control his IDDM. This also allows the family a period of time in which adjustments can be made in the home prior to the patient's return. Some chronic illnesses, such as spinal cord injury, require a prolonged period of therapy after hospitalization for the acute injury, in which almost all skills that the patient has learned have to be relearned and reintegrated into their life style. In contrast, the patient in Case 6-2 was discharged after 5 days of hospitalization after learning the techniques of insulin injection, when to adjust his insulin dose, self-blood glucose monitoring, what to eat, and when to exercise. Two weeks after his hospitalization, the patient was doing well, injecting himself with insulin twice a day, and maintaining good blood glucose control as evidenced by his self-blood glucose monitoring.

CLINICAL MANAGEMENT

Case 6-3. A 63-year-old female nurse presented to a family practice clinic with longstanding NIDDM. Over the past 2 months she had made frequent visits complaining of fatigue, weight loss, and frequent urination. Tests of her blood sugar consistently showed blood glucose values over 300 mg/dl. Because of these high blood glucose readings, the physician had progressively increased her insulin dosage, almost doubling it over the past 2 months. Despite this increase, the patient's blood glucose on the day of her most recent visit was 321 mg/dl.

The physician expressed his concern to the patient by stating that since outpatient treatment over the past 2 months had not brought her NIDDM under better control, he felt that the best option would be to admit the patient to the hospital. The patient initially resisted the idea but eventually consented and was admitted.

The physician began his treatment of the patient by using her last outpatient insulin dosage that he had recommended. Unfortunately, on that dosage the patient became very hypoglycemic after the first injection and mildly hypoglycemic after the second. The physician then readjusted the insulin dose so that over the next 2 to 3 days the patient's blood sugars came under good control, using about three-quarters of her most recent outpatient insulin dosage. The physician realized that the patient's failure to adequately control her blood sugars was probably caused by noncompliance.

Rather than confront the patient directly with his suspicions, the physician expressed confusion to the patient that he did not understand how she could be so easily controlled in the hospital on lower dosages of insulin but yet not be very well controlled as an outpatient on higher dosages of insulin. The patient then explained to the physician that she worked the night shift at the local hospital and so often ate most of her food at night when she received her smallest insulin dose. She was easily controlled in the hospital because she ate most of her food during the day after her biggest injection of insulin. The nurse also told the physician that she was much more concerned about having an attack of hypoglycemia than achieving tight control. She was comfortable if most of her blood sugar readings were under 200 mg/dl.

The physician then acknowledged the patient's concern and, when the patient was discharged, switched her morning and evening doses of insulin so that she received most of her insulin dose in the evening. He also gave up his goal of tight glucose control (most blood sugar under 140 mg/dl) in favor of the nurse's less stringent goal. With those changes, over the next year, the patient returned with blood sugars in the 140–180 range without any episodes of hypoglycemia or symptoms suggestive of hyperglycemia.

Clinical management is that process during which physicians and patients collect information, set goals, and develop plans to optimize the health of the patient. It is particularly important to note the two words *"and patients."* Physicians practicing from a strictly biomedical model, in which the management plan automatically flows from the diagnoses of certain diseases and certain disease-specific parameters, often forget these two critical words. Noncompliance is often the result. Clinical management plans not only need to be "disease specific" but "patient specific" as well (Brody, 1980).

Taylor, Gordon, and Ashworth's study entitled "A Systems Perspective on Clinical Management" is one of the earliest studies of the clinical management process (Taylor, Gordon, & Ashworth, 1984). Taylor and colleagues examined the content of the conversation that occurred between 24 physicians and their diabetic patients, using a structured interview, videotaping of some office visits, and content analysis. This analysis revealed that more than 90% of the statements that physicians and patients made about the management process fell into one of four areas: systems assessment, goal setting, management plan, and tactical implementation.

Systems Assessment

Systems assessment is that phase of the clinical management process in which physicians try to determine the patient's current disease status and what events have taken place since the patient's last visit. Taylor *et al.* noted that during this phase physicians often begin by madly thumbing through the patient's chart in an effort to refresh their memory of the patient's condition. Typically, physicians will assess both subjective and objective criteria related to the patient's disease. Examples of some of these criteria are shown in Table 6-2.

With the realization that diseases and their treatments not only affect disease-specific parameters but other areas of patient functioning, doctors are beginning to assess those "quality of life" issues as well. Tarlov (1983) has recently stated that the new challenge of medicine in the coming years may be not only to continue medicine's concentration on the prevention of death and prolongation of life but also to maintain or improve the ability of the patient to function. Ware (1984) has proposed a patient functioning framework by conceptualizing five areas that should help physicians assess the many diverse components of quality of life. They are (1) disease-specific factors, (2) personal functioning, (3) psychological distress/well-being, (4) general health perceptions, and (5) social and role functioning.

Disease-specific factors are those measurable symptoms and physiological perimeters associated with the disease in question. **Personal functioning** is defined as the performance and the capacity to perform the kind of task that most people do daily, including self-care, ambulation, physical activities, sexual functioning, and cognitive functioning. **Psychological functioning** refers to the emotional state of the patient. **General health perceptions** refer to the individual's perceptions of his health. These perceptions are usually based on the previous three areas of patient functioning. Even though they are associated with those areas of patient functioning, Ware felt that general health perceptions were sufficiently independent to justify a separate category. **Social and role functioning** is defined as the person's ability to perform activities associated with his or her role in society, including employment, school work, housework, and family tasks and roles. Often, a few questions to the patient on how the disease or the treatment is affecting his or her life are sufficient to uncover concerns that the physician and patient should address.

If any change in the patient's disease state is noted, then the physician will also need to assess why that improvement or deterioration occurred. A deterioration would not be unexpected in a disease with a progressively deteriorating natural history, but if the natural history of the disease is such that treatment interventions should result in an improvement and one did not occur, the physician needs to question his or her diagnosis, see if other factors that might affect the disease state have arisen, determine if noncompliance is occurring, or determine if there are other aspects of the patient's life, such as a stressful family or job situation, that might have affected the patient's quality of life. Additionally, because many chronic illnesses are associated with complications that have profound effects on the patient's functional status, physicians should screen for those complications when assessing the patient. For example, diabetes mellitus

Table 6-2
Criteria Typically Assessed in Selected Chronic Illnesses

Chronic illness	Subjective criteria	Objective criteria
Arthritis	Joint soreness Functional limitation	Joint swelling and erythema Sedimentation rate
Asthma	Shortness of breath Frequency of attacks	Respiratory rate Wheezing Peak expiratory flow Arterial blood gas
Congestive heart	Shortness of breath Orthopnea Ankle swelling	Weight Rales Ankle edema Heart size on chest x ray
Diabetes mellitus	Fatigue Polyuria Polydypsia Polyphagia	Fasting blood glucose value Glycosolated hemoglobin
Hypertension	None	Blood pressure
Ischemic heart	Chest pain Frequency of attacks	ECG changes on an exercise stress test Coronary angiography
Lung cancer	Shortness of breath Chest pain	Diminished breath sounds Tumor size on chest x ray Metastasis on bone scan
Peptic ulcer disease	Abdominal pain Nausea and vomiting Bleeding	Finding on upper gastrointestinal endoscopy Hematocrit Test for blood in the stool

is associated with retinopathy (blindness), nephropathy (kidney failure), and peripheral vascular diseases (leg pain as a result of ischemia). Lastly, attempting to estimate the patient's prognosis—how long the patient is likely to live and what complications are likely to develop in the future—is also a task that is performed during the system's assessment.

It is important to realize that the physician is not the only person conducting a systems assessment. Patients also, prior to the visit, conduct a systems assessment on themselves. Often the reason for the patient's visit is that the patient's own systems assessment has not yielded any information that could result in an intervention that would improve the health of the patient or has resulted in an intervention that has had no effect.

Finally, it is imperative for the patient and physician to agree on the nature of the problems that exist in order to proceed to the next step. This is important because patients will often have erroneous but powerfully held beliefs about their illness that may cause conflict over future management decisions. Bass *et al.*, in a study of 193 patients with nonrespiratory symptoms such as headaches, low back pain, or abdominal pain, noted that resolution of the patient's symptoms in 1 month was associated with agreement between the patient and the physician about the nature of the problem (Bass, Buck, Turner, Pickie, Pratt, & Robinson, 1986). Thus, physicians should spend time with patients to insure that both agree about the nature of the problem and, if multiple problems exist, which one to work on first in order to optimize the patient's health.

Goal Setting

After the assessment phase, the physician and the patient move into the goal-setting phase during which both begin to determine realistically what improvements can be made in the patient's condition. This is the phase in which physicians put the most time and thought, as evidenced by it being the area with the highest percentage of physician statements, 39%. Also, it is the area that is a direct reflection of the physician's medical values. For example, should physicians keep diabetic patients under tight or loose control? Should physicians treat patients with mild hypertension?

Even though patients tend to give less thought to the goal-setting phase than physicians, this phase is also a clear reflection of the patient's values. Often diseases or their treatments involve trade-offs that the patient must consider. For example, Mengel, Connis, Gordon, and Taylor (1988) have found that IDDM patients beginning insulin pump therapy show a significant deterioration in family social activities compared with a control group of patients on conventional insulin therapy. Mengel *et al.* hypothesized that many IDDM patients may not want to start insulin pump therapy, even though it does bring their blood sugars under better control, because they are unwilling to suffer the loss of family social functioning that instituting pump therapy entails. Thus, if a goal to achieve better control over a chronic illness is to be set, then specific trade-offs that the patient will have to make should be identified and considered by both the physician and the patient.

The importance of physician and patient agreement during goal setting has been shown in several studies. Marteau, Johnston, Baum, and Bloch (1987) studied 65 children with IDDM and their parents to see if there were significant differences between the goals of the doctor and those of the parents. Marteau and colleagues did find very significant differences in goals between parents and physicians, with physicians being much more concerned with preventing the complications of IDDM through improved glucose control. Parents were much more concerned with preventing episodes of hypoglycemia. Interestingly, the degree of diabetic control the child achieved was much more closely associated with the parents' goals. Marteau *et al.* suggested that physicians should negotiate with the parents of a diabetic child to make their goals explicit and to work with them to try to achieve not only their own goals but the physician's goals as well. Becker, Abrams, and Onder (1974) showed that there was much less sabotage of treatment activity if goals were mutually agreed on by both the patient and the physician on a rehabilitation unit.

An example of physician–patient disagreement over treatment goals is described in Case 6-3 where the physician would have preferred a goal of tighter glucose control than the patient. Quill (1983) has recommended that when such disagreements occur, the physician should be as flexible and creative as possible to individualize the care of the patient, but not so flexible that he or she violates his own sense of ethnics or medical values. Quill recommends negotiation, defined as a "process between two persons who have relatively equal power willing to be influenced by one another." Quill emphasizes that during this process it is important to identify the needs and desires of the patient and then try to achieve a workable compromise in which both the patient and the physician feel that a positive outcome will result. Quill also cautions that some patients may not be up to this approach because they are either too ill physically or too immature psychologically.

If both the patient and the physician are interested in negotiating goals, then Quill recommends a contract be formed. A contract is an "explicit bilateral commitment to a well-defined course of action in which both parties gain." Quill emphasized that in formulating this contract there are four assumptions: (1) that both parties are responsible, the physician for medical expertise and the patient for the effect of the disease and its treatment on his life, (2) both parties come to the arrangement under a consentual, not an obligatory, arrangement in which trust is necessary, (3) both are willing to negotiate, and (4) both must gain from the arrangement.

In their book *Getting to Yes,* Fisher and Ury (1981) emphasize the importance of "principled" negotiation in achieving an agreement. They state that typically negotiations are over "positions," what the parties should or should not do, rather than over the interests, needs, hopes, or dreams of the parties involved. Often when negotiations occur over positions, participants feel that they are locked into those positions and must "save face" rather than negotiating a mutually acceptable agreement. Face-saving, blaming, and delaying tactics are the norm in negotiations over positions. Clearly, such a negotiation strategy would not be very effective in the medical setting in which the patient and the physician must form a relationship in which they are trying to optimize the patient's health. Physicians, in negotiating with patients, should focus on interests rather than positions.

Fisher and Ury also emphasized that it is important to consider the other party, in this case the patient, in negotiating. First, the perceptions and emotions of the patient should be acknowledged and dealt with as separate issues apart from the negotiation. The physician should have the capacity to step into the patient's shoes, acknowledge and attempt to understand his or her own perceptions of the patient's difficulties, and not react emotionally, for example, in anger or frustration, when the patient appears to be behaving emotionally him- or herself.

Goals or judgments about the attainment of goals should be based on objective standards. Thus, an appropriate goal for a diabetic patient would be to try and achieve more than 80% of her blood sugars under 180 mg/dl. It would probably not be wise for the physician and patient to set a vague subjective goal, as it would be difficult for both the patient and the physician to agree if the goal has been reached. An objective criterion allows a standard independent of the will of either the patient or the physician and may serve to diffuse future disagreements as to whether a goal was achieved or a specific treatment was effective.

Management Plan

After specific achievable goals have been set, then the patient and the physician move into the management plan phase in which a general approach to the care of the patient is formulated. Unfortunately, physicians don't spend a lot of time in this phase, as to them it seems to flow naturally from the goal-setting phase. Nor do physicians spend enough time either eliciting patient's opinions about the various possible intervention options or explaining to the patient the details of a particular intervention.

Patients, however, consider this phase to be particularly important, as evidenced by the high proportion of their responses that were categorized within the management plan phase. Patients frequently come to doctors after an intervention they have devised for themselves has failed or to obtain something, e.g., prescription drugs, that they cannot attain themselves. Additionally, many patients are aware of past medical interventions used on them that were ineffective or, worse, harmful. Such patients will often exercise a healthy skepticism toward the doctor's recommended intervention unless it is explained in great detail.

There are two questions that a physician must answer for every patient during the management plan phase. (1) Is there an effective intervention that would help achieve therapeutic goals? (2) If multiple effective interventions are available, which one should be used?

The first question is often surprisingly difficult to answer. Roper, Winkenwerder, Hackbarth, and Krakaner (1988) have acknowledged that there simply are no scientific data available on the effectiveness of many interventions, even many that are used widely in medicine, or the data available are from studies that are flawed scientifically. Physicians may not know how to critically evaluate the medical literature to determine if a particular intervention was from a flawed study. Also, physicians often overdiagnose and thus overintervene in medical problems because they don't think probabilistically and are afraid of missing rare but serious diagnoses. Sometimes physicians apply an intervention that works with one particular disease to another disease state or type of patient because they think the two diseases arise from similar pathophysiological processes. Unfortunately, generalizing interventions to similar but unrelated conditions usually does not work.

The gold standard for deciding whether an intervention actually does more good than harm in a particular clinical setting and how effective that intervention is in achieving therapeutic goals is the double-blind, placebo-controlled, randomized clinical trial (Pocock, 1983). In such a trial an intervention, such as a new medication, is compared against an ineffective placebo to control for the effects of time and attention on outcome. Often medical diseases will resolve on their own accord without any intervention. Likewise, diseases may respond to a "placebo effect" simply because the physician may be paying more attention to the patient. Double-blinding refers to the fact that neither the patient nor the physician knows to which treatment group the patient belongs, so that outcomes are not subject to the bias inherent in that knowledge. Often, if the patient or physician knows that he or she is in the active therapy group, he or she will subjectively exaggerate the effects of the treatment. A trial is randomized in order to insure that the two treatment groups are similar on a number of variables that might significantly affect the outcome of the trial. Criteria have been published that will enable interested physicians to assess randomized controlled trials adequately (Sackett *et al.*, 1985).

The second question is also difficult to answer. If multiple interventions are available for a particular medical problem, then physicians often turn to cost-effectiveness analysis to determine which intervention would be least costly but still effective in a particular setting (Sox *et al.*, 1988). Cost-effectiveness analysis compares different management strategies in terms of the cost per unit of outcome, where the outcome is life saved, quality of life improved, or complication rate decreased. Cost-effectiveness analyses are often very complex. Many different costs must be quantified and benefits determined.

Often the results of the cost-effectiveness analysis also vary depending on the value the patients place on the various costs and benefits to be gained. In other words, the patient may be willing to take a more costly drug if it would mean he would have a lower chance of experiencing side effects, even though the cost-effectiveness analysis of the two drugs may reveal that a less expensive, more side-effect-causing drug is equally effective and more cost-effective. When applying the results of a cost-effectiveness analysis to a particular patient, it is important for the physician to scientifically critique such studies while taking the patient's own values into consideration.

Finally, each physician must determine his or her own therapeutic threshold (Farrow, Wartman, & Brock, 1988). That is the point at which the physician thinks a disease state should be treated. Scientific studies help to determine the best place to begin treatment; for example, studies have shown that a diastolic blood pressure of over 90 mm Hg or a cholesterol of over 240 mg/dl should receive some form of therapy (Hypertension Detection and Follow-up Program

Cooperative Group, 1983; National Cholesterol Education Program Expert Panel, 1988).

Unfortunately, many therapeutic threshold studies are not carried out for a long enough time period to determine if short-term gains may be made at the expense of long-term morbidity or mortality. For example, giving rheumatoid arthritis patients oral steroid medication may provide some short-term benefits, less sore joints, unfortunately at the expense of greatly increased morbidity from the complications of long-term steroid use. Additionally, trials often do not measure all the outcomes that would be important for the patient and physician.

Several studies support the idea that the patient should be actively involved during the management plan phase. Greenfield, Kayslan, Ware, Yamo, and Frank (1988) conducted a randomized controlled trial on 59 adult diabetic patients using assistants who encouraged patients to negotiate medical decisions with their physicians. These assistants encouraged patient involvement by utilizing the patient's own medical chart and reviewing it with him or her in a standardized fashion before their visit. Videotape analysis of these doctor–patient interactions reveal that these patients were twice as effective in obtaining medical information from the physicians than the patients in the nonintervention group. After 6 months the degree of glucose control achieved by the patients in the intervention group was significantly better than that achieved by the nonintervention group. Likewise, Uhlmann, Inui, Pecorado, and Carter (1988), in a study of 51 NIDDM patients, showed that some measures of compliance were higher if the doctor responded to the patient's request. The investigators noted that 75% of the requests dealt with treatment options, whereas 25% of the requests concern psychosocial issues.

Thus, designing an effective management plan requires not only the contribution of the physician but the active participation of the patient. The physician needs to be reasonably comfortable that the interventions recommended to the patient will do more good than harm while achieving the therapeutic goals that both have set. The patient then needs to weigh the options based on their own feelings about the potential risks and benefits of each intervention. Working together, the patient and physician can then construct a plan that will have the best chance of improving the patient's life while minimizing potential ill effects.

Tactical Implementation

After deciding that an intervention is necessary and what the therapeutic options are, the physician and patient then enter the tactical implementation phase. In this phase they decide on the specifics of the intervention, when it is to be applied, how it is to be applied, where it is to be applied, how to monitor progress, if and when other health care professionals need to be involved, if and when other members of the patient's family need to be involved, and when follow-up should occur. For example, the physician may have decided for a patient with newly diagnosed NIDDM that appropriate options to discuss with the patient would include dietary therapy, insulin injections, oral hypoglycemic agents, and an exercise program. If the patient and physician decided during the management plan phase that they would pursue dietary therapy and drug treatment with an oral hypoglycemic agent but not insulin injections or exercise therapy, then during the tactical implementation phase the specifics of those two interventions would be negotiated.

A combination of scientific information and the patient's own values is needed to make an effective decision during the tactical implementation phase. For example, the physician may feel that the patient described in the above paragraph should be placed on a 2200-calorie diet in order to effectively control blood glucose values, but if the patient also desired to lose weight, then the physician could modify the number of calories to insure adequate weight loss as well. Additionally, the physician could describe the characteristics of the available oral hypoglycemic agents and then negotiate a selection based on cost and compliance issues.

Physicians should be able to create a variety of options for the patient during the tactical implementation phase. It is often difficult for physicians to create numerous options for the patient, as physicians often fixate on their favorite way to deal with a particular problem. For example, the physician in Case 6-3 typically prescribed the largest dose of insulin in the morning with a smaller second dose in the evening. This clearly was not appropriate for the patient, as she was a nurse who ate most of her food during her night shift.

Unfortunately, physicians also do not spend a great deal of time on this phase of the clinical management process. Patients, however, are very concerned about the tactical implementation phase and desire a great deal of knowledge about the specifics of their interventions and education on how treatments will affect their overall health, life style, and functional status.

The involvement of other family members is also critical during this phase. For example, involving the family member who prepares the meals for an NIDDM patient is an obvious example of the importance of family involvement when trying to optimize the patient's health. Failure to involve the family meal preparer might result in an ineffective intervention simply because the meal preparer does not know how to prepare the foods in such a way as to ensure that the caloric limits of the patient's diet are not exceeded.

The physician can also serve as a source of encouragement and suggest strategies that will aid the patient in carrying out the specifics of the plan. A study by Guyatt, Pugsley, Sullivan, Thompson, Berman, Jones, Fallen, and Taylor (1984) in 43 patients with chronic obstructive pulmonary disease and congestive heart failure showed that simple encouragement by the physician increased these patients' performance on a 6-min walking test similar to the magnitude of performance improvement gained from drug use alone. Thus, the physician's own encouragement and support can have literally the same effect on some outcomes as medications. Likewise, physicians can recommend behavioral strategies or contracts that will help the patient perform the necessary behaviors associated with the intervention, such as taking medicines, exercising appropriately, and staying on a diet.

Follow-Up

Even though decisions as to follow-up were not a formal part of the management process described by Taylor *et al.*, this is a critical phase in the clinical management process. The reason for this is simple: often, despite the best efforts of the physician and patient, a therapeutic plan will not result in an improvement in patient health. By following up with a patient when appropriate, a physician can request information as to the effectiveness of a therapeutic plan and make changes if the plan is not as successful as was hoped. Likewise, the effect of the plan on the patient's life can be assessed. If the patient failed to carry out parts of the plan, then reasons for that failure can also be assessed, such as unrealistic goals, medication side effects, or a failure on the part of the patient to integrate the steps of the plan into his or her life style. Tactics to improve the effectiveness of the new therapeutic plan can then be instituted, such as utilization of less costly interventions, behavioral strategies such as involvement of family members to increase social support, or devising more realistic therapeutic goals.

The frequency of follow-up should be determined based on the natural history of the disease in question and the doctor's feeling of how frequently he or she should monitor the patient and support the patient in his or her efforts to optimize their health. The patient's own desire for follow-up should also be taken into account.

PATIENT COMPLIANCE

Case 6-4. A 38-year-old male presented to a physician's office for the first time for a complete physical examination. The physical examination revealed that the patient was obese with a blood pressure of 180/110 mm Hg. The physical exam and subsequent laboratory tests did not reveal any secondary cause for this patient's high blood pressure. Blood pressure readings taken every day for the next 3 days continued to reveal high values.

After having obtained the necessary work-up to rule out secondary causes of hypertension, the doctor made the diagnosis of essential hypertension. The patient agreed with this diagnosis and after learning about the potential complications of high blood pressure agreed that he should be placed on medication. After discussing medication options that were available, the doctor and patient agreed that an angiotensin-converting enzyme inhibitor would probably be the best choice. The doctor and patient also negotiated a weight loss diet and an exercise program. The doctor asked the patient to return in a week to assess the patient for side effects of the medication.

One week later the patient returned with no complaints. His blood pressure of 160/95 mm Hg. Because the full benefits of antihypertensive therapy are usually not reached for 2 to 4 weeks after initiation of therapy, the doctor was satisfied with the progress the patient was making; so was the patient. The doctor asked the patient to return in 1 month.

One month later the patient returned with an elevated blood pressure of 175/105 mm Hg. His weight was down 4 lb from his previous visit, and he had begun a walking program. The doctor was perplexed because the patient's blood pressure had been decreasing so well but now appeared to have returned to its previous high value. When the doctor expressed his confusion to the patient, the patient said, "Oh, I'm not taking those any more,

Doc. You only prescribed 30 tablets, and since the prescription didn't have a refill, I figured that was all I needed to take."

Case 6-5. A 22-year-old single mother of two presented to a clinic with complaints of pelvic pain of 3 days' duration associated with fever and a purulent vaginal discharge. The diagnosis of pelvic inflammatory disease was quickly made, a work-up for other sexually transmitted diseases was initiated, and the patient consented to antibiotic therapy.

As was his practice, the physician prescribed a form of tetracycline that could be taken twice a day (tetracycline usually needs to be taken four times a day), figuring that twice-a-day therapy would improve patient compliance. He prescribed the drug using the trade name of the medication. The patient also consented to receive a shot of a different antibiotic that would insure the death of other organisms that cause pelvic inflammatory disease, organisms that were not well treated by the oral antibiotic the physician prescribed. The patient left satisfied that her infection had been treated, agreed to ask her male partner to come in for treatment, and actually liked her new physician since he treated her "very nicely."

Unfortunately, the patient returned 3 days later with continued complaints of pelvic pain, fever, and purulent vaginal discharge. Her physician was initially angry with the patient, figuring that the patient had not been compliant with her oral medication. When he confronted the patient with his suspicions, the patient was initially confused and stated that she didn't need the oral antibiotic as she had been given a shot in the office by the physician. She explained to the physician that she had tried to get the antibiotic filled anyway, but that it cost $42 for a 10-day supply, a prohibitive amount given her meager budget. The physician realized that he had not explained the necessity of two antibiotics for the treatment of pelvic inflammatory disease and also realized that if he had prescribed the generic variety of the oral antibiotic, the cost would have been much less for a 10-day course. Unfortunately, on reexamination the patient was in such bad shape that she required treatment with intravenous antibiotics in the hospital.

The problem of noncompliance is a vexing one for physicians. First, the definition of what constitutes noncompliance is not always clear. Does noncompliant behavior include those patients who simply refuse to follow medical instructions, or is it just those patients who agree with medical advice but who for whatever reason cannot follow the instructions of their physicians? For the purposes of this chapter, the latter definition of noncompliant behavior is used. Second, although it is hypothesized and has been proven in some studies that noncompliance prolongs illness, increases time lost from work, increases the complication rate from chronic disease, and increases health care costs (Ammirato, 1989), it is clear that noncompliant behavior does not always result in a poor outcome for an individual patient (Eraker, Kirscht, & Becker, 1984). For example, noncompliance with a medication that causes an adverse side effect in some patients, such as the use of propranolol in the treatment of hypertension causing fatigue and impotence in some patients, may actually yield beneficial results for some patients, particularly in the short term. Third, compliance is not easily predicted based on the sociodemographic characteristics, personality, or disease state of the patient (Hefferin, 1979). In fact, those factors seem to influence compliance behavior only marginally if at all. Fourth, compliance is difficult to measure (Eraker *et al.*, 1984). Simply asking a patient if he or she is compliant with a treatment plan may not always yield a valid answer, as the patient may be embarrassed or afraid to tell the truth. Objective measures, such as drug levels, are not available for all medications and are influenced by many other variables besides the intake of medication. Counting the patient's pills when he returns for a follow-up visit or asking him to keep a drug diary is too time consuming and inconvenient for most physicians and patients.

What is clear about noncompliance is that it is widespread (Ammirato, 1989). It is estimated that 20% of patients won't even fill their prescriptions, even for acute infections. Fifty percent of patients who were diagnosed as hypertensive will not be taking their medications 1 year later. Ten percent of all hospitalizations are estimated to be for noncompliance, and 23% of nursing home admissions are similarly estimated to be for noncompliance. Given the widespread prevalence of noncompliance and its hypothesized link with adverse health outcomes, what can physicians do to improve compliance by their patients to therapeutic plans?

First, physicians can assess four factors that often lead to noncompliance. These factors can be thought of as the "four Ms" of noncompliance: misunderstandings, motivation, medication, and money (Jonas & Bauer, 1989).

Misunderstandings

Misunderstandings, either the physician's or the patient's, are quite common in medicine. Case 6-4 illustrates a common misunderstanding that occurs frequently. In this case the patient had received the diagnosis of hypertension, a condition that requires lifelong medical therapy. However, the patient misunderstood this requirement, probably because it was not adequately explained by the physician. Similarly, in Case 6-5, the patient did not understand that she needed two antibiotics; again this critical idea was not communicated by the physician, and so she felt safe in not obtaining the expensive oral antibiotic.

Such misunderstandings can be avoided if the physician takes the time to educate the patient on what disease the patient has and why the prescribed therapy is needed. Although general knowledge on the patient's disease appears to have little relationship with compliance, specific knowledge as to what the patient has and what he should do and why does appear to improve compliance (Eraker *et al.*, 1984). Likewise, specific instructions delivered in a simple clear language, rather than the technical medical terminology most doctors use, seems to improve compliance. Instructions should be formatted based on the following principles:

1. Instructions delivered first are remembered best.
2. Instructions that are emphasized by being mentioned two or three times are recalled best.
3. The fewer instructions that are given, the more are remembered.

4. If complex instructions are given to the patient, such instructions should be written, or the patient should be asked to repeat them back to ensure understanding.

Motivation

Motivation can be defined as the desire to perform a task or carry out a therapeutic plan. Physicians often assume that patients are very motivated to optimize their health, and indeed they are most of the time. However, such a simple notion does not recognize the complexity of human motivations, nor does it recognize the fact that motivations often are conflicting. Optimizing health is not always the first priority of patients.

Researchers have found that the patient's motivation for a particular therapeutic option generally depends on his or her health beliefs: (1) the patient's perception of his or her susceptibility to a particular disease or complication, (2) the severity of the disease both clinically and socially, and (3) the benefits or barriers derived or encountered if treated (Eraker *et al.*, 1984). This health belief model has been useful in predicting noncompliance in patients on antihypertensive therapy, cholesterol therapy, and yearly immunization with influenza vaccine.

Viewed from this model, it is particularly easy to see why patients treated with antihypertensives have such a high rate of noncompliance. Hypertension is an asymptomatic disease that causes little if any loss in the patient's quality of life. Complications of hypertension occur years after the diagnosis and can be denied psychologically by the patient, similar to the way smokers don't really feel they will ever get lung cancer.

Physicians can help motivate patients to follow therapeutic plans by discussing their health beliefs, formulating shorter-term goals, such as normalizing blood pressure rather than preventing the complications of hypertension, instituting treatment regimens that have a low incidence of side effects, and utilizing contingency contracting, which are discussed below.

Medication

The two most obvious characteristics of the medication that affect compliance are frequency of dosing and side effects. In a summary of 26 studies examining dosage schedule, Greenberg (1984) showed significantly improved compliance with once- or twice-a-day dosing compared with three- or four-times-a-day dosing. This fact alone may explain the widespread noncompliance with antibiotics, even though most are used to treat acute conditions for short periods of time, as most antibiotics require three- or four-times-a-day dosing. Physicians who wish to improve patient compliance should attempt to find medicines that can be dosed once or twice a day.

Likewise, medication side effects can lead to noncompliance. Croog, Levin, Testa, Brown, Bulpitt, Jenkins, Klerman, and Williams (1986) conducted a multicentered, randomized, double-blind, clinical trial among 626 men with hypertension to determine if captopril, methyldopa, or propranolol have significant effects on quality of life. Their study showed that patients taking captopril reported fewer side effects and a greater improvement in overall general well-being when compared to the other two treatment options. The investigators also showed that the frequency of side effects in all of the three treatment options was related to the patient withdrawing from therapy.

Failing to give the patient some perspective on the frequency of side effects may result in the patient prematurely discontinuing therapy simply because he or she becomes frightened after reading about all the possible side effects either in the package insert or in the *Physician's Desk Reference*. In a study of patients with rheumatoid arthritis, patients were presented with the risks and benefits of an unknown medication (Epstein & Lasagna, 1969). The risks of the unknown medication were spelled out in great detail. Many of the patients refused the medication even after it was revealed to be aspirin. Many patients are risk avoiders, such that when they learn of all the potential side effects of the medication, no matter how rare many of those side effects may be, they will prematurely discontinue or even refuse a potentially beneficial medicine. Physicians can improve compliance by presenting an accurate perspective on the frequency of side effects, particularly to patients who are risk avoiders.

Regimens that are of long duration, dependent on life-style alteration, and inconvenient also have higher rates of noncompliance than those that are of short duration, simple, and convenient (Eraker *et al.*, 1984). Physicians can help patients simplify their regimen by attempting to discontinue medication that may no longer be useful, by helping the patient integrate the medication into his or her life style by using events the patient experiences every day to trigger the patient to take the medicine, and by suggesting the use of pill boxes that contain a daily supply of medicine, so the patients do not become confused as to whether they have taken their medicine for that day or not.

Money

As illustrated in Case 6-5, the financial resources that the patient has can be a critical factor in aiding or hampering compliance. The expense of medication is not the only important cost; the cost of office visits and laboratory tests can also play a role in noncompliance with medical follow-up. Thus, even though it is often uncomfortable for physicians to discuss financial issues with a patient, such a discussion may improve patient compliance, as less expensive treatment options are often available such as generic pharmaceuticals.

What is probably most help for patients is to have some notion of the cost of treatment options when they are being discussed by the physician. For example, the patient in Case 6-5 could have been presented with three treatment options with regard to her oral antibiotics, all of which are equally effective in the outpatient management of pelvic inflammatory disease. Those options are: (1) generic tetracycline, 500 mg four times a day, \$5–8 for a 10-day course, (2) generic doxycycline, 100 mg twice a day, \$10–15 for a 10-day course, and (3) nongeneric doxycycline, \$30–50 for a 10-day course. Given such a presentation, with an explanation for the necessity of two antibiotics in the treatment of pelvic inflammatory disease, the patient may have selected a less expensive option but would have been much more likely to comply. Even though the physician in this case tried to improve patient compliance by prescribing a twice-a-day oral antibiotic, he ultimately failed because he did not take into account the cost of the treatment regimen.

Other Determinants of Compliance

The context of the patient's care greatly influences patient compliance. The term "context of care" refers to the many relationships that have an effect on the patient's health, including the doctor–patient relationship, family relationships, and relationships between physicians and other members of the health care team. Although these contextual issues receive greater treatment in subsequent chapters, a few issues deserve mention.

Compliance has been shown to increase if the patient is satisfied with his or her visit with the physician and to decrease if the visit is perceived as being short or impersonal (Eraker *et al.*, 1984). Communication between the physician and patient that is clear and direct, eliciting all important issues, improves compliance (Ross & Phipps, 1986). Power struggles between the patient and the physician in which both are trying to negotiate from a fixed position rather than from their own interests decrease patient compliance. Lack of family support has been shown to decrease compliance (Eraker *et al.*, 1984). Finally, a communication pattern between members of the health care team in which all pertinent information is not shared and goals are not agreed on leads to confusing messages being given to the patient and also decreases compliance.

Strategies to Improve Compliance

If the physician suspects the patient to be noncompliant, the physician should first review in his or her own mind the patient's adjustment to the chronic illness, the specifics of the clinical management process, particularly the characteristics of the therapeutic plan, and whether the patient agrees on each facet of that plan, the "four Ms" of noncompliance (misunderstandings, motivation, medication, and money), and factors in the context of that particular patient's care that may be affecting the patient's ability to comply with the therapeutic plan. If in thinking about the patient's situation the physician feels that a particular issue is important, then an open-ended discussion on that particular issue should be begun. If no particular issues come to the physician's mind, then the physician can begin a general discussion with the patient by expressing his dismay or confusion that the therapeutic plan is not working and asking the patient whether he or she has any idea or reason why the plan is not effective. Such an open-ended discussion will usually reveal a facet of the plan that the patient either does not understand or with which he or she disagrees. It is important to remember during this discussion that the physician should try not to blame the patient or become angry because the plan is not working. Such blaming can only result in either power struggles or dissolution of the doctor–patient relationship.

Should an open-ended discussion not reveal any particular reasons why the therapeutic plan is not working, then some authorities have recommended behavioral or contingency contracting as a way to improve patient compliance. A contingency contract has been defined by Steckle and Swain (1977) as "a contract in which compliance behavior is followed by a satisfying state of affairs," "stamping in" the necessary behavior. The compliance behavior that is necessary to follow the therapeutic plan should be measurable and described in realistic terms. Both the physician and the patient should agree that the treatment goals and progress toward those goals should be monitored not only by the physician during frequent office visits but by the patient using self-monitoring of whatever parameters the patient and physician feel are appropriate. Those parameters should be objective and should be recorded at agreed-on times. A time limit should be placed on the contract so that it is not open-ended. Finally, the rewards should be pleasurable for the patient and not harm the patient's disease state. Proven successful rewards include money, books, or free time. Free office visits are also a reward that some patients find valuable. The rewards do not necessarily have to come from the physician, however. For example, the patient may collect a pot of approximately $100 of his or her own money before the contract begins, and then the physician or an interested third party distributes that money back to the patient in $5 increments as intermediate goals are met.

Management Failures

There are clearly times when legitimate disagreements remain between the patient and the physician or when every strategy that the physician feels comfortable trying has not resulted in an improvement in the patient's health. Such situations are often highly frustrating for physicians, as their professional self-image has a great deal to do with their ability to aid ill patients in improving their health. This professional self-image not only is a product of the physician's own sense of responsibility for his or her patients but also results from collegial reinforcement. Physicians almost uniformly admire colleagues who can dramatically improve the health of their patients, for example, through the use of an impressive surgical procedure or a new counseling technique. Such effectiveness is usually rewarded both subtly and outright in the form of respect among colleagues, an increase in patient referrals, honoraria at lectures, and nomination for physician awards.

Two strategies are important to consider if nothing else works. First, the physician can shift into a mode in which the simple stabilization of the patient's illness becomes the goal (Eraker *et al.*, 1984). Using this approach the physician can also set limits as to what facets of the patient's care he will manage. Other options that the patient should consider can be suggested, but a formal therapeutic plan need not be constructed. The physician can simply try to preserve the relationship in the hopes that some day a formal therapeutic plan can be devised that will improve the patient's health, meanwhile taking care of other illnesses that the patient may develop. The other option that many physicians employ in this situation is to obtain consultative help from other professionals. Physicians are not infallible, and there are times when factors that might improve the patient's health are overlooked. Consultation with other professionals, if the patient agrees, can be very useful in finding problems that might have been overlooked.

Finally, if all else fails, or if there is such a disagreement between the patient and the physician that the doctor–patient relationship has been harmed beyond repair, termination of care should be considered. Termination of care is not a process that should be considered lightly; however, there are instances in which such conflict develops between the patient and the physician that the patient may indeed receive better care from another physician. Although physicians do not often want to come from behind their cloak of professionalism and admit that their own personality quirks might affect the care they deliver to patients, such instances are clearly documented in the medical literature (see Chapter 8). Likewise, patients also do not want to admit that they too have unique personalities that may result in conflict within the doctor–patient relationship. Clearly, if such a phenomenon is occurring, a "parting of the ways" may be best for both parties.

If this decision to terminate care has been made, then a strict process should be followed in order to ensure that the patient obtains quality care from another physician. This process will also protect the physician against charges of abandonment. First, the physician should either invite the patient in for a visit in which the issue of termination is discussed and document that discussion in the chart or send a letter to the patient specifying why the physician feels that termination is best, offering to find a new physician for the patient, and providing a specified time period, usually a month, during which the physician will care for the patient should any emergencies arise. The letter should be sent by certified mail so that the physician will know if the letter has been received by the patient. A copy of the letter should be placed in the patient's chart. If the patient has no comments, then the termination process can proceed.

Often a patient feels that there are reasons why termination should not happen. The physician can then listen to the patient's reasons and determine if any are substantive enough to change his or her mind. Sometimes when patients realize that their physician is serious about termination, new information is revealed that may enable the formulation of a therapeutic plan and may mend the distressed patient–physician relationship. In contrast, sometimes the termination process only serves to increase the conflict between the patient and physician. In those circumstances, the process should proceed according to plan.

It is important to note that physicians should not use the threat of termination liberally in order to get patients to comply with the therapeutic plan. Such threats, if idle, often work for only a short period of time and may result in a significant decrease in the physician's case load. Termination should only be considered if the physician feels that a continued relationship with the patient will be detrimental either to the patient's health or to his or her own caretaking abilities.

CONCLUSIONS

Managing patients with chronic illness can be one of the most challenging tasks for physicians. This challenge not only stems from our lack of knowledge in the clinical management area but also arises because chronic illnesses vary as to onset, course, outcome, and degree of incapacitation such that managing a patient with a chronic illness literally becomes a unique experience with every patient.

Chronic illnesses are also quite challenging for patients and their families. Overcoming the fear of a diagnosis during the prediagnostic phase, adjusting to the demands of a chronic illness once a diagnosis has been made, and integrating the management plan into the patient's life style, actively managing the illness during the chronic phase, and finally adjusting to the terminal phase of the illness are all challenges that must be met by any patient with a chronic illness. Fortunately, physicians can be very instrumental in aiding patients in meeting the challenges of each phase of a chronic illness by an appropriate clinical management process.

The clinical management process of Taylor *et al.* can be divided into four phases: systems assessment, goal setting, management plan, and tactical implementation. During the systems assessment phase the physician measures not only disease-specific parameters but other areas of patient functioning to include personal functioning, psychological functioning, general health perceptions, and social and role functioning. Next, specific realistic goals are set by the physician and the patient through a process of negotiation. Once goals have been determined, therapeutic options that might meet those goals can be explored during the management plan phase. During tactical implementation, options are selected that will best meet the patient's goals while exacting a minimum of harm on the patient's life style. Appropriate follow-up is important to assess the effects of the plan on the patient's life. Should the plan not meet therapeutic goals, the plan should be redesigned.

During each phase of the clinical management process patients and family members who are important to the management plan should be involved. Physicians should spend time with the patient and his or her family in order to gain agreement on the nature of the problems facing the patient, negotiate mutually acceptable goals, provide enough information on therapeutic options to enable patients and their families to make wise decisions, and provide specific education necessary to implement the therapeutic plan. Failure to work with the patient to gain agreement on all aspects of the therapeutic plan may result in noncompliance.

Noncompliance has emerged as the most vexing problem for physicians who care for patients with chronic illnesses. Although it is not easily defined, measured, or predicted, it is clear that noncompliance is widespread and probably exacts a toll on patient health. If a physician suspects noncompliance, the physician should discuss with the patient difficulties the patient may be having in adjusting to the illness, review the clinical management process, and then assess specific factors associated with noncompliance, such as misunderstandings, motivational difficulties, medications, and money. Physicians should assume a nonjudgmental stance, realizing that blaming the patient for difficulties in complying with the therapeutic plan may result in short-term gains but over the long term will accomplish little and may harm the doctor–patient relationship. Contextual issues, such as the doctor–patient relationship itself, family relationships, and relationships between physicians and other members of the health care team should also be examined.

If open-ended discussion does not reveal any reasons for the patient's noncompliance, then contingency contracting can be attempted to improve compliance. If contingency contracting fails, then physicians can try to stabilize the patient's illness as well as they can or can consider terminating the doctor–patient relationship with that particular patient. Termination should not be considered lightly but clearly has a place in medical practice when the physician feels that a continued relationship with the patient will only be detrimental either for the patient or for his or her own caretaking abilities.

As stated earlier in this chapter, the clinical management of a patient with chronic illness is most closely tied with the notion of the "art" of medical practice. Although systematic scientific investigations of the clinical management process are beginning, the science of clinical management is still in its infancy. In the future, better-defined clinical management strategies will be available to aid physicians in improving the health of their chronically ill patients. Until that time, physicians can gain a great deal of professional and personal satisfaction from involving themselves in the lives of their chronically ill patients.

CASES FOR DISCUSSION

Case 1

Mrs. Maloney is a 52-year-old white female who presents to your clinic with complaints of polyuria, polydipsia, polyphagia, and fatigue of 2 months' duration. A random blood sugar obtained in your clinic was 220 mg/dl. Two fasting blood sugars obtained over the next week were 162 mg/dl and 185 mg/dl, respectively. Because of these blood sugar results you make the diagnosis of NIDDM and ask Mrs. Maloney to return for a visit.

1. Mrs. Maloney has returned to your clinic and is waiting for you. How would you break the news to Mrs. Maloney that she has diabetes, and then what would be your strategy during the next several minutes of conversation with Mrs. Maloney?
2. Mrs. Maloney seems somewhat shocked by the diagnosis and seems to withdraw a bit. Realizing her emotional needs, you reassure her and suggest that she begin a trial of oral hypoglycemics. You make this decision because you believe that the better able you are to restore your diabetic patient's blood sugar to normal, the fewer long-term complications will develop. Mrs. Maloney simply nods her head at your suggestions, saying she will try. However, 2 weeks later, at her follow-up visit, she has continued symptoms and is not taking any of her medicine. What would be your strategy at this point?
3. You discover that Mrs. Maloney does not want to take pills. How would you negotiate a solution to this dilemma?
4. After 3 months of diet therapy, Mrs. Maloney's fasting blood sugar is still over 140

mg/dl. Additionally, she has not lost much weight. What would be your strategy at this point in time?

5. How would your management strategies change if Mrs. Maloney also had hypertension and heart disease? How would it change if you learned that Mrs. Maloney's mother died of renal failure secondary to IDDM?

Case 2

Ed is a 6-year-old with sickle cell anemia. Before moving to your town and entering your practice, he had been hospitalized 20 times for pneumonia and sickle cell crises. He is shy but cooperative. Except for mildly icteric sclera and a palpable liver edge, he is fairly healthy looking. His mother barely speaks, seems to know little of his history, and watches you warily. She doesn't seem to know if he has ever been on folate and remembers giving Ed penicillin occasionally. She doesn't seem to know much about preventing or mitigating crisis with proper hydration.

1. What chronic illness phase is Ed in? Is he doing well?
2. How can you help Ed during this phase of his chronic illness? What do you think are the most important things to do?
3. The mother seems uncertain, withdrawn, and intimidated. How would you involve her in Ed's care?
4. You schedule a return visit for Ed and his mother in 6 weeks after explaining how you could be reached if problems arose. You prescribe penicillin and folate daily. Ed presents 2 weeks later to the emergency room (ER) in mild crisis. He is treated and referred back to you. The ER doctor says that Ed has not been taking his medicine. Now what?

Case 3

Susan is a 32-year-old married woman expecting her third child. She is due in 4 months. You have asked her several times to stop smoking, but she continues to smoke two packs a day. She reasons that her other two kids turned out OK, so why bother? Since the birth of her last child she has developed essential hypertension. When this pregnancy was diagnosed you asked her to stop her diuretic and started her on methyldopa, 250 mg po tid (three times a day). The past two visits her blood pressure has been 140/85 and 150/80 at a time in pregnancy when blood pressures should fall relative to her initial level. These values are slightly greater than her initial values.

1. What phase of the clinical management process are you in? What are you going to do in that phase to increase your chances of a successful outcome?
2. What goals and interventions are you thinking about for Susan? How will you discuss those goals and interventions with her? Do you think Susan will agree with you?
3. Susan's next visit was scheduled for 2 weeks to recheck her BP, but she wasn't able to come because of car problems and sitter problems. When you next see her, she is 7 months along, and her blood pressure remains as before; her uterine size is small for that predicted by dates and an early (accurate) ultrasound. What do you do now?

4. Toward the end of Susan's pregnancy her blood pressure gets harder to control. You feel that it is important to ask her to stop working as a sales clerk. You explain the need to be off her feet all day, but she insists that she must keep working until she delivers. You are worried about placental insufficiency and fetal impairment, and she is worried about keeping her job. Do you see any way to resolve this issue?

Case 4

Mr. Zelnik is a 52-year-old white male who presents to your office after learning that his cholesterol is 245 mg/dl, a result he obtained at a neighborhood health fair. Mr. Zelnik is very worried that he might be predisposed to heart disease given this high cholesterol and wants something done about it immediately. He has heard that a very good new drug has just been released onto the market that will lower cholesterol promptly. He would like you to place him on that drug even though he knows that it is very costly.

1. Do you have misgivings about Mr. Zelnik's desire to try a cholesterol-lowering agent at this time? If so, what concerns do you have?
2. You order a repeat fasting cholesterol on Mr. Zelnik, which returns 220 mg/dl. How would that change your management strategy? If the repeat fasting cholesterol returned 280 mg/dl, how would that change your strategy?
3. Because Mr. Zelnik is slightly obese, your favorite strategy for treating such patients with mildly elevated cholesterol is diet and exercise. You manage to convince Mr. Zelnik that he should attempt these two interventions first, and he begrudgingly goes along with you. Three months later, however, Mr. Zelnik returns still overweight, still requesting to be put on the cholesterol-lowering agent. What would be your strategy at this time?
4. Would your strategy change if Mr. Zelnik also had a family history of heart disease and was a smoker?

Case 5

Mary Jane and Charlie Jones are middle-aged adults, married, and living independently. They both have cerebral palsy and are confined to their wheelchairs. They seek your care because they are "fed up" with their prior doctor. On the first visit you learn they both smoke, that Mary Jane has problems with her menstrual periods and has gastritis as well as mild arthritis, and that Charlie has a seizure disorder, arthritis, and uncontrollable tremors of all extremities.

1. What type of chronic illness is cerebral palsy? How would this affect your initial strategy for the Joneses?
2. What will your initial management strategy be?
3. About 2 weeks later you are having lunch at a neighborhood deli when you see something bouncing toward you in the center of one of the four lanes. You realize it is Charlie rolling backwards in his chair, propelling himself with one foot. He does not wear a helmet. What concerns will you address at his next visit?
4. Having discussed Charlie's behavior with him, you don't expect further problems. One week later, you are called late one night because Charlie is seizing in the ER.

When you get there, you find out he has a scalp laceration and abrasions. Once he is stabilized, what will you do to improve things?

5. While you are sewing Charlie up, Mary Jane reveals that they are most scared of being institutionalized again. How will you handle this new information?

RECOMMENDED READINGS

Rogers, C. S., McCue, J. D., & Gal, P. (1987). *Managing chronic disease.* Oradell, NJ: Medical Economics Book Co.

This is an excellent text on the medical management of common chronic illnesses. Other issues important to the management of patients with chronic illness, such as compliance, are also covered, but not in as much depth.

Chilman, C. S., Nunnally, E. W., & Cox, F. M. (1988). *Chronic illness and disability.* Newbury Park, CA: Sage Publications.

The editors of this text have asked experts in the field to write chapters on the impact of chronic illness on patients and their families. Chapters are extensively referenced and are well written.

Fisher, R., & Ury, W. (1981). *Getting to yes: Negotiating agreement without giving in.* New York: Penguin Books.

Although not directly on negotiation between patients and their physicians, this slim book contains a great many "pearls" for physicians interested in learning the fine art of negotiation.

CHAPTER 7

Health Maintenance

Gregory H. Blake

Case 7-1. The last appointment of the afternoon for a busy physician is a "well-baby" examination on 4-month-old Jonathan. Jonathan's family has moved into the community following his birth to allow his father, Peter, to begin a new job at a local industry. Jonathan's mother, Sue, is a 24-year-old housewife. Both parents are present for the exam.

Sue relates that Jonathan, her only child, had an uneventful antenatal course and delivery. He received his last examination 2 months ago, and they were told he was normal. Sue reports that no problems have occurred since Jonathan's last examination.

After conducting a physical examination on Jonathan, who is normal for his age, the physician begins to give some anticipatory guidance to both Peter and Sue concerning Jonathan. However, from the parents' expressions the physician senses that questions remain.

The physician asks, "What questions do you have?"

Sue responds, "Doctor, I'm so glad Jonathan is all right, but are you sure everything is OK?"

"In what way do you feel something is wrong?" the physician asks.

Sue, in a low tone, responds, "My older brother, Josh, died 2 months ago from colon cancer. He had always been healthy, but then suddenly he was found to have cancer. He only lived a short time. I don't want anything to happen to Jonathan." Fighting away tears, Sue looks toward the floor.

The physician responds that Jonathan is well at this time and expresses sympathy for the stress Sue and Peter are feeling.

Sue asks, "What can we do to insure that Jonathan won't get colon cancer like my brother?"

Peter, after placing his hand on Sue's shoulder, asks, "Doctor, with Josh having colon cancer, what is the likelihood Sue could get cancer? What do we need to do to screen Sue for cancer? Are there changes we need to make in our life style to protect Sue from getting cancer?"

INTRODUCTION

The questions being asked by Peter and Sue pose dilemmas for both physicians and patients. Physicians are not able to predict with absolute certainty who will get a disease in spite of knowing the patient's relative risk for that disease. Furthermore, many factors that increase the patient's risk for disease, such as age, gender, and family history, cannot be modified. Given these unmodifiable risk factors and the difficulties in interpreting scientific and epidemiologic data that suggest relationships between modifiable risk factors and health, how should physicians proceed when confronted with patients who may be at high risk for a disease?

Physicians can use tests to screen for diseases in high-risk patients. However, even these seemingly valuable tools have potential difficulties. Prior to requesting a test, the physician must consider the sensitivity and specificity of the test in predicting the presence or absence of a disease. If a test with low sensitivity is negative, the result may be a false negative. If the test is positive but the specificity is low, then the result may be a false positive. Also, screening for a disease with a long latent phase or a disease that lacks an effective and acceptable treatment may only increase the patient's anxiety should the screening test be positive.

The physician must consider whether the test is really a marker for the disease in question, or whether it is associated with another process that occurs concurrently with the disease. An example of this phenomenon is the relationship between low cholesterol and colon cancer. Some studies examining this association support a causal relationship, but others suggest that low cholesterol values occur as a consequence of the disease itself (Rose & Shipley, 1980; Williams, Sorlie, Feinleib, McNamara, Kannel, & Dawber, 1981; Winawer, Flehinger, Buchalter, Herbert, & Shike, 1990). If the latter is true, then current efforts to lower cholesterol are appropriate. But if a low cholesterol value places one at risk for colon cancer, then by attempting to lower cholesterol levels we are trading one problem (arteriosclerosis) for another.

The physician is also at risk for experience bias. If a physician took care of a few patients with a low serum cholesterol at the time that colon cancer was detected, then he would likely regard cholesterol as a valid screening test for cancer. Anecdotal information and experiences create illusions for the physician that may cause physicians to support a particular practice or procedure even though it may not be scientifically justified. This is not to say that a physician's experience should be discounted, but it should be evaluated in light of known facts and the natural history of the disease in question.

In order to weigh appropriately clinical evidence and anecdotal experiences, physicians must utilize both clinical and epidemiologic criteria. In 1965, Hill outlined epidemiologic criteria to guide health care providers in determining whether a causal association exists between a risk factor and an illness. For a causal association to exist, the following criteria must be satisfied: (1) the strength of the association must be statistically significant and not a product of design or statistical error; (2) the frequency of the disease must increase with exposure to the factor; (3) exposure to the factor must precede the disease; (4)

findings must be consistent among studies; (5) the risk factor's role in the disease must be biologically plausible; (6) study findings should not conflict with the known natural history of the disease; and (7) there must be a specificity of association between the factor and the disease (Hill, 1965). Once these criteria are satisfied, screening protocols and preventive measures can be developed for those at risk.

This chapter provides information to assist physicians in wrestling with health maintenance questions. First, it is necessary for the physician to understand the categories of prevention and how to integrate health maintenance activities into a medical practice. The physician must appreciate the obstacles the patient has to hurdle to participate successfully in health maintenance activities and recognize the personal costs both he and his patient face when formulating a health maintenance contract. Most importantly, the physician must realize that before any recommendations can be accomplished by the patient, they must also become personal goals for that patient.

CATEGORIES OF PREVENTION

As depicted in Case 7-1, all individuals are concerned about the health of those they love. To understand fully what health means to the patient and in turn to be able to recommend a health maintenance program, the physician must learn the patient's personal health goals. Although an individual's definition of health may be nebulous, each individual may be considered as migrating along a wellness continuum (Fig. 7-1). Wellness is more than the absence of disease but takes into account physical, emotional, and social functioning as well as risk potential. From birth, individuals need a degree of "wellness" to accomplish the goals and tasks they set for themselves. At some point along this continuum, they will contract a disease. Initially, the disease may have a latent or asymptomatic period where only a few signs, usually subtle, will indicate its presence. Then symptoms of the illness will develop, prompting the patient to seek medical attention. At this time the patient's physician labors to help the patient cure or at least control the disease and prevent complications. At some point, the accumulation of disease factors and natural aging result in the death of the patient.

Primary prevention involves those activities that, if successful, will block

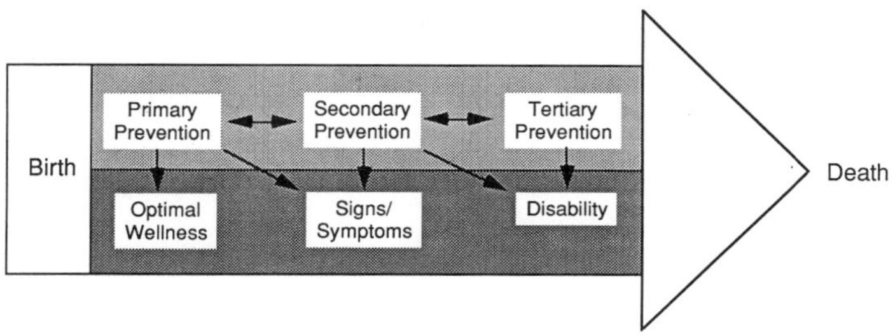

Figure 7-1. Wellness continuum.

the clinical manifestations of the disease process. Health education activities are primary prevention activities if they are applied to individuals without known disease. Immunizations are also examples of primary prevention; for example, oral polio vaccine, if given shortly after birth, prevents the development of polio during childhood.

Those procedures employed by a health care provider to detect a disease process in its latent or asymptomatic phase are considered secondary prevention activities. Examples of this include the use of mammography to screen for asymptomatic breast cancer, obtaining a Papanicolaou (Pap) smear to detect early cervical cancer, and hemoccult screening of stool to detect colon cancer. Secondary prevention is also called "screening."

Once a disease produces symptoms, tertiary preventive medical measures are employed. These activities are designed to prevent complications of the disease and promote restoration of functional status. Control of diabetes mellitus with insulin injections is an example of tertiary prevention. Providing dietary information to lower cholesterol and sodium intake in a myocardial infarction patient would also be a tertiary preventive activity.

Case 7-2. Paula is a 42-year-old executive secretary who presents to her physician for an annual examination. Paula reports no acute illnesses since her last blood pressure examination 6 months ago. Three years ago she was placed on a diuretic for mild hypertension. She relates no symptoms suggestive of side effects from that medication. She does admit it is hard for her to maintain the prescribed low-sodium diet and exercise program because of pressures at home and at work. She does not smoke cigarettes or drink alcoholic beverages.

Paula's physician based her physical examination on routine health maintenance recommendations for her age and her diagnosis of hypertension (Table 7-1).

Vital signs: Height 5′8″; weight 175 lb; blood pressure standing 155/92 mm Hg, lying 150/90 mm Hg; pulse 80 beats per minute

Neck: Carotids equal without bruits; no thyroid nodules or enlargement

Lungs: Normal to inspection, percussion, and auscultation

Breasts: No abnormalities noted during inspection and palpation; no axillary adenopathy

Heart: No normalities to inspection, palpation, percussion, or auscultation

Abdomen: No abnormalities noted during inspection, auscultation, and palpation

Pelvic: Normal external genitalia, vaginal, cervical, and bimanual exams; rectovaginal exam confirmed the bimanual exam, and the stool was negative for blood; a Pap smear was obtained

From the medical history and physical examination, the physician con-

Table 7-1
Adult Health Maintenance Flow Sheet, Ages 18 to 49 Years[a]

	Age																														
	18	19	20	21	22	23	24	25	26	27	28	29	30	31	32	33	34	35	36	37	38	39	40	41	42	43	44	45	46	47	48	49
Blood pressure	•		•		•		•		•		•		•		•		•		•		•		•		•		•		•		•	
Serum cholesterol	•				•				•				•				•				•				•				•			
History of tobacco use	•		•										•										•									
Weight	•				•				•				•				•				•				•				•			
dT booster							•										•										•					
Fecal occult blood													•	•									•		•		•		•		•	
Pap smear		•	•		•		•		•		•		•		•		•		•		•		•		•		•		•		•	
Breast examination	•		•		•		•		•		•		•		•		•		•		•		•		•		•		•		•	
Mammogram																							•		•		•		•		•	
Eval osteoporosis risk																													•			
Education																																
Use of seat belts	•				•				•				•				•				•				•				•			
Self exam of skin, oral cavity, testes	•				•				•				•				•				•				•				•			
Breast self-examination	•				•				•				•				•				•				•				•			
Teach to record postmenopausal bleeding																													•			

[a]Reprinted with permission from Frame (1986).

cluded that Paula's blood pressure was not under ideal control, and her weight was too high.

Based on these impressions, several recommendations were offered to Paula to improve her risk profile. Given her desire to lower her blood pressure toward normal without adding medication, a 2-g-per-day sodium diet and a weight control program were offered (Moore, 1985; Weinberger, Cohen, Miller, Luft, Grim, & Fineberg, 1988). Techniques to reduce stress including an exercise program were discussed. Paula contracted to begin a walking program and to reenter the weight control class offered by the hospital.

In addition to the Pap smear, Paula was advised to have several other screening tests performed. To help assess her risk of ischemic heart disease, a serum cholesterol was drawn. She was scheduled for a screening mammogram (breast cancer) and given three guaiac cards to test for occult blood in her stool (colon cancer).

Paula's physician discussed the value of Paula periodically examining her own skin and oral cavity for nodules and other changes suggestive of cancer. He provided her with information on breast self-examination. Methods of accident prevention, such as the use of seat belts, were discussed. After all of Paula's concerns were addressed she was given a follow-up appointment in 1 month for a blood pressure check and discussion of the screening results.

In this case, the physician utilized primary, secondary, and tertiary preventive medical practices. The physical examination revealed no signs of ischemic heart disease, so efforts at weight reduction and stress management were primary prevention. Discussion of other risk factors causing ischemic heart disease such as tobacco smoking and cholesterol control were also primary prevention, as was the recommendation to use seat belts. Secondary prevention was accomplished by obtaining the Pap smear, mammogram, serum cholesterol level, and stool samples to be tested for occult blood. Because Paula already had an elevated blood pressure, the counseling about the 2-g sodium diet was tertiary prevention. Since a reduction in stress and a loss in total body weight are capable of lowering blood pressure, these recommendations would also be considered tertiary prevention.

THE HISTORICAL PRECEDENCE FOR HEALTH MAINTENANCE

Today the majority of health care providers are involved in providing tertiary preventive medical care for patients with established diseases. However, the value of primary prevention has not gone unnoticed by past health care providers. Four thousand five hundred years ago, the Chinese Yellow Emperor wrote:

> Hence the sages did not treat those who were already ill: they instructed those who were not yet ill. To administer medicines to diseases which have already developed is comparative to the behavior of those who begin to dig a well after they have become thirsty, and of those who begin to cast weapons after they have already engaged in battle (Veith, 1949).

The foundation for the early teachings in preventive health also came from religious precepts and tenets from respected authorities. The *Bible* contains many public health instructions intended to protect the Jewish nation from disease. Sanitation, nutrition, methods for waste disposal, and the control of contagious disease are referenced in *Leviticus*. The validity of one of these passages has been confirmed by cholesterol researchers during this century. *Leviticus* 3:17 states, "It is a perpetual statute throughout your generations in all your dwellings: you shall not eat any fat or any blood" (The Lockman Foundation, 1960).

Up until the 20th century, interest in prevention centered around public health issues: water supply, sewage disposal, working conditions, and living arrangements. The major events directly affecting health were famines, epidemics, and episodic acute and chronic infectious diseases. The diseases at the top of mortality tables in 1900 were infectious diseases (Table 7-2). Poor social conditions, including crowding, unsanitary water supplies, and poor waste disposal kept these diseases at the top of the mortality tables until the public health innovations of improved sanitation, chlorinated water supplies, improved sewage disposal techniques, and improved living conditions reduce mortality from these infectious diseases. Later, greater availability of food supplies and knowledge of adequate nutrition continued to improve the overall living standard.

During the 20th century a shift in the leading causes of death started by improvement in sanitation and continued by the development and widespread use of antibiotics occurred. Chronic noninfectious diseases surpassed the infectious diseases as leading causes of death as people lived longer (Table 7-3). These diseases are caused by multiple risk factors often having complex interrelationships. Ischemic heart disease is associated with cigarette smoking, hypertension, and hypercholesterolemia (Kannel, Castelli, Gordon, & McNamara, 1971; Kannel, Dawber, Sorlie, Revotskie, & Wolf, 1976). If two or more of these major risk factors exist together, the incidence rate rises synergistically. With obesity, an elevated blood sugar, a sedentary life style, hypertriglyceridemia, a positive family history for heart disease, and type A personality each being independent minor risk factors, the issue of how to prevent ischemic heart disease becomes quite complex (Breslow & Buell, 1960; Cady, Gertler, Gottsch, & Woodbury, 1961; Carlson, 1960; Epstein, 1964, 1965; Kannel, Kagan, Dawber, & Revotskie, 1962; Mann & Inman, 1975; McDonough, Hames, Stulb, & Garrison, 1965; Rosenman, Jenkins, Brand, Friedman, Straus, Wurm, 1975; Taylor, Klepeter, Keys, Parlin,

Table 7-2
Leading Causes of Death, 1900, Mortality Rates/100,000 People per Year

Disease	Rate	Percentage of total death
1. Pneumonia and influenza	202.2	11.8
2. Tuberculosis (all forms)	194.4	11.3
3. Diarrhea, enteritis, intestinal ulceration	142.7	8.3

Table 7-3
Leading Causes of Death, 1983, Mortality Rates/100,000 People per Year

Disease	1983 Rate	Percentage of deaths	1900 rate	Percentage of deaths	1900 rank
1. Heart disease	276.2	38.2	137.4	8.0	4
2. Cancer (malignant)	169.0	21.9	64.0	3.7	8
3. Cerebrovascular disease	54.1	7.7	106.9	6.2	5
Total		67.8		17.9	

Blackburn, & Puchner, 1962; Manson, Colditz, Stampfer, Willett, Rosen, Monson, Speizer, & Hennekens, 1990).

Cancer is the second leading cause of death in this country. Just as shifts in the overall leading cause of death occurred, a change in the leading causes of cancer mortality also occurred (Table 7-4). Each of these cancers is associated with several risk factors. Lung cancer is associated with cigarette smoking, atmospheric pollution, asbestos exposure, and occupational exposure to various metals and chloromethyl ethers (Selikoff & Hammond, 1978; Wynder, 1980; VanHoutte, Salazer, Phillips, & Asbury, 1983). A high-fat diet, radiation exposure, and a positive family history are risk factors for the development of breast cancer (Cole, 1980; Keys, Bakemeir, & Salov, 1983; Grobstein, Cairns, Berliner, Broitman, Gampbell, Gussow, Kolonel, Kritchevsky, Mertz, Miller, Prival, Slaga, Wattenberg, & Sugimura, 1982; Land, 1980, Wynder, 1972). Colorectal cancer is related to a low-fiber diet, a positive family history of colorectal cancer, and predisposing medical problems such as ulcerative colitis, adenomatous polyps, and villous adenomas (Grobstein *et al.*, 1982; Morton, Poulter, & Pandya, 1983). The etiology of prostrate cancer is unknown (Frank, Keys, & McCune, 1983). Each of these carcinomas has other, less-well-documented risk factors.

Hypertension, diabetes mellitus, alcohol consumption, smoking, and preexisting heart disease are known risk factors for cerebrovascular diseases (Heyman, Karp, Heyden, Bartel, Cassel, Tyroler, Cornon, Hames, & Stuart, 1971; Kannel *et al.*, 1976; Kessler, 1971; Gill, Zezulka, Shipley, Gill, & Beevers, 1986; Welin, Svardsudd, Wilhelmsen, Larsson, & Tibblin, 1987). Additionally, an elevation in serum lipids and obesity are minor risk factors for strokes.

Because these diseases are chronic and noninfectious in origin, control is

Table 7-4
Leading Causes of Cancer Mortality by Sex, 1930 and 1986

	Male		Female	
Rank	1930	1986	1930	1986
1	Stomach	Lung	Uterus	Lung
2	Colorectal	Colorectal	Stomach	Breast
3	Prostate	Prostate	Breast	Colorectal

Table 7-5
Risk Factors for Current Mortality Leaders

Disease predisposition	Activity	Nutrition	Substance ingestion	Genetic	Other
Heart	Sedentary life style	Hypercholesterdemia, obesity, hyperglycemia	Cigarette smoking	Positive family history	Type A personality, hypertension, diabetes mellitus
Cancer					
Lung			Cigarette smoking		Asbestos exposure, metal exposure, chloromethyl ethers, pollution
Breast		High-fat diet		Positive family history	Radiation
Colorectal		High-fat diet, low-fiber diet		Positive family history	Inflammatory bowel disease, polyps
Cerebrovascular		Serum lipids, obesity, hyperglycemia	Cigarette smoking	Positive family history	Heart disease, diabetes mellitus, hypertension

not possible with traditional public health strategies. Risk factors for these mortality leaders are overwhelmingly byproducts of our personal life styles and our genetic makeup (Table 7-5). For these reasons, the emphasis in preventive practice shifted in the 1920s to more individual interventions. Gould, an oculist, brought the concept of the periodic health examination to the United States from Europe. Dr. E. L. Fisk, a physician affiliated with the Metropolitan Life Insurance Company, created the Life Extension Institute, where he carried out yearly physical exams (Charap, 1981). The periodic health exam, designed to identify illness in its early stages, soon became a part of mainstream medical practice. The early popularity of these examinations was based on the discovery of physical defects in a majority of assumed healthy individuals who were examined.

However, since most of these discovered defects were within the normal spectrum of health in the population or of minor consequence, the periodic health examination failed to reduce the incidence of the major causes of death. After decades of unquestioned, uncritical acceptance by the medical profession and public of the general periodic health examination for the asymptomatic, apparently healthy person, the American College of Physicians' Medical Practice Committee concluded that prevention and early detection of disease could be better accomplished through a selective approach based on the age and sex of the patient (Medical Practice Committee, American College of Physicians, 1981). Their conclusions were based on the studies of Frame and Carlson, Breslow and Somers, The Canadian Task Force on Periodic Health Examination, and those of the American Cancer Society.

Frame and Carlson in 1975 reviewed 36 diseases selected on the basis of "incidence and prevalence, progression with and without treatment, risk factors associated with development of disease, and availability of screening tests" (Frame & Carlson, 1975). They evaluated screening tests for those diseases based on a set of criteria (Table 7-6). Following their analysis, they concluded that examination procedures should be selected in relation to the age and sex of the patient. Breslow and Somers in 1977, using their "Lifetime Health-Monitoring Program," described health goals and professional services suitable for ten different age groups based on eight clinical and epidemiologic criteria (Breslow & Somers, 1977). In 1979, the Canadian Task Force reported on 78 major preventable conditions affecting Canadians (Spitzer, 1979). The Task Force recommended health protection packages based on the life stages of the patient. The

Table 7-6
Screening Criteria Used by Frame and Carlson (1975)

1. The condition must have a significant effect on the quality and quantity of life.
2. Acceptable methods of treatment must be available.
3. The condition must have an asymptomatic period during which detection and treatment significantly reduce morbidity or mortality.
4. Treatment in the asymptomatic phase must yield a therapeutic result superior to that obtained by delaying treatment until symptoms appear.
5. Tests that are acceptable to patients must be available at reasonable cost to detect the condition in the asymptomatic period.
6. The incidence of the condition must be sufficient to justify the cost of screening.

Table 7-7
Adult Health Maintenance Flow Sheet, Ages 50 to 81 Years[a]

	Age																														
	50	51	52	53	54	55	56	57	58	59	60	61	62	63	64	65	66	67	68	69	70	71	72	73	74	75	76	77	78	79	80	81
Blood pressure	•		•		•		•		•		•		•		•		•		•		•		•		•		•		•		•	
Serum cholesterol	•				•				•				•				•				•											
Weight	•				•				•				•				•				•				•				•			
dT booster					•										•										•							
Fecal occult blood	•	•	•	•	•	•	•	•	•	•	•	•	•	•	•	•	•	•	•	•	•	•	•	•	•	•	•	•	•	•	•	•
Pap smear	•		•		•		•		•		•		•		•		•		•		•											
Breast examination	•	•	•	•	•	•	•	•	•	•	•	•	•	•	•	•	•	•	•	•	•	•	•	•	•	•	•	•	•	•	•	•
Mammogram	•	•	•	•	•	•	•	•	•	•	•	•	•	•	•	•	•	•	•	•	•	•	•	•	•	•	•	•	•	•	•	
Eval osteoporosis risk	•				•																											
Education																																
Use of seat belts	•				•				•				•				•				•				•				•			
Self exam of skin, oral cavity, testes	•				•				•				•				•				•				•				•			
Breast self-examination	•				•				•				•				•				•				•				•			
Teach to record postmenopausal bleeding	•				•				•				•				•				•				•				•			

[a]Reprinted with permission from Frame (1986).

Table 7-8
Schedule of Recommended Visits for Children[a]

	Birth–6 months				Infancy					Preschool		School age		Adolescence	
	<1 mo	2 mo	4 mo	6 mo	9 mo	12 mo	15 mo	18 mo	24 mo	2–4 yr	5–6 yr	7–9 yr	10–12 yr	13–15 yr	16–18 yr
History															
Initial interval	•	•	•	•	•	•	•	•	•	•	•	•	•	•	•
Measurements															
Ht./wt.	•	•	•	•	•	•	•	•	•	•	•	•	•	•	•
Head circumference	•	•	•	•	•	•	•	•	•						
Blood pressure										•	•	•	•	•	•
Sensory screening															
Vision	S	S	S	S	S	S	S	S	S	S/O	O	O	O	O	S
Hearing	S	S	S	S	S	S	S	S	S	S/O	O	O	O	O	S
Developmental behavioral assessment	•	•	•	•	•	•	•	•	•	•	•	•	•	•	•
Physical exam	•	•	•	•	•	•	•	•	•	•	•	•	•	•	•
Lab tests/diagnostic procedures															
Hereditary/metabolic screen	•												•	•	
Immunization		•	•	•			•	•			•			•	
Tuberculin test					•	•	•	•	•	•	•	•	•	•	•
Hct/Hgb					•	•				•			•		
Urinalysis									•	•	•				
Anticipatory guidance	•	•	•	•	•	•	•	•	•	•	•	•	•	•	•
Initial dental referral										•					

[a]Reprinted with permission from American Board of Family Practice (1989). •, to be performed; S, subjective by history; O, objective by a standard testing method; (shaded •), performed within this time interval.

frequency of test administration varied according to age and sex. Finally, in 1980, the American Cancer Society recommended nine tests and procedures that were effective in reducing the morbidity and mortality of cancers based on evaluation of the potential costs, risks, and benefits of these tests. These procedures were also grouped by patient age and sex (American Cancer Society, 1980).

From these original studies, many newer recommendations have been made. These recommendations cover both the pediatric and adult populations. Some standards include anticipatory guidance as well as screening recommendations based on patient age and sex (Tables 7-1, 7-7, and 7-8). Each set of recommendations may vary depending on the weight their evaluating committee placed on the information evaluated and the criteria used, although most used criteria similar to Frame and Carlsons'. As can be seen from Table 7-6, these criteria incorporate both clinical and epidemiologic principles. They also recognize the role economics plays in any mass screening program. These criteria, however, leave many ethical and legal questions unanswered.

OBSTACLES TO HEALTH MAINTENANCE ACTIVITIES

Prior to discussing how to incorporate health maintenance procedures into medical practice, we must consider obstacles to successful incorporation. The initial obstacle is the physician. He must be aware of the importance of health maintenance and understand how to successfully assist his patient in preventing diseases. A second obstacle is the patient. The physician must recognize that each person brings a unique personality into the doctor–patient relationship, and each person ultimately determines whether medical recommendations will be followed. The third obstacle is the societal environment that fosters risk factors that health maintenance programs are attempting to control.

The Physician

The physician, convinced that preventive and screening methods are beneficial, runs the risk of being viewed as a "nag" by his patients. If screening procedures lack strong support as a screen or risk reducer, then the physician must consider potential ethical conflicts. Is his loyalty to the procedure a result of its effectiveness or a mechanism to bring extra income into his practice? Furthermore, even for procedures having strong clinical and epidemiologic research supporting their value as screening tools, performing such screening procedures takes time away from treating patients with more acute and chronic illnesses.

Poor reimbursement can be a barrier for physicians performing preventive medicine activities even though research evidence supporting the role for prudent nutrition, exercise, and the elimination of tobacco and alcohol abuses in promoting improvements in health is accumulating. Aerobic exercise increases HDL-cholesterol and decreases blood pressure, total serum cholesterol, LDL-cholesterol, VLDL-cholesterol, triglycerides, glucose, and uric acid (Cooper,

1982). Increase in HDL-cholesterol with the resultant decrease in total cholesterol reduces the risk for ischemic heart disease (Gordon, Castelli, Hjortland, Kannel, & Dawber, 1977). A study of 16,936 Harvard men revealed that the death rate steadily declined as weekly exercise energy expenditure increased from 500 to 3,500 kilocalories per week. The increase in life expectancy attributable to exercise by age 80 was more than 2 years (Paffenbarger, Hyde, Wing, & Hsien, 1986). A study of 10,224 men and 3,120 women indicated that higher levels of physical fitness appear to delay all causes mortality, primarily through lowered rates of cardiovascular disease and cancer (Blair, Kohl, Paffenbarger, Clark, Cooper, & Gibbons, 1989). As a result of lengthy investigations, the American Heart Association endorses a dietary cholesterol intake of only 300 mg per day (Grundy, Brown, Dietschy, Ginsberg, Goodnight, Howard, LaRosa, & McGill, 1989). Furthermore, The National Research Council recommends a reduction of dietary fat from 40% to 30% of total calories; inclusion of whole grains and vegetables high in carotenoids; limitation of cured, pickled, or smoked meats; and limitation of alcohol to reduce cancer risk (Grobstein *et al.*, 1982). In spite of these findings and recommendations, government programs and private insurance carriers poorly reimburse physicians when they take the time to educate patients about the above evidence and support patients in their attempt to reduce their risk.

A physician's involvement with health promotion may also be demoralizing. A failure to recognize the obstacles faced by the patient and the patient's personal responsibility for his own health may result in the physician accepting too much responsibility for his patient's health. The physician may become frustrated with the perceived ineffectiveness of health maintenance interventions he recommends if his expectations are not met. Repeated failures may result in the physician decreasing his involvement in health promotional activities. Furthermore, the physician may blame the patient for his or her inability to comply, resulting in a further breakdown of the doctor–patient relationship.

The Patient

Patient obstacles also contribute to the failure of health maintenance endeavors. Barriers to patient compliance can be either medical or nonmedical. Nonmedical barriers include smoking, inactive use of leisure time, obesity, blue collar employment, and lack of spouse support. When patients are asked why they quit an exercise program, an inconvenient or inaccessible program location, lack of time, work conflicts, and poor spouse support are most commonly listed (Dishman, 1987; Oldridge, 1982). However, studies have revealed that sedentary people have as much weekly leisure time as exercisers, and those listing distance from a facility as a reason for dropping out actually lived closer to the facility than exercisers did (Gettman, Pollock, & Ward, 1983; The Perrier Study, 1979). Even among post-myocardial-infarction patients who were prescribed an exercise program, only 29% remained active 2 years later, with another 17% reporting they were training on their own (Sanne, 1973). If patients with an identified health problem for which an exercise program is prescribed are unable to comply, how can nonmedical barriers to prevention be overcome by those patients who do not have overt health problems?

Many programs have been designed to help smokers stop using tobacco. The recidivism rate at 1 year is approximately 80% (Hunt, Barnett, & Branch, 1971). This is not to say that smoking cessation programs lack value; on the contrary, they have helped thousands quit smoking while improving their individual health status, thereby reducing risk and health costs. Unfortunately, people begin and continue smoking for personal and social reasons other than their health; therefore, successful smoking cessation programs must be individualized.

Dietary weight reduction programs utilizing various modalities have been developed. Stunkard and McLaren-Hume reviewed eight outpatient programs in 1959 and found that only 25% of grossly overweight people lost 20 lb and only 5% lost 40 lb over the life of the program (Stunkard & McLaren-Hume, 1959). In 1979, Wing and Jeffery reviewed outpatient weight reduction programs utilizing anorectic or hormonal drugs, exercise, diet, and behavior therapy as their primary technique. They observed that the average weight loss was 12 lb; 20% of clients were able to lose 20 lb, and an average program attrition rate was 16%. Behavior therapy produced the best maintenance of weight losses (Wing & Jeffery, 1979). Thus, outpatient weight reduction programs that optimize patient compliance utilizing behavioral techniques have the best chance of long-term success.

Other patient barriers to physician-sponsored preventive activities exist. Once patients become aware of their health risks, they may not seek information and counseling solely from reliable sources. The lack of consensus among health care experts in many areas of health maintenance and prevention allow preventive health ideas and regimens to flourish without adequate scientific investigation supporting their claims of benefit. Many of the fad diets and wellness programs available today are examples of these activities. On the other hand, many patients view physicians' recommendations as sacrosanct. For that reason, physicians themselves may encourage patient involvement in questionable health maintenance activities through their overzealous enthusiasm for preventive medicine. Patients may become demoralized if the suggested preventive medicine regimens fail to live up to their expectations.

Societal Environment

Environmental influences are physical features capable of producing accidents or other injuries to human bodies. Societal influences are social trends and values that may modify life styles. These factors are often not under the direct control of the individual. If health maintenance activities are ultimately to succeed, then the detrimental elements of the societal environment must be controlled.

Some insults to health occur quickly in the form of accidents, whereas others such as heart disease result from chronic excesses or deficiencies. Accidents from electrocution, falls, drowning, wounds secondary to weapons, and motor vehicle accidents affect people of all ages. However, among children, adolescents, and young adults, accidents are the number-one cause of mortality and morbidity. Some of these accidents are not preventable, but others, such as a motor vehicle accident while under the influence of alcohol, result from personal habits. For these reasons, physicians must emphasize to children and young adults the value of swimming lessons, houseproofing to prevent falls and ingestions, and the appropriate care and use of firearms.

The mortality leaders in America have not always been byproducts of an individuals' life styles. Our human ancestors did not need an organized wellness program to maintain their mental and physical well-being. Destructive personal habits such as smoking were not widespread. Personal activity levels were high, as modern labor-saving devices were nonexistent. Commonly eaten foods were high-fiber vegetables and breads. The largest meals tended to be breakfast or lunch rather than the evening meal.

Today the typical American is surrounded by modern conveniences from automobiles to electric toothbrushes. Many American eat a large percentage of their meals at restaurants. These meals tend to be high in fat, cholesterol, and sodium and low in fiber content. The demands of our modern society often necessitate the evening meal being the family's social hour. Thus, the evening meal frequently contains the largest number of calories consumed that day. The "rapid-paced," aggressive life style of America's affluent society has fostered a new awareness of stress and "burnout" in many occupations.

The incidence of substance abuse involving both socially acceptable tobacco and alcohol consumption and other illegal agents is high. One reason for the high consumption of tobacco is the current high level of advertising, often aimed at adolescents or special groups such as athletes, women, and blacks. With tobacco companies sponsoring athletic events, art festivals, and other cultural activities, it is little wonder that substance abuse is difficult to control. Until society can effectively limit substance abuse, chronic illness resulting from substance abuse will continue to plague America.

HEALTH MAINTENANCE ACTIVITIES

Efforts in primary prevention involve both public health measures and individual doctor–patient encounters. Public health strategies have a place in increasing the public's awareness of unhealthy habits and affecting societal changes. The efforts made by The National Cattleman's Association and The National Live Stock and Meat Board to decrease the quantity of saturated fat in meat sold at market and retailed to customers attest to the efforts made by physicians acting socially (Berglung, 1989; Breidenstein & Williams, 1987). Further, the availability of blood pressure monitors in pharmacies allows the public the opportunity to gauge their own health status. Health fairs provide useful information by offering clinical or laboratory evaluations, such as cholesterol levels, that allow individuals the opportunity to identify their own risk factors. However, some danger exists in simply diagnosing medical problems without offering good follow-up to ensure proper treatment of newly discovered risk factors.

Many physicians choose to be actively involved in organizations that promote primary prevention. Some serve as consultants to the American Heart Association or to other nonprofit medical organizations. Physicians often speak to public school assemblies, local governmental body meetings, and other civic organizations in favor of health promotional activities. One such organization,

Doctors Ought to Care, focuses on problems of alcohol abuse, tobacco abuse, drug abuse, need for immunizations, and nutrition. They are involved in "counteradvertising" directed against advertising techniques used to attract the public to harmful substances such as tobacco and alcohol.

There are many ways to incorporate health maintenance into the practice of medicine. Many physicians weave health maintenance activities into their patients' visits for acute and chronic illnesses. Flow sheets listing screening procedures and anticipatory guidance can be valuable tools to aid the physician in integrating such activities into practice. Physicians who receive monthly feedback reports of their compliance with preventive care protocols have been shown to increase their compliance rate from 10–15% at base line to 50%. Further, if physicians receive specific reminders at the time of each patient's visit of appropriate health maintenance items, the improvement was even greater (Tierney, Siu, & McDonald, 1986). Often busy practitioners will refer health maintenance activities to nurses or physician assistants, thereby freeing themselves for more acute medical care.

Physicians need to incorporate health maintenance and preventive medicine activities into their practices in a manner that will strengthen the doctor–patient relationship. Once an individual is identified to be at risk for a disease or becomes interested in his own health risk profile, the physician has the opportunity to raise the issue. Once the presence of a risk factor is documented, the physician must present the therapeutic options to the patient, recognizing the uniqueness of the patient's personality and situation. The key to a successful program is to individualize the recommendations presented to the patient. To do this, the physician must understand the patient's personal goals, and other significant factors utilized by the patient in making decisions. These factors may include personal strengths and weaknesses, prior health history, and significant events and relationships in the patient's life.

It is important for the physician to negotiate the health maintenance program with the patient. This will help ensure the patient's acceptance of recommendations and allow the patient's personal strengths to be utilized. These negotiations may result in the patient being referred to another health care provider, or the primary physician may choose to manage the program through either individual or family intervention. Each method offers advantages depending on the individual's personality and situation. If the patient is a member of a family, several medical problems or a single problem common to another family member may be addressed by the same intervention. The following cases illustrate methods of incorporating health maintenance into medical practice.

Case 7-3: An Individual Health Maintenance Program. John is a 35-year-old dentist who has been a patient with a physician for 1 year. During a routine examination John tells the physician that he has smoked cigarettes since dental school. He only smokes at home because he feels smoking around his patients would not be appropriate. He has tried to quit before, but the stress of his job always got the best of him, and he restarted. John is married with two children. His wife does not smoke.

John has identified a health risk. It is important for the physician to agree with John that smoking is a health hazard and to make a clear and unequivocal statement of the reasons why. John should be asked if he would consider attempting to quit smoking again. At this point, understanding John's goals, strengths, and weaknesses would help the physician design a smoking cessation program. The physician can use this information to strengthen John's resolve. The physician can also express to John the positive prognostic factors for success (having a prior failure in smoking cessation) and describe what he should avoid (quitting during a very stressful time) in his effort to successfully quit smoking (Ockene, Benfar, Nuttall, Hurwitz, & Ockene, 1982).

If John agrees to try to quit smoking, the physician should discuss appropriate techniques and ask him to set a quit date. If John is willing to quit smoking but uncertain about setting a quit date, then the physician should ask him if he would make another appointment with his wife. At this visit, the physician can explore the options and encourage John to set a quit date. Once John sets a quit date, the physician should give John a smoking cessation booklet. Additionally, a prescription for a nicotine-containing chewing gum may be helpful in overcoming the symptoms associated with nicotine withdrawal.

The physician should see John prior to the quit date. At this time, he will relate maintenance strategies, discuss relapse contingencies, and obtain a contract for individual and partner involvement. It is important that a regular schedule of follow-up visits be established for the purpose of solving any problems John is having. If John is unsuccessful after several attempts, then he should be referred to a formal smoking cessation program.

As can be seen from the above case, the better the doctor–patient relationship, the more likely John will be able to quit smoking. If the physician understands John's goals well, he can provide him with suggestions on how best to withdraw from his tobacco addiction and still satisfy his personal needs. If he doesn't know John's goals and strengths, the suggested smoking cessation program may appear impersonal and standardized. The more contact the physician and John have, the better are John's chances of success. Thus, it is important for the physician to keep in close touch with John. This technique is summarized in Fig. 7-2 (Becker, Steinbauer, & Doherty, 1985).

Case 7-1 (continued): A Family Health Maintenance Program. The case presented at the beginning of the chapter provides an excellent example of how a family intervention might be beneficial. Peter and Sue have a common health concern, Jonathan's risk for colon cancer. A strategy that will meet the needs of both parents may succeed in meeting family needs. To accomplish this the physician needs more information concerning the health of both parents before the program can be outlined. Also, family goals, stressors, and history need to be explored. When this information is obtained, the physician can design a wellness program that can address the concerns of Peter and Sue.

For example, assume Peter smokes and Sue is 15 lb above her ideal body weight. Both Peter and Sue desire to be in better physical condition so they can better enjoy Jonathan's childhood. Combining this information with the knowledge that dietary fat is a risk factor for colon cancer, a wellness prescription can be written. The program would include a balanced diet for the family, in which the percentage of saturated fat in the family diet is lowered. Peter and Sue would be encouraged to engage in a physical activity that is enjoyable to both, such as walking, swimming, or cycling. The increased aerobic exercise may lead Peter to ask how he can quit smoking because smoking will limit his physical activity and be a detriment to Jonathan's health (U.S. Department of Health and Human Services, 1984). By integrating preventive medicine recommendations, family cohesion can be increased, and patient compliance can be improved. Secondary prevention activities such as stool guaiac screening for occult fecal blood and a schedule of flexible sigmoidoscopies for Sue would also be a part of the program (Fig. 7-3).

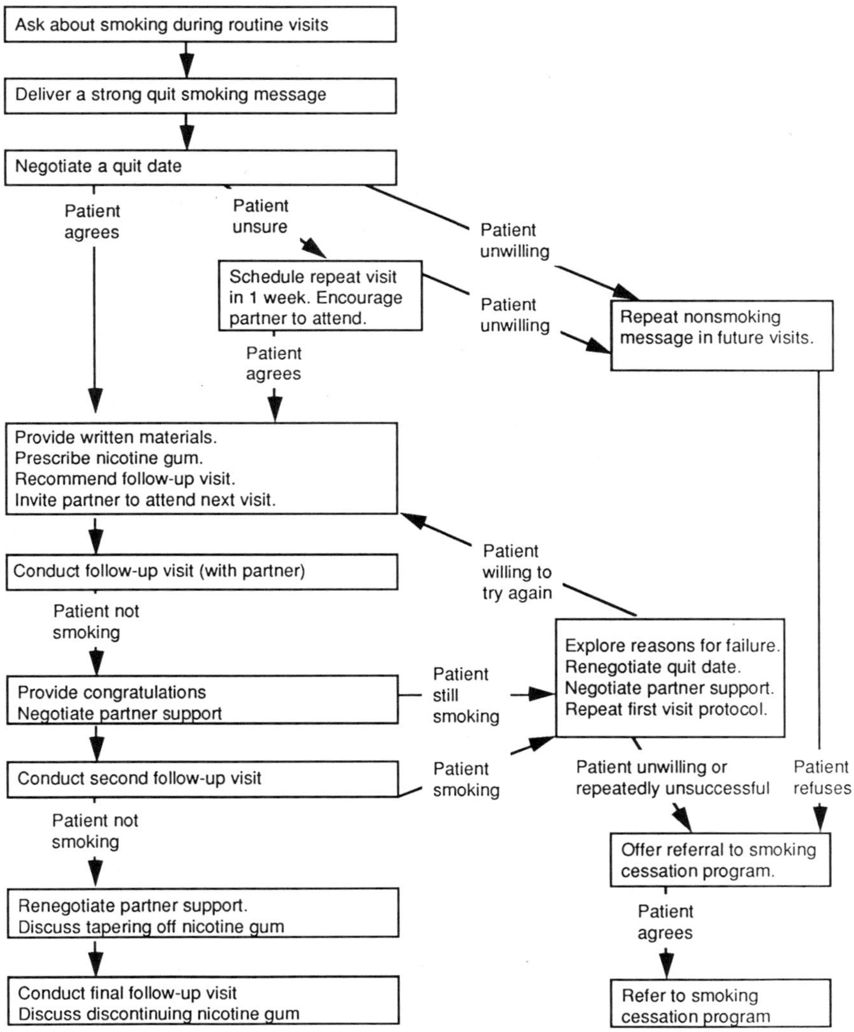

Figure 7-2. A smoking cessation protocol. Reprinted with permission from Becker *et al.* (1985).

Case 7-4. The A. B. Smith family made an appointment to see a new physician. The family consisted of Adam Smith, 40 years old; his wife Carol, 34 years old; their three children, John, 12 years old, Sarah, 6 years old, and Scott, 16 months old; and Carol's mother Connie, 65 years old. They desired to establish a relationship with a physician and have complete medical evaluations performed. Their health profiles are described below.

Adam is an executive for a local industry. He reports no acute medical problems. He drinks five glasses of wine or vodka and water each week with an additional six-pack of beer on the weekend. For the last 15 years Adam reports smoking $1\frac{1}{2}$ packs of cigarettes per day. His past medical history is significant for irritable bowel syndrome. His father died of a myocardial infarction at age 45. Adam's physical examination is remarkable for a height of 6′2″ and a weight of 245 lb.

Carol is a mother and housewife who teaches aerobic dancing at a local health club. She is a nonsmoker and only drinks socially. She describes no acute problems and reports a negative past medical history. Her father died of colon cancer 4 years ago. Her physical examination is unremarkable.

John will begin the seventh garde in September. He looks forward to playing athletics and making new friends. John reports no acute medical problems, and his past medical history is significant for an appendectomy at

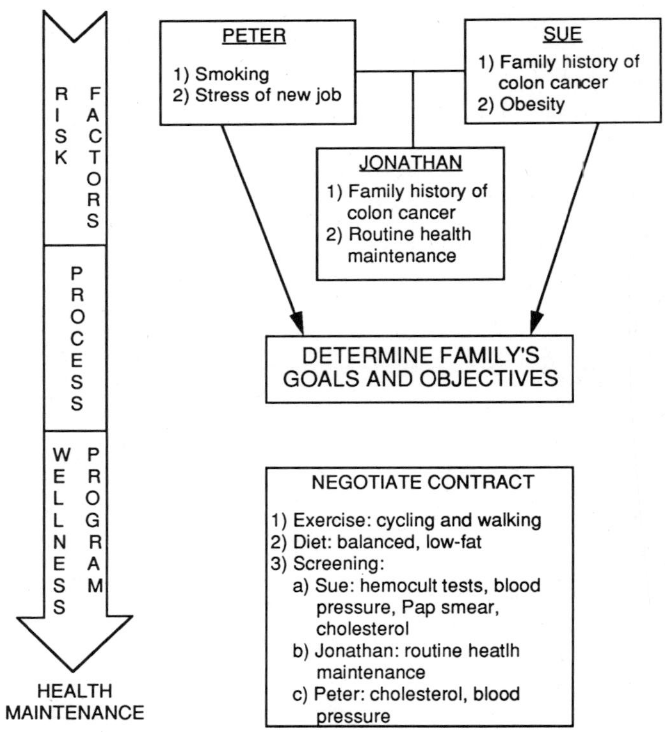

Figure 7-3. The development of a family health maintenance program for Peter, Sue, and Jonathan.

Table 7-9
Health Maintenance Program for Smith Family

Names	Medical problems	Risk factors	Recommended health maintenance	Recommended health program
Adam	Irritable bowel	Alcohol use Tobacco use Obesity Stress at work Family history of heart disease	Blood pressure checks q 2 years Serum cholesterol Fecal occult blood Instruction in seat belt use Instruction in testicular and skin self-exam	Balanced diet Exercise program Smoking cessation program Alcohol abuse program Stress reduction program
Carol		Passive smoking Family history of colon cancer	Blood pressure checks q 2 years Serum cholesterol Fecal occult blood Tetanus booster Pap smear Breast examination Instruction in seat belt use Instruction in breast and skin self-exam	Balanced diet Exercise program
John		Passive smoking Family history of colon cancer		Balanced diet Exercise program
Sarah		Passive smoking Family history of colon cancer Asymptomatic bacteriuria		Balanced diet Exercise program
Scott	Recurrent otitis media	Passive smoking Family history of colon cancer		Balanced diet Exercise program
Connie	Diabetes mellitus Hypertension	Passive smoking Obesity	Blood pressure checks q 2 years Serum cholesterol Fecal occult blood Instruction in seat belt use Instruction in breast and skin self-exam Mammogram	Balanced diet Exercise program

age 7. He denies alcohol, tobacco, or drug usage. His physical examination is normal.

Sarah began school last year. She is currently healthy without complaints. One year ago she was found to have a urinary tract infection. Her growth parameters and physical examination were appropriate for age.

Scotty is an active child who has had two cases of otitis media within the last 8 months. His growth parameters and physical examination are appropriate for age.

Connie moved in with the Smiths after the death of her husband 4 years ago. She reports having diabetes mellitus for the last 5 years. This condition is currently controlled by diet. For the last 3 years, her blood pressure has been reported as slightly elevated. Her family history is unremarkable. Physical examination was significant for a blood pressure of 155/90, height of 5′6″, and weight of 155 lb. No other abnormalities were noted.

In this case, the physician is faced with managing six individuals who possess different but somewhat related risk profiles and problems (Table 7-9). Many problems are unique to a single individual. The anticipatory guidance for Scott, Sarah, and John are good examples of this uniqueness (Table 7-10). Although the topic to be discussed is the same, the specific content will be different depending on the child's age, gender, and developmental stage. For example, the discussion of physical and sexual growth with John, an adolescent, will be different from the issues pertinent to Sarah. Also since John is an adolescent, some topics may best be covered by John and the physician without the rest of the family being present.

However, the Smith family collectively shares several risks and problems. These areas may best be handled through an integrated wellness prescription. Adam could improve his health by losing weight, beginning to exercise, and

Table 7-10
Anticipatory Guidance for Smith Children

John	Sarah	Scott
Screens		
Height	Height	Height
Weight	Weight	Weight
Blood pressure	Blood pressure	Head circumference
Vision screen	Vision screen	Vision screen
Hearing screen	Hearing screen	Hearing screen
Tetanus immunization	Urinalysis	Hematocrit
Anticipatory guidance		
Nutrition	Nutrition	Nutrition
School	School	Accidents and safety
Accidents and safety	Accidents and safety	Toilet training
Substance abuse	Substance abuse	Family adjustments
Sexual development	Sexual development	Development
Peer relationships	Social development	Dental cleansing
Exercise/sports	Peer relationships	Immunizations
Venereal disease	Television use	

quitting tobacco usage. Carol can lower her colon cancer risk by modifying the amount of saturated fat in her diet. Connie needs a balanced diet appropriate for her diabetes mellitus and high blood pressure management. Since the children also need balanced diets for their growth and development, all the family could be encouraged to adopt a balanced diet, which would be mutually beneficial.

Exercise is beneficial for controlling weight and helpful in managing both diabetes mellitus and hypertension (Lowenthal & Broderman, 1983; Felig, 1983). Thus, a combined regimen could assist both Adam and Connie. Carol and the children already are involved in exercise-related activities. If a common leisure-time aerobic activity could be found for the whole family, then the family might grow together interpersonally as well as in overall health.

In order to accomplish this program, the physician must allow all family members to participate with him in designing the prescription. Before the program will succeed, each family member must be willing to work together for the good of the whole family. This can be accomplished by allowing the Smiths to maximize their individual strengths while minimizing their collective weaknesses. The physician provides expertise, guidance, and encouragement in this process and supports their efforts through follow-up medical visits and secondary preventive evaluations.

CONCLUSIONS

The cornerstones of health maintenance activities are primary, secondary, and tertiary prevention. The goal of primary prevention is to modify an individual's life style such that the risk of developing a certain disease is lowered. Secondary prevention encompasses procedures to detect the presence of certain diseases before they are clinically apparent so appropriate therapy can be provided. A physician's effort at limiting the complications of a disease once symptoms develop is tertiary prevention.

Mechanisms for improving health through prevention have been advocated by health care providers throughout history. At the turn of this century, chronic noninfectious diseases replaced acute infectious diseases as our nation's mortality leaders. Unlike the old mortality leaders, these new leaders are caused by many factors that often act synergistically to increase the patient's risk of disease. Improved sanitation, nutrition, and other public health projects, which controlled the acute infectious diseases of the past, are not able to prevent these chronic disease processes. For this reason, the emphasis in prevention has shifted from major public projects to more individual interventions.

The prevention and detection of disease is accomplished through a selective approach based on the age and sex of the patient. Whether a disease is preventable is determined by analyzing the disease's incidence and prevalence, progression with and without treatment, risk factors associated with development of the disease, and the availability of screening tests. For the diseases meeting the criteria for prevention, anticipatory guidance and screening procedures based on patient age and gender are developed for use by both primary and specialty care physicians.

The physician, the patient, and the social environment can serve as obstacles to the successful incorporation of health maintenance procedures into medical practice. Poor reimbursement for preventive medical activities and the demoralizing impact of patients who fail to accept personal responsibility for their health may lead physicians to decrease their involvement in health promotional activities. Patients have the ultimate responsibility for their health, yet, for both medical and nonmedical reasons, many patients fail to comply with their physician's recommendations. Our societal environment can be an obstacle to health promotion by encouraging activities and attitudes that actively promote a disease's development and progression.

Physicians can encourage health maintenance activities not only through individual doctor–patient encounters but through public health activities as well. Physicians' support of national health directives within their communities promotes health maintenance. Many nonprofit organizations engaged in primary prevention desire physician assistance in their programs. Through these activities the physician maintains an awareness of health promotion and models the importance of wellness to his or her patients.

Health maintenance and preventive medical activities are an integral part of medical practice. Within their practices, physicians can promote health maintenance by carrying out appropriate screening measures and counseling their patients to improve their life style. These activities can be accomplished in a single doctor–patient encounter or through a family-directed health promotion program. Such encounters serve as an effective means of improving the patient's quality of life and decreasing the cost of health care. For health maintenance activities to be effective, the physician must recognize the uniqueness of each doctor–patient interaction and strive to individualize each patient's wellness program beginning with established guidelines. The physician must consider obstacles that impede patient success and work with the patient and his or her family to overcome the costs each faces in developing a successful health maintenance program.

CASES FOR DISCUSSION

Case 1

John is a 26-year-old airline pilot. He is married with one child. John made his initial appointment because his company recently adopted a nonsmoking policy. John has smoked cigarettes for the last 8 years. He has never tried to quit smoking and feels that it would be very stressful for him to quit. He relates no other medical problems at this time. His physical examination is within normal limits.

1. Is John at risk for developing diseases from his smoking? Which diseases?
2. What other historical information would help you in addressing John's concerns?
3. How could you encourage John to quit smoking? Outline a smoking cessation program for John.

Case 2

Mary is a 32-year-old housewife. Mary visits you for symptoms suggestive of a urinary tract infection. Mary states that she has been in good health;

however, she has not seen a physician since the birth of her second child, 3 years age. Mary states that she smokes a half pack of cigarettes per week and is a social drinker. Her mother currently has breast cancer, which is being treated with chemotherapy. Her father died of a myocardial infarction at age 56. Physical examination is significant for tenderness over the bladder. Urinalysis noted numerous white blood cells per high-power field and 10–15 red blood cells per high-power field (findings consistent with a urinary tract infection). After prescribing appropriate therapy for her suspected urinary tract infection, you discuss health maintenance activities with Mary.

1. What types of office visits can you use to bring up health maintenance issues?
2. What other historical information would be important to appropriately manage a health maintenance program for Mary?
3. What secondary prevention procedures are indicated?

Case 3

Elizabeth is a 2-year-old female. Elizabeth was brought to you for a well-child examination. Her mother relates a history of two ear infections, at 17 months of age and at 1 year of age. Elizabeth has a good appetite and is currently being toilet trained by her mother. Elizabeth's mother relates a family history of diabetes mellitus and states that she smokes one pack of cigarettes per day. Physical examination is appropriate for a 2-year-old female.

1. How should Elizabeth's examination be constructed in order to perform necessary health maintenance activities?
2. What are some primary prevention maneuvers that are appropriate for Elizabeth?
3. What are some secondary preventative medicine techniques that are appropriate for Elizabeth?

Case 4

The Hayes family consists of Joe, who is 27 years old, Terry, who is 24 years old, Michael, who is 3 years old, and Karen, who is 4 months old. The Hayes family has just moved to your community. They have come in, as a family, to see you. Joe is a bricklayer and relates no health problems. He was a high school football player but has no current exercise program. He smokes two packs of cigarettes a day and drinks a six-pack of beer per week. Joe's history is significant for colon cancer in his mother. Physical examination is significant for height of 6′0″, weight of 175 lb, and rhonchi on chest examination (consistent with bronchitis).

Terry is a secretary at the high school. She graduated from junior college with an associate degree in business. She is a nonsmoker and is actively involved in aerobic dancing. Physical examination is significant for height of 5′6″, weight of 135 lb, and flat feet.

Michael and Karen are in good health without current symptoms. There immunizations are up to date.

1. What risk factors does each family member have?
2. How would you design a family intervention targeted at those risk factors?
3. What are the primary and secondary preventive factors in your health maintenance program?

Case 5

Dr. Harvey is a 60-year-old physician who has been practicing in a metropolitan area for the last 45 years. He has a clinical appointment at a local medical school and currently serves as chief of staff at a community hospital. Dr. Harvey is an advocate for health maintenance activities in his community. He was one of the first physicians to incorporate primary and secondary preventative medical activities into his practice.

Mr. Twity is a 67-year-old long-time patient of Dr. Harvey. He has valued Dr. Harvey's approaches to health maintenance. Mr. Twity has smoked two packs of unfiltered cigarettes per day. He saw Dr. Harvey 10 days ago with a cough and fever. A chest x ray revealed a lung mass suggestive of carcihnoma in his right lung.

Dr. Harvey asked Mr. Twity to come to his office for a follow-up visit. After relating the situation to Mr. Twity, Mr. Twity asked,, "How did this get missed? For the last 10 years we have been actively involved in health maintenance activities. If a chest x ray had been taken yearly, would it have discovered the tumor earlier?"

1. How should Dr. Harvey respond to Mr. Twity's questions?
2. What should Dr. Harvey do in the future with patients, such as Mr. Twity, who continue to smoke despite efforts of primary prevention?
3. How should Dr. Harvey approach Mr. Twity's care in the future?

RECOMMENDED READINGS

Last, J. M. (1986). *Public health and preventive medicine.* Norwalk, CT: Appleton-Century-Crofts.

Last provides a comprehensive review of public health methods, communicable diseases, environmental health, behavioral factors affecting health, and noncommunicable and chronic disabling conditions. A discussion of health care planning, organization, and evaluation is included.

O'Donnell, M. P., & Ainsworth, T. (1984). *Health promotion in the workplace.* New York: John Wiley & Sons.

O'Donnell and Ainsworth provide a review of health promotion as it applies to the workplace. He discusses program design and the role of external institutions in health promotion decision making.

Riegelman, R. E., & Povar, G. J. (Eds.). (1988). *Putting prevention into practice: Problem solving in clinical prevention.* Boston: Little, Brown.

This book contains a collection of chapters on preventive medicine topics relevant to primary care in which the authors expertly utilize the tools of clinical decision making to decide if an intervention is indicated and, if so, what intervention. A series of study questions, with answers at the end of the book, help the reader to learn important concepts.

Sheridan, D. P., & Winogrond, I. R. (1987). *The preventive approach to patient care.* New York: Elsevier.

The authors provide a thoughtful discussion of prevention from the perspective of the life cycle. Additional chapters on health promotion topics, such as nutrition, exercise, etc., are provided to support their incorporation into clinical practice.

U.S. Preventive Services Task Force. (1989). *Guide to clinical preventive services: An assessment of the effectiveness of 169 interventions.* Baltimore: Williams & Wilkins.

This report reviews the scientific evidence for 169 preventive interventions for 60 of the most important diseases and health issues. Recommendations are grouped into screening, counseling, and immunizations according to the age, sex, and risk factors of the patient. Recommendations are then summarized by age group on pocket-sized plastic cards, so that the task force's recommendations can be easily integrated into practice.

PART III

Relationships in Clinical Practice

Those "ties that bind" can have a profound effect on the health and clinical care of patients. Although relationship issues have been previously ignored by traditional biomedicine as irrelevant, recent research clearly demonstrates the importance of relationships, especially the doctor–patient relationship, to the health and care of patients. Arising from many perspectives and theoretical models, this research also indicates that physicians, if they take relationship information into account when formulating a therapeutic plan with patients, can to a much greater degree improve the patient's health or at least come to a better understanding of the action constraints affecting the patient's health.

CHAPTER 8

The Doctor–Patient Relationship

Kathryn E. H. Reilly

Case 8-1. A 24-year-old pharmacy student consulted a new physician for a cold that had been "hanging on" for several days. She had a runny nose, cough, sore throat, and occasional low-grade fever. She had final exams coming up in a few days and wanted to feel better as soon as possible. After taking a careful history and doing an examination, the doctor explained to the patient that she had an upper respiratory tract infection and that there was no medication that would cure her immediately. The patient and physician discussed treatment options that were available to her, including rest, cough syrups, and decongestants. The patient agreed to try these over-the-counter remedies and to call back if her symptoms worsened or did not go away in a few more days.

INTRODUCTION

In many ways the relationship between a physician and a patient is unique. Most patients want to establish a long-term relationship with a physician, with the expectation that the doctor will be able to assist them with their physical and emotional problems. Patients expect to bare not only their fears and pains to the physician but also their bodies, to a degree that is unmatched in any other professional relationship. Patients have expectations of their physicians in return: expectations that the physician will listen to their problems carefully, diagnose the cause of their problems, and cure or ameliorate them if possible. Additionally, patients have the expectation that their physicians will always treat them with respect and that their confidences will be respected.

The doctor–patient relationship is in many ways similar to that of any professional relationship. Patients expect to call their physician and receive help, just as they expect to call their car mechanic and get their car fixed. They expect to be treated courteously and expediently in both situations. However, there are distinct differences between the doctor–patient relationship and other professional relationships. There is an implicit and explicit expectation of confidentiality on the part of the physician and his staff. In addition, each patient expects to be evaluated and treated as an individual. No patient wants to be "the interesting patient in the next room" or "just one of the diabetics that doesn't take of herself."

Unfortunately, some patients have unrealistic expectations of their physicians, for example, that physicians should never make a mistake. This expectation of perfection is, of course, impossible to achieve. Unfortunately, although patients may recognize that their expectations are unrealistic in the abstract, they may not comprehend the unrealistic nature of their expectations when their care or the care of their family is involved.

The advantage of these demanding patient expectations is that physicians are allowed to understand and to share large portions of their patients' lives. The joy of watching a child grow from the time of delivery or of caring for a family through good times and crises is immensely rewarding.

Patients are individuals with distinct wants, needs, and expectations. Some patients will be very likable and easy to treat. Others fill doctors with dread every time their names appear on their schedule. Some patients make their doctors feel great after each office visit; others leave their physicians feeling hopeless and helpless. If physicians can maintain an awareness of their responses to individual patients as well as classes of patients, they will begin to understand some of the causes of these responses. For example, one physician may dread seeing patients who have incurable diseases. Alternatively, a particular patient may remind a physician of a family member or close acquaintance from the past with whom the physician did not get along well. Another patient may have personal characteristics such as poor hygiene that a physician finds unpleasant. The patient who leaves the physician feeling great usually likes his physician and is more likely to follow the physician's suggestions. This same patient may have characteristics that remind the physician of someone in his past whom he liked and respected. The patient who leaves the physician feeling depressed is often quite depressed himself, with a deep sense of hopelessness that life will never get better.

Understanding one's responses to particular kinds of patients can help physicians to improve their ability to help them. Awareness of their reactions to patients will also help physicians understand when a patient is behaving in an inappropriate manner. The patient who is inappropriately attempting to obtain addicting drugs to maintain a habit or the seductive patient can be detected by a physician who is attentive to the feelings aroused in him or her by the patient.

The recognition of one's responses to patients can also assist the physician to see each patient as a person, worthy of respect and dignity, who has problems and characteristics that separate him from all others. Once a patient becomes a person, rather than a set of diseases to be cured or problems to be solved, it is easier to like and care for him or her. Respect for the patient's situation can also be enhanced when the physician understands the patient's social and personal context. The mother who calls her child's doctor because he is sick but then is unable to comply with a request to have the child come to the office because she has no transportation is no less concerned about her child than the middle-class mother who arrives at the office within minutes of the call. She just may not have the resources or social support she needs to get to the doctor's office. It is sometimes hard for physicians, who live in a middle-class environment, to "put themselves in the other person's shoes," but being able to do so enhances the quality of medical care provided to patients.

The importance of the relationship between doctor and patient has only recently begun to be systematically studied. The first to publish widely was Michael Balint, a Czechoslovakian psychoanalyst who worked with British general practitioners in the 1950s (Balint, 1957). Balint's area of interest was the doctor–patient relationship and the way the relationship affects both physician and patient. One of Balint's observations was that the interaction between the patient and the physician was, by itself, a potent therapeutic and diagnostic tool. Balint emphasized that merely asking the patient questions was not sufficient for accurate diagnosis. The physician also needs to diagnose the whole patient; for example, is the patient's sore throat the reason for the visit, or is it a ticket that allows access to the physician to discuss something else entirely. Balint observed that the doctor–patient relationship could function like a drug to promote a therapeutic response. As with any other drug, the doctor can change the dosage, frequency, and strength of the relationship to achieve the therapeutic goals required.

This chapter reviews recent research on the doctor–patient relationship and provides a framework for future learning. Hierarchical models of health care are discussed first. These models vary from one in which the physician is the sole decision maker and the patient is the recipient of the doctor-directed action to one of mutual participation in which the doctor and patient are partners in the quest for health. Next, unconscious feelings that both patients and physicians experience during their encounters and their effects on the relationship are discussed. Last, determinants of patient satisfaction with health care encounters are covered, together with ways to use this information to improve health care encounters.

HEALTH CARE MODELS

Case 8-2. P.T., a 25-year-old man with a 10-year history of insulin-dependent diabetes mellitus (IDDM), was extremely knowledgeable about his disease. He monitored his blood sugar four times daily and gave himself injections with regular insulin as indicated by his blood sugar readings. When he became sick with viral gastroenteritis, he continued to monitor his blood sugars but was unable to control his vomiting and diarrhea and so became dehydrated. His regular physician was out of town, so he was seen by another physician who immediately placed him in the hospital for intravenous fluid therapy. As the day passed, P.T. became increasingly concerned since no blood sugar readings were being taken and he had not received his normal doses of insulin. He expressed his concerns to the nurse, who told him that no orders had been written for blood sugar testing. Additionally, she refused to call the physician for those orders. P.T. became increasingly concerned overnight such that by the next morning, he was frantic.

When the "substitute" physician rounded the next morning, he expressed his concerns vocally. The physician told him that he (the physician) was an expert in diabetic care and that he did not appreciate having his orders questions. P.T. continued to insist that his blood sugar was too high and that he needed supplemental insulin. When the physician finally agreed to have P.T.'s blood sugar test run just to "satisfy" him, the blood sugar value returned much higher than it should have been. The doctor treated the high blood sugar but continued to refuse to acknowledge the patient's expertise and concerns. P.T. was accustomed to being an active participant in his health care. Unfortunately, when he became sick and required hospitalization, he was forced to work with a physician who was not comfortable with a more participatory model.

All of us, both patients and physicians, have an idealized picture of how health care ought to be conducted. For most people, this model is a composite of early experiences with their personal physician, doctors they have seen on television or in the movies, and aspects of their own personality that affect their interaction with people in general. In addition to the technological changes that have occurred in medicine during the last 40 years, significant changes have also taken place in the conceptual model of the doctor–patient interaction. Forty years ago, most patients regarded the doctor as an authority figure to be obeyed without question. It is not uncommon to find patients who had major surgery 20 or 30 years ago who never understood why the surgery was necessary or even what was done during the surgery. When they are asked about the surgery, their general response is, "The doctor said I needed it, and in those days we didn't ask questions." Another example is the almost routine performance of circumcisions on infant boys in the 1950s. Mothers signed the consent form with the other hospital admission papers, assuming that the operation was necessary since the doctor had recommended it. It is no longer implicitly accepted that the physician should be all powerful and that the patient should respect that power and obey the physician unquestioningly.

Many patients are now demanding more participation in their care and in the decision making about that care. Brody recently suggested that a total redefinition of power within the doctor–patient relationship is needed (Brody, 1988). It is usually supposed that allowing the patient to have more power in the relationship means that the physician by definition has less (a zero-sum game). Brody proposed that if both physicians and patients share power, the total amount of power available in the relationship actually increases. Thus, both patient and physician are "empowered" by such power sharing.

Szasz and Hollender (1987) have described three basic models of the doctor–patient relationship. The first and earliest models historically is an "activity–passivity" model in which the physician's role is to do something to the patient and the patient's role is to be the passive recipient of the physician's action. This is similar to the interaction between a parent and an infant, with the parent actively caring for the infant and the infant passively accepting the parent's care. In modern medical practice, this model is practiced in limited circumstances in which the patient is unable to participate, such as anesthesia or acute trauma. The second model, termed "guidance–cooperation," is the model of a generation ago. In this model, the physician tells the patient what to do, and the patient cooperates. This interaction can be seen as equivalent to the relationship between a parent and a child. This is the interaction style of Case 8-1 in which the patient consults with the physician, acknowledging the physician's superior knowledge and skill, and implicitly agrees to follow the physician's orders in order to return to a state of health. This interaction style is common in cases of acute illness, when the patient's major concern is to find a cure for his disease so that he can resume a normal life. In this model, "treatment" refers to whatever the physician does. The success of the interaction as seen by the physician is measured by the degree to which the patient complies with the physician's advice.

The third model is termed "mutual participation." In this model, the physician helps the patient to help himself improve his health. Both parties bring important knowledge to the interaction, which is used to formulate strategies that will allow the patient to achieve his health goals. This adult–adult interaction is favored by patients who want to take care of themselves. In chronic diseases, such as diabetes mellitus, this model is both effective and necessary, since optimal adjustment to and management of a chronic disease requires the patient to become an expert on his or her own health needs. Other types of patients are interested in participating in their own health care. The emphasis on improving health through diet and exercise and the news media's ever-increasing number of medical "self-help" articles have led to an increasing awareness on the part of the general public that people can and should be involved in health care and health care decision making.

There is a tendency to feel that the "activity–passivity" model is the most primitive, the "guidance–cooperation" model more advanced, and the "mutual participation" model the most advanced model and the one that all physicians should employ all the time. This conception is too simplistic. Not all clinical situations are appropriate for mutual participation. The doctor treating a comatose patient in the emergency room cannot discuss the treatment with the patient. However, once the treatment has been successful, it would be equally inappropriate for the interaction to remain "activity–passivity." It is also not appropriate to feel that a given model is the "right" one for all office situations. Many patients, particularly the elderly, are more comfortable with a doctor–patient relationship that corresponds to the "guidance–cooperation" model. Although it may be possible over time to encourage these patients to accept more responsibility for their health care, movement to a more mutual participation model cannot be assumed and may not always be appropriate. It is crucial that doctors and their patients work in the same model if the health care interaction is to be satisfactory for both parties.

It would be unfair to assume that the doctor in Case 8-2 never used the "mutual participation" model of health care, although that certainly could be true. The incongruity between the physician's style and the patient's desires unfortunately resulted in significant anxiety and frustration for both patient and physician. Additionally, effective communication about medical management of the current problem was impaired. Although P.T.'s blood sugars were ultimately controlled and he recovered uneventfully from his illness, the lack of congruence between his model of health care and the physician's model was a source of "disease" for both of them. It is possible to imagine a different outcome in this situation, one that would have left both physician and patient feeling more satisfied. If the physician had acknowledged P.T.'s expertise in managing *his* diabetes mellitus and had functioned as a consultant for the acute problem, the dehydration, he would have accomplished the same result much more easily, with less anguish (Solowiejczyk & Baker, 1981).

There is no magic formula that can ensure an optimal doctor–patient interaction. Even physicians who prefer to use the "mutual participation" model for health care find that certain situations exist in which this model does not work well. LeBaron *et al.* studied the responses to physician style among women undergoing therapeutic abortions (LeBaron, Reyher, & Stack, 1985). The same physician adopted either a paternalistic or an egalitarian style with randomly selected patients who underwent an elective abortion. These investigators found that patients who were cared for paternalistically had less discomfort, less stress, and perceived the doctor as warmer and more supportive. The authors postulated that although patients may prefer to be active participants in routine health care or if they have a chronic illness, during crisis situations they need and prefer more guidance.

As was mentioned above, both patients and physicians have an internalized model of ideal health care. When those models conflict, it may be impossible for the doctor–patient interaction to be completely effective. A patient who wants to receive information that will allow him to manage his illness will not be satisfied with a prescription and a "pat on the head." Another patient who has learned to be dependent on physicians for all health care instructions will be uncomfortable and unable to accept a significant role in decision making. Patients have ultimate control in this situation, since they can and do search for and find a physician whose model matches their own. Thus, every physician's practice is made up of a majority of patients who are comfortable with that physician's style of practice. Physicians, as a result, may decide that theirs is the most effective of all possible styles. The more flexible a physician can be in modifying his approach to meet the needs of each patient and each situation, the more effective he will be as a physician.

The doctor–patient relationship is not static. Either party, the patient or the physician, may elect to attempt to change the contract under which the relationship has been conducted. A patient who has been seen for episodic care, who has not wanted to "mutually participate" in that care, may want to become more involved in decision making after developing a chronic disease. Or the physician may have experimented with increasing the involvement of patients in their own care and want more of his patients to assume that responsibility. In either case, the negotiation of the new relationship will present a strain for both parties. The magnitude of the strain depends on the flexibility that each possesses and how strong the desire to continue the relationship is.

It is certainly not always possible to change the relationship so that both doctor and patient are satisfied, particularly when the doctor and patient have known each other for a long time. When it is not possible to alter the relationship so that both are satisfied, the patient usually seeks another source of medical care. However, this solution is not available when it is the physician who is feeling that change is necessary. If the doctor does feel that a change in the relationship is necessary but the patient refuses to make those changes, the physician will need to decide whether or not to terminate the doctor–patient relationship. The decision to terminate the relationship is usually made because the physician feels incapable of providing adequate medical care to the patient. An example is given in Case 8-3.

Case 8-3. A 16-year-old adolescent had insulin-dependent diabetes mellitus for 6 years. At the onset of the disease she and her mother had been quite compliant about treatment. They monitored her blood sugars regularly and made regular visits to see her physician. Over time this compliance decreased. The patient missed several scheduled appointments and was admitted to the hospital three times within 6 months for diabetic ketoacidosis. After prolonged discussion during the last of these admissions, the physician realized that the patient was not likely to change her behavior. The physician in turn felt that he could not continue to care for the patient despite his liking for her and his feeling that she was unlikely to get better care in another setting. He wrote a letter to the patient stating that he could no longer care for her, described the reasons why, and suggested options that were available to her for future care. The physician felt that the patient needed to take some responsibility for her own care, and his level of discomfort over her neglect of her own health ultimately made it impossible for him to continue as her physician.

When the reason for termination of the doctor–patient relationship is not a medical–legal one, the physician can directly discuss the problem with the patient, informing him that because of their differences the patient might be more comfortable with another physician caring for him. This suggestion may prompt the patient to consider negotiating with the physician about the matters in question if he does not want to change doctors.

EFFECTIVE DOCTOR–PATIENT INTERACTION

Case 8-4. A 62-year-old music teacher was continually dissatisfied with her physicians. She refused to go back to several who were fine doctors because the doctors and their office staffs all called her by her first name. Rather than confront these physicians directly, she chose to find another physician. This "doctor shopping" ceased when she found a physician who routinely called all patients by their surnames.

Mutual respect is the foundation on which a good, therapeutic doctor–patient relationship is built. It is vital to demonstrate to the patient the same amenities that one would to another person in any social situation. Respect includes such things as knocking on the door before entering a patient's room, introducing oneself by both name and title or purpose (it is uncomfortable for both the patient and the medical student or resident when he or she is mistaken for the phlebotomist or a nurse), and ensuring as much privacy as possible for the patient during the interview and exam (Platt & McMatch, 1979). It is important to address the patient by name and to use a title such as Mr. or Mrs. plus the surname unless the patient is a child. Many people, like the patient in Case 8-4, do not accept being called by their first name by medical personnel, although a few may prefer it. It is much safer and conveys a feeling of personal concern to avoid using first names, unless the patient requests one to do so.

Although the above actions will set the stage for an effective interaction, the need for respect continues throughout the entire interview and exam. The patient must be certain that the physician is paying attention to him and understanding his story and concerns. Understanding or supportive statements that communicate "I am with you" or "I am listening to you" dramatically facilitate communication. Conversely, continuous note taking and chart reading suggest to the patient that the physician is not paying attention, whether or not that is actually true. Unfortunately, it is tempting, particularly early in clinical training, to spend some time looking at the patient's chart during the interview, the chart representing a medical "security blanket." Unfortunately, reading the chart also acts as a barrier to communication, preventing eye contact and observation of nonverbal communication. Although supportive statements are generally useful in communicating to the patient that the physician is attending to him, Beckman and Frankel report that such statements inserted during the patient's opening statement lead to loss of information about the patient's concerns and may directly lead to "Oh by the way" questions as the doctor is leaving the room (Beckman & Frankel, 1984). In 74 patient encounters, the patient was allowed to express all of his concerns without interruption in only 23% of the cases. In the remaining 77% of encounters, the physician interrupted the patient after a mean of 18 s and took control of the visit by asking closed questions. Beckman found that any utterance that encouraged elaboration on a previously expressed concern inhibited expression of subsequent concerns. Continuers such as "I see," "go on," and "uhn-huh" facilitated completion of the patient's list of concerns. Beckman's report emphases the importance of using open-ended questions, particularly during the early part of the interview.

Open-ended questions, with attentive listening by the physician, allow the patient to take control of the interview. Closed questions wrestle control of the interview away from the patient. This can have the undesirable effect of suppressing important information and thus may prevent the physician from obtaining a complete description of the patient's problem.

Case 8-5. A second-year medical student was about to do her first history and physical exam on a hospitalized patient. Although the course rules precluded examining the chart prior to the exam, nothing was said about using other sources of information. So when the patient's nurse volunteered volumes of verbal information about the patient, the student listened and took notes. When she actually saw the patient, her questioning strategy was to elicit the information that she already had written down. She asked only closed questions, allowing the patient to respond only with yes and no. The physical exam, too, was focused on the patient's known medical problem. Unfortunately, the patient's main problems were completely different from what the nurse had reported. The student completely failed to obtain the pertinent history.

It is unfortunately easy for physicians to lead patients into telling the story that they expect to hear. In an effort to save time, physicians often take control of the interview too soon and end up with inaccurate or incomplete information that ends up wasting time in the long run. Word usage is important too. Medicine has a language of its own that allows unambiguous communication between professionals. Use of medical jargon when talking to patients can lead to confusion, however. For patients who are unwilling to confess that they do not understand the jargon, use of medical phrases can even lead to misleading information being communicated. For example, even a simple word such as "void" is frequently misunderstood to mean, for example, "avoid" or "defecate." More importantly, the physician's ability to make a diagnosis and to effect change in the patient's condition is contingent on both the patient and physician understanding what the other is saying. Avoiding medical jargon becomes increasingly difficult the longer a person is a physician. Practicing the ability to explain medical concepts using nonmedical terms is an extremely important part of becoming an effective physician.

It seems intuitively obvious that a patient who is satisfied with his encounter with a physician will be more likely to comply with instructions and more likely to return. Unfortunately, it is not easy to define the attributes of an encounter that will lead to increased patient satisfaction. However, there are some strategies that the physician can use to increase patient satisfaction with each encounter. Not surprisingly, patients will be more satisfied when they "get what they came for." Mothers attending an acute care pediatrics department were significantly more satisfied when they learned what was wrong with their children (Francis, Korsch, & Morris, 1969). One of the parents' goals in bringing their children to the clinic was to learn the cause of their illnesses. When this goal was not attained, they were dissatisfied with the encounter regardless of the outcome of the illness itself.

Other investigators have found that patients are more satisfied when they express their request for medication early in the encounter (Carter, Inui, KuKull, & Haigh, 1982). The expression of desire for medication early in the visit allows the doctor and the patient to discuss and negotiate about the patient's need for the medicine. Since medication has many different meanings for patients (a means of mastery over illness, nurturance by the physician, or a reminder that something is wrong with the patient), early and complete discussion about the medications desired by the patient can improve the patient's understanding about why medications are required or not (Barsky, 1983).

In much the same way, discussion fairly early in the visit of what the patient hopes to achieve from the visit can improve both the patient's satisfaction and the physician's sense of fulfillment (Lazare, Eisenthal, & Wasserman, 1975). At times it is not immediately obvious why a patient has come to see a physician, and at other times the patient's stated reason for coming is misleading or oversimplified.

Case 8-6. A 26-year-old factory worker visited his wife's physician with a complaint of having had a cold for several days. He had not had any fever but had a constant cough that had been preventing him from sleeping well. He was also quite fatigued. He expressed a desire not to be placed on any medications, since he had experienced reactions to numerous antibiotics. At that point, the physician felt confused, since in his experience people who came for such minor complaints usually were looking for a "magic bullet" to make them better again. He was feeling quite impotent, since he was unable to think of anything to suggest to the patient other than rest and fluids. He excused himself from the room briefly and, after thinking for a few minutes, returned to ask the patient what he hoped to obtain as a result of the office visit. The patient explained that he had been off work for 3 days and needed a note from the doctor excusing his time off from work in order to go back to work. Additionally, he was still quite fatigued and not quite ready to return. After this explanation, the physician was able to write the note the patient needed, since he agreed that the patient did require a few more days of convalescence. Both patient and physician ultimately felt that the encounter had been successful.

Lazare suggests that the best time to elicit the patient's request is after the patient has expressed his chief complaint and the clinician has understood the scope of the problem. Patient and physician can then enter into a negotiation, which Lazare sees as the "coming together between the patient who is formulating what he thinks he needs and the clinician who is formulating what he thinks is clinically important" (Lazare *et al.*, 1975). This coming together allows the patient to feel that he has truly been heard and will probably lead to greater compliance with prescribed treatment.

Patients want their physicians to treat them as people. The stereotype of the surgeon operating on the "gallbladder in room 419" is very real to people. Thus, patient satisfaction increases when physicians ask questions about family and social situations and when there is social continuity (Is your husband feeling any better since you were last in?) from one visit to the next (Weinberger, Greene, & Mamlin, 1981). Neglect of social amenities by the physician can adversely affect the whole doctor–patient relationship.

Case 8-7. A 56-year-old housewife was being seen for the first time. When the physician asked her why she was there, she stated that she was shopping for a new doctor. She has been seeing her old doctor for about 10 years and had no complaints with the medical care that she had received. But she felt that he "was beginning to take her for granted." Specifically, she was upset that he took phone calls from others while he was seeing her, but she had to wait for him to return her phone calls. It also seemed to her that he was spending less time with her and seemed less concerned about her as a person. So she had decided to find a physician who would treat her in a more caring manner.

The physical relationship between patient and physician is also important. Weinberger found that patient satisfaction decreased with increased distance between the patient and the physician during the interview (Weinberger *et al.*, 1981). Emotional distance can also be affected by the physician's posture during the interview. The doctor who leans against the wall or leans back in the chair conveys a lack of interest in the patient's problems and is much less likely to achieve a good interaction than a physician who looks and acts interested in the patient. It is also difficult for spontaneous interaction to occur when one party is "towering" over the other. For example, a doctor making rounds in the hospital who stands over the patient for a minute or two only indicates to the patient that he has no time for trivial concerns or questions. The doctor who instead sits by the patient's bedside appears more relaxed; although he may spend no more time than the busy physician, he will be more likely to invite pertinent questions from his patients, who will feel that their concerns have been heard.

Dissatisfied patients are not likely to remain patients of the physician who has caused the dissatisfaction. In addition, it has been postulated that a satisfied patient will be compliant, whereas a dissatisfied patient will be noncompliant with physicians orders and suggestions. In fact, this theory does appear to be true for the most part, although Francis found that even highly satisfied patients were not always compliant, and highly dissatisfied patients were sometimes compliant (Francis *et al.*, 1969). Since poor compliance by patients is a major source of frustration for physicians, any changes that can be made in the doctor–patient interaction that would increase compliance would be beneficial.

DIFFICULT PATIENTS

Case 8-8. M.J., a 45-year-old woman, has been seen at the family medicine clinic for several years. A resident has cared for her for the past $2\frac{1}{2}$ years. He describes the patient as extremely anxious and unable to give a coherent history. He at times feels that the patient gives an incomplete, inaccurate history on purpose. Her symptoms are vague. He is further frustrated because he is unable to make a diagnosis or construct a therapeutic approach that would benefit the patient. During rare occasions when he is able to define an appropriate therapy, the patient is unable to comply. "She has no resources, no money for medicines, no brains to understand, and no family support," he states. The root of the resident's frustration with this patient was her inability or unwillingness to take responsibility for herself.

It is an interesting exercise to ask physicians about difficult patients; almost without exception, physicians are immediately able to describe the difficult patient's history and personal characteristics in precise detail. For example, a third-year family practice resident described the patient in Case 8-8 spontaneously in a discussion about the topic of difficult patients.

Physician frustration, as described in Case 8-8, is a common reason that patients are perceived as difficult. Schwenk *et al.* asked 22 family physicians to select difficult patients from their practices and to evaluate each patient according to the applicability of 40 behavioral and physical characteristics (Schwenk, Marquez, Lefever, & Cohen, 1989). The physicians rated a total of 205 difficult patients. Two factors were identified as common to these patients who were perceived as difficult: medical uncertainty, characterized by particularly vague, difficult to describe, undifferentiated medical problems, and interpersonal difficulty, reflected in a perceived abrasive behavioral style. When the physicians were asked to rate the importance of various motivations for practicing medicine, the primary motivations were satisfaction derived from solving medical problems and the desire to help people. Thus, the physicians' primary satisfactions in practicing medicine were not able to be achieved in interactions with these difficult patients, leaving the physicians feeling frustrated. Difficult patients create a dissatisfied feeling in the physician, with frustration being the base of at least part of that dissatisfaction.

Although difficult patients share a common characteristic of experiencing undifferentiated medical problems, their abrasive behavioral styles come in many guises (Groves, 1978). The *overtalkative* patient is difficult, particularly for inexperienced interviewers. This patient answers every question, even those that are clearly "yes/no" questions, with paragraphs of information. Some of these patients may be unable to focus their answers because of mild dementia or other brain dysfunction. Other patients who are overtalkative need to be sure that you understand their problem exactly. Direct questions, rather than open-ended ones, can help the interviewer to get the information needed. Courteous interruptions, followed by another direct question, may be helpful. However, some patients will continue to express themselves, regardless of the interviewer's attempts. In this case, the interviewer should try to relax, accept the problem, and enjoy the interaction.

Angry patients are fairly common. Some angry patients are demeaning or sarcastic; others are demanding, aggressive, and hostile. Some remain silent during the interview or make remarks that are condescending. The interviewer may feel resentment, anger, threatened authority, impatience, or frustration as a result of the patient's obvious anger. In order to deal effectively with the angry patient, the interviewer needs to understand the source of the patient's anger. The patient who is angry because he has an incurable disease will require different intervention than a patient who is angry about something that happened while he was in the waiting room. Confrontation is a useful technique when the patient seems angry. "You sound very angry" or "You're obviously angry about something; tell me about what is wrong" are approaches that allow the patient to express his or her anger without becoming defensive. If the patient is angry about something that you can not do anything about, an awareness of the problem will help the interviewer to avoid further antagonizing the patient.

An *aggressive* patient attempts to control the interview and the course of his treatment. This patient is easily irritated and may fly into a rage when not allowed to have things his way. However, if allowed to have his way, this patient is generally quite pleasant. In general, it is helpful to avoid areas of conflict early in the interview and to attack the areas of potential conflict later when rapport has been established. A subset of the aggressive patient group is the *demanding* patient. This patient makes demands on everyone, using intimidation and guilt to force others to meet his needs. Recognizing that this is occurring and addressing it with the patient is infrequently effective. Limit setting by the medical staff, when carried out consistently, can help to limit this problem.

The *help-rejecting* patient can be extremely frustrating. This patient has usually seen many other physicians, who have all failed to discover what is wrong and how to cure it. When a symptom is relieved, another symptom appears to take its place. These patients may be extremely depressed, using their symptoms as a tool to enhance their relationship with the physician. These patients can sometimes be helped if the physician can accept their symptoms and provide gentle reassurance and support, without trying to "fix" them by eliminating their symptoms.

The *insatiable* patient produces similar problems for the physician. This patient is never satisfied. He or she has many questions and is never satisfied with the explanations provided by the physician. When confronted with an insatiable patient, the physician can use a closing statement that is definite, such as "We have reached the end of our time today. I will see you again in 2 weeks" or "Our time for today is up. I will refer your concerns to your doctor."

There are certainly other abrasive behaviors that patients can exhibit that make them difficult for physicians. Each physician over time develops techniques for managing these behaviors. In many cases, the key problem is identifying what the specific behavior is that is creating the difficulty. Self-awareness and introspection can assist the physician to identify why the patient he sees as "difficult" is just that.

UNCONSCIOUS INFLUENCES

Case 8-9. A young family physician who had just finished her residency and opened a practice was consulted by a 65-year-old man who had mild hypertension. He told her that he had chosen her for his physician because she came from an area of the country of which he was fond. The patient stated that he was only interested in care for his hypertension, and only "on his terms." He did not want to change medications and was not interested in dietary advice about sodium restriction or about lowering his high cholesterol. His office visits were constructed by him to be social calls in which his blood pressure was checked and prescriptions were written.

At first the young physician was accepting of this approach, but as she gained more confidence in herself, she began to put pressure on the patient to come in for a general physical examination. After several months, the patient did come in for a physical exam but would not allow her to do a rectal exam. On his next visit, the patient informed her that he would no longer be seeing her and that he was switching to another woman physician in the same practice.

As the physician thought about the patient after he left her practice, she realized that he had been treating her as a child, and that she had responded to him in much the same way that she would have responded to her own father, by not confronting him or going against his wishes. The relationship could not withstand the strain of the physician's growing clinical competence and her unwillingness to continue her role as the unquestioning daughter. If the physician had been more perceptive during this patient's initial visits, she could have discussed with the patient their differing goals. She and the patient could then have negotiated what would be included in his medical care. Perhaps the outcome would have been the same, but there would have been a better chance that the doctor–patient relationship could have been maintained, with both parties being in agreement on the rules of the relationship.

Understanding descriptive models of health care can help a student or physician understand the interpersonal interactions that occur with patients. Unfortunately, this understanding, combined with good training in interviewing techniques and medical decision-making skills, is not enough to ensure that every interaction with a patient will go well. Both the patient's response to the doctor and the doctor's response to the patient are affected by many factors including prior life events and relationships and acute emotional disturbances.

The psychoanalytic term for a patient's emotional response to the physician is transference. **Transference** can be conceptualized as the shift of emotions from past experience (especially emotions from childhood) to the present doctor–patient relationship. Transference occurs in all doctor–patient interactions, the patient attributing characteristics and attitudes to the physician that are not possessed by that physician. Transference can be either negative or positive. Positive transference can leave both the patient and the physician feeling warm and nurtured. Negative transference, in which the physician is perceived in negative terms by the patient, can utterly disrupt the doctor–patient interaction. Negative transference causes the physician to feel disliked. Negative transference can be a general response to physicians as a class or can be a reaction to an individual physician (Kvale & Dayringer, 1987; Stein, 1980, 1985c).

Transference is particularly likely to be important when a patient has a chronic disease the management of which requires a long-term relationship with a physician. An elderly person will frequently view her physician (especially a young physician) as being like one of her children. In a positive relationship, the physician is seen as a good and caring child from whom the elderly person can gain strength and a sense of dependence. When the patient's needs are not gratified, the physician can be seen as a bad or uncaring child (Kvale & Dayringer, 1987).

The physician's unconscious response to the patient has been termed **countertransference.** During countertransference, the physician's feelings toward people from the past are transferred to the patient. Countertransference is also extremely common and can cause the physician to misinterpret, overlook, or misjudge the significance of information obtained from the encounter with a patient. Thus, countertransference can lead to errors of judgment, without the physician even being aware that errors are occurring, as in Case 8-9. The physician's acceptance of the role given to her by the patient ultimately prevented her from feeling comfortable with the care that she was providing. When the physician becomes aware of countertransference, he can become much more effective in delivering medical care by consciously avoiding the errors that it can cause and by using it as important information about the patient and the relationship.

Mengel has reported that loss of physician effectiveness occurs when previous experiences from the physician's family of origin closely resemble aspects of the patient's problem (Mengel, 1987c). To study this phenomenon, Mengel asked experienced physicians to discuss difficult cases and then collected information about each physician's family of origin. He found that in cases where the physicians were particularly frustrated, they frequently had developed alliances with the patient or other family members that closely resembled alliances within their own families of origin. Conflicts developed between the physicians and the patients or their families in areas that were similar to conflicts that had occurred in the physicians' own families. Other characteristics such as secret keeping, assuming too much responsibility for a case, or avoiding conflicts also led to physician ineffectiveness and frustration. These alliances, conflicts, and transferred family rules prevented the physicians from being able to act as agents of change in the patient's system. Instead, the physicians inadvertently functioned to maintain dysfunctional systems, leading to therapeutic ineffectiveness.

In Case 8-9, the physician was ineffective in part because of her family-of-origin issues. Her father expected all of the women in his family to conform to his wishes without question. She had developed a habit of passively acceding to his wishes, although she also actively rebelled at times. The relationship between the physician and her father was distant and maintained in part by her obedience. Thus, when her patient, who was close to her father in both age and medical problems, treated her as a child, she responded in a manner similar to the way in which she would have responded to her father, by not confronting or negotiating areas of conflict. This resulted in dissatisfaction and ineffectiveness within the doctor–patient relationship, as the patient would not allow a necessary exam and eventually left the physician's practice. Although this is speculative, a less passive initial stance by the physician might have resulted in a better outcome.

As can be appreciated, unconscious responses by both physician and patient affect the interaction between them. It is impossible to avoid transference and countertransference. They are inevitable, since each of us has within our memories an organized repository of feelings and experiences onto which we try to fit new feelings and experiences. This reference is so deeply embedded in our psyches that we try to fit all new feelings and experiences into it, even when the fit is not a close one. Thus, patients see the physician as a composite of all the physicians that they have encountered as well as the nurturers they have experienced, whereas the physician responds to the patients with attitudes and actions that were learned from past relationships. Although it is not possible to avoid these responses, it is crucial to learn to recognize them and to be able to understand the responses when they occur. Recognition of transference, countertransference, and family-of-origin issues allows the clinician to use them as a tool for clinical understanding to increase therapeutic effectiveness (Stein, 1985c).

One clue to the presence of an unconscious response to a patient can be a poor interview performance. The physician may find himself feeling unsatisfied after such an interview, with a sensation that something was left undone. Smith analyzed videotaped interviews conducted by medical students and residents and found that the most common unconscious error was avoidance of difficult subjects such as death, disability, and loneliness (Smith, 1984, 1986). The next most common unhelpful behaviors were passivity (failure to control the interview), detachment (avoiding relating to the patient), overcontrol (inappropriate interruption, changing the subject, and directing the interview), and overly pleasing behavior (being overly social and reassuring). The reasons for these behaviors were primarily fears the physicians experienced: fear that the patient would be harmed, that they would lose control of the interview, or that the patients would not like them. These unconscious fears prevented the physicians from interacting effectively with their patients.

Gorlin has discussed reactions that physicians have toward patients and suggests methods for dealing with those responses once they are recognized (Gorlin & Zucker, 1983). For example, he suggests that avoidance of a patient with a terminal illness can be surmounted when the physician understands his feelings, analyzes why he feels the way he does, and, if possible, discusses those feelings with colleagues. In other cases, such as feeling unable to meet a patient's needs, he suggests referral to a colleague more experienced in the patient's problem.

Another unconscious response to patients is stereotyping. All physicians have a picture in their minds of the ideal patient. The patient who superficially meets his stereotype will usually be perceived as being more intelligent, more trustworthy, and in general a better patient (Johnson, Kurtz, Tomlinson, & Howe, 1986). The unsoundness of basing clinical judgments on physical appearance or other superficial criteria is obvious.

Although conscious exploration of responses to individual patients is an important skill for each physician to attain, many physicians have found that group discussion of difficult or troubling relationships is an effective means of understanding their feelings. Michael Balint, the psychoanalyst mentioned earlier in the chapter, organized a group of general practitioners who met monthly to discuss difficult cases. One practitioner presented a difficult case in depth, after which the group analyzed the situation, including the practitioner's own emotional response. Many family practice residencies have adopted "Balint" groups as a mechanism to teach young physicians the skill of self-analysis. Physicians who have experienced Balint groups while in training frequently search out similar opportunities during their practice years.

Case 8-10. A female resident, a regular participant in a Balint group, presented a case concerning an elderly couple who refused to behave as the physician felt they should. She felt that she understood both their medical problems and their social concerns and circumstances. Despite her attempts at meeting their concerns, both husband and wife had elected to see another physician. After the group discussed the case for an hour, the physician understood that her desire to make this couple happy had caused her to make concessions regarding their care that may not have been appropriate. Even now, when they had communicated their plan to seek another physician's care, the resident expressed concerns about how quickly they would seek out that care. She could recognize that she wanted to take more responsibility for these patients than was realistic and appropriate for a physician. Recognition of this pattern allowed the resident, over time, to decrease her overinvolvement in certain patients as she learned to foster self-responsibility in those patients.

Another type of group for physicians focuses on behavior patterns derived from experiences in the family in which the physician was raised. Careful exploration of the dynamics of a physician's family of origin has been found to greatly improve awareness of emotional and behavioral relationships. Family systems theory states that a person's ability to maintain his objectivity within a clinical encounter is dependent on how well he has been able to differentiate from his own family of origin (Bowen, 1972). The more differentiated a physician is, the less he becomes emotionally reactive to the clinical situation and thus the better able he is to accomplish therapeutic goals. Mengel and Mauksch have recently described a group training experience utilizing family-of-origin techniques (Mengel & Mauksch, 1989).

CONCLUSIONS

This chapter is an introduction to a very complex subject: the doctor–patient relationship. The concepts presented can help physicians to understand what occurs within that very special relationship. Negotiating the "model" of health care that is comfortable for both the physician and the patient, understanding transference/countertransference issues, improving communications, and showing respect for the social needs of patients will not only decrease "doctor shopping" and improve compliance but will increase the physician's ability to appreciate the distinctness and individuality of patients and enhance his enjoyment of clinical medicine.

CASES FOR DISCUSSION

Case 1

Dr. R.J. is a 34-year-old male family practice resident who regularly participates in his residency's Balint group. Today he presents the case of a 57-year-old male alcoholic whom he has been following for about 6 months. The patient has abnormal liver enzymes, which indicate modest liver dysfunction, and high blood pressure, which is controlled fairly well with medication. The patient has failed to modify his alcohol intake despite an apparently clear understanding about the effect of continued drinking on his liver. Dr. J. is presenting the patient because he finds to his amazement that he likes his patient in spite of his uncontrolled alcohol intake. Dr. J. states that he usually dislikes alcoholics intensely.

1. What experiences in Dr. J.'s past might there be that would explain his dislike of alcoholics?
2. Would your opinion change if you knew that his religion was extremely opposed to drinking alcohol? If his father was an alcoholic?
3. What characteristics of this patient might have altered Dr. J.'s perception of him?

Case 2

A 45-year-old man is seeing you for follow-up of his high blood pressure. Because of an emergency that has delayed you, he has been waiting 90 min to see you. When you enter the room, he will not look at you and barely responds to your greeting. You assume that he may be angry because of the long wait, so you begin to apologize for the delay. He interrupts you to state that yes he is angry about waiting, but that what he is really angry about is how he was treated by your receptionist. He states that she was rude to him when he first arrived at the office and that he could hear her laughing and joking while he was waiting. Other patients who arrived at the office after him were seen by you and left the office before he was even called to be seen. He says that he will never return to see you and that your whole operation is poorly run.

1. How would you pacify this patient? Is pacification indicated?
2. How would you conduct the rest of the office visit?

Case 3

A 2-year-old boy who has been your patient since birth is admitted to the hospital for the fourth time in a year with asthma. His parents are quite good about giving him his medication. You are convinced that the reason that he has had so much trouble with his asthma is that both parents smoke heavily. You have been unable to alter this behavior by repeated counseling. You also recognize that you have a strong bias against parents smoking in front of their children and worry that this bias is affecting your ability to deal with this problem effectively.

1. What strategies might you use to (a) convince the parents that smoking is affecting the child's health and (b) change their behavior if they cannot or will not stop smoking?
2. Does it matter if a physician is strongly biased against certain behaviors and communicates that to patients?

Case 4

A 35-year-old well-dressed woman is scheduled for a complete physical examination. When you look at her chart, you notice that you have seen her once before, approximately 1 year previously, when she was experiencing some stress at work. You prescribed a mild tranquilizer at that time, but it had not been helpful. When you enter the room, the patient obviously expects you to remember her and her problems. She begins immediately to tell you what a wonderful doctor you are. She continues that she is confident that you will be able to find a cure for her problems, which center around "stress." After praising you to the point that you are certain that she desires drugs, she launches into a rambling history of stress at home, at work, and with a grown son. You feel trapped.

1. How can a physician discriminate between drug-seeking behavior and a legitimate need for psychoactive medication?
2. Is it acceptable to prescribe psychoactive mediation for a patient you think is drug addiction prone, if you think he or she has a problem that would be helped by them?
3. How can a physician find time to analyze his or her feelings of uneasiness during an office session?

Case 5

You are the chief resident in family medicine at a small community hospital. Recently, you have begun to feel inordinately fatigued and unable to complete your work effectively. You have had blood work done in the hospital lab that indicates that your liver functions are abnormal. You realize that you should consult another physician about your illness but are reluctant to do so because of the size of the hospital and the medical community.

1. Is this resident's concern about confidentiality realistic? Would his disease process make a difference in the appropriateness of his concern; i.e., would it be different if he thought he had mononucleosis versus hepatitis versus AIDS?
2. Should physicians identify a personal physician? If so, what characteristics would be important? Should physicians be hospitalized in "their" hospital or in a hospital in which they are not known?

EXERCISES FOR PRACTICE

The best way to develop strategies helpful in interacting with difficult patients described in this chapter is to practice such strategies on real or simulated patients. These exercises build on the exercises for practice from Chapter 3 in that further experience is obtained in patient interviewing, this time with difficult patients. If real or simulated patients are not available, then role-playing a medical encounter can be equally effective.

During the role-play, one student should play the difficult patient, one the physician, and one should observe the interview. The "patient" should "make-up" a difficult patient scenario (overtalkative, demanding, hostile, passive, etc.), or a short clinical vignette can be supplied by the instructor. The "physician" then interviews the "patient," trying to obtain a focused medical history, utilizing the strategies described in this chapter. After the interview, both the "observer" and the "patient" provide feedback to the "physician" on his or her interview style and use of strategies to improve the interaction with difficult patients. The roles among the group of three students then change, and the process repeats as time allows.

RECOMMENDED READINGS

Balint, M. (1957). *The doctor, his patient and the illness.* New York: International Universities Press.

This old but excellent exposition is a superb introduction to the process and benefits of Balint groups.

Stein, H. F. (1985). *The psychodynamics of medical practice: Unconscious factors in patient care.* Berkeley: University of California Press.

In this book, Stein describes how countertransference can affect the care physicians give patients. Written in a clear, elegant style with plenty of "real-life" examples, this book is also appropriate for the beginning student.

Stein, H. F., & Apprey, M. (1990). *Clinical stories and their translations.* Charlottesville, VA: University Press of Virginia.

An ethnographic description of the ways that practitioners unconsciously distort the stories of patients and their families.

Stoekle, J. D. (Ed.) (1987). *Encounters between patients and doctors.* Cambridge, MA: MIT Press.

This book is an excellent collection of readings on the doctor–patient relationship, including an excellent historical overview of the doctor–patient relationship by Stoekle himself.

CHAPTER 9

The Family System

Mark B. Mengel

Case 9-1. A 16-year-old girl with insulin-dependent diabetes mellitus (IDDM) has been admitted almost monthly to the hospital with severe diabetic ketoacidosis. While in the hospital, her diabetes is always brought under rapid control, and she is maintained on low doses of insulin. However, after she leaves the hospital her insulin requirements gradually increase. These larger doses have little effect on her diabetic control, and she is eventually admitted back into the hospital again.

In order to determine the reasons for this patient's frequent attacks of diabetic ketoacidosis, a more thorough assessment is carried out including an evaluation of personal and family characteristics. During the interview with the patient, she appears to be a nice, cooperative adolescent, not at all rebellious, with very concerned parents who desperately want to help their daughter control her IDDM. An interesting interaction pattern is noted during the interview, in which every time the patient is asked a question, one or both of the parents provide the answer. Questions about potential stressors, strains, or conflicts within the family yield the answer that there are none, except for their daughter's IDDM. In asking what the parents do to help their daughter with her IDDM, the mother reveals that she still gives the patient her shots, monitors her blood sugars, and adjusts her insulin dosages not actually on the basis of the monitored blood sugar results but because she just "knows" how the girl's blood sugar behaves in certain situations and adjusts the insulin accordingly. When suggestions are made that the patient might be of an age where she could manage her own IDDM, the parents state flatly that would be impossible.

INTRODUCTION

Family systems medicine is a subdiscipline of medicine dedicated to the investigation of how the family affects the health of its individual members. Even though past practitioners of the art of medicine, such as Hippocrates, clearly recognized that psychosocial factors influence a patient's health, the field of family systems medicine really began in the late 1940s with the convergence of three historical developments (Christie-Seely & Crouch, 1987). The first development occurred when physicians, especially psychiatrists in the mental health arena, and other health professionals and researchers, particularly social scientists and epidemiologists, recognized and then performed research studies documenting that family factors, such as structure, marital status, communication patterns, and loss of a spouse, affect an individual's health, both mental and physical. The second development was the creation of a theoretical framework and body of knowledge describing the ways that problems form within families and how change can occur by treating not just the individual but individuals and their families together in therapy. This movement was begun and perpetuated by a group of family therapists, many of whom have established their own schools of therapy. The third and latest development that has encouraged the formation and development of family systems medicine occurred within organized medicine. That development was the birth and growth of family practice, which arose in response to public and private pressure resulting from dissatisfaction with the increasingly specialized nature of medical care. Family practice adds to its ancestral base of general practice by being a primary care discipline that includes within its purview not only the individual patient but their families as well.

These three historical developments have contributed to the field of family systems medicine in a number of ways. First, physicians and other health care professionals have conducted research showing that family factors have profound influences on the health of individual family members, including general outcomes such as mortality and morbidity as well as more specific outcomes associated with cardiovascular disease, hypertension, diabetes mellitus, asthma, pregnancy, obesity, compliance behavior, mental health issues including schizophrenia and depression, and substance abuse, including alcoholism (Campbell, 1986). Second, family therapists have developed a strong theoretical base arising from general systems theory and powerful therapeutic techniques that have encouraged practitioners to observe and treat whole families (Hoffman, 1981). Third, family physicians and therapists have worked hard to integrate research and therapeutic techniques within primary care practice to enable physicians to gain further improvements in patient health through inclusion of the family in the care of their patients (Doherty & Baird, 1983). Thus, it is clear to many practicing physicians that including the family in the context of patient care helps physicians to diagnose and treat their patient's illnesses more effectively.

Given the above strides in the field of family systems medicine, the goals of this chapter are to (1) develop an understanding of the family as a system, (2) understand several family systems terms that describe family dynamics and interaction patterns, (3) develop an understanding of how the family system can affect the health of its individual members, (4) develop the skills to conduct a family assessment, and (5) develop an understanding of how to include the family within an individual patient's therapeutic plan.

The biomedical model has been the dominant concept of medical care during the 20th century. This model's central principle is that disease arises from organic dysfunction within a specific organ that is not voluntary and is not affected by anything external to the patient. Thus, a disease such as atherosclerotic heart disease can be readily explained by the biomedical model as dysfunction of the heart secondary to arteriosclerotic plaque narrowing coronary arteries. Physicians using this model restore health by attempting to reverse the organic dysfunctions that causes disease, for example, bypassing clogged coronary arteries during open-heart surgery.

No one can dispute the great strides medicine has made utilizing the biomedical model. However, many health care providers and their patients have come to realize that the biomedical model is not the whole story. Standard biomedical treatments that are supposed to correct dysfunctional aspects of a patient's physiology do not always restore health. In 1977, George Engel critiqued the failures of the biomedical model by providing examples in which the biomedical model failed to improve patient health. He then proposed a new model of health, the biopsychosocial model, in which disease is viewed within the context of the patient's life. Engel went on to provide examples of how viewing the patient "biopsychosocially" enabled the physician to diagnose and treat conditions when a strict biomedical orientation was ineffectual.

Although the merits of the biomedical versus the biopsychosocial approach are still hotly debated, the resulting tension has spawned two models of how family factors can affect individual health, the socioepidemiologic approach and the systems approach.

The Socioepidemiologic Model

The socioepidemiologic model is derived from an infectious disease model of health in which a disease agent, such as a virus, bacteria, or fungus, infects a susceptible host. Disease depends not only on the quantity and virulence of the disease agent but also on host factors that affect susceptibility, such as genetic predisposition, malnutrition, etc. The late epidemiologist John Cassel adapted this infectious disease model to study the effect of social factors on health (Cassel, 1976). Cassel studied social factors such as stressors, those social events that lowered host resistance to disease agents, and social supports, those events that buffered the effects of stressors or actually improved host resistance to disease agents, in his research. His work examining the effect of stress and social support on pregnancy outcomes supported this model (Nuckolls, Cassel, & Kaplan, 1972). In his study of 340 primiparous women followed throughout their pregnancy, Cassel and co-workers found that among women with a large number of prepregnancy and antepartum stressors, those with low social support had three times the chance of having an adverse pregnancy outcome as those with high social supports.

Some investigators feel that social support not only acts to buffer the effects

Table 9-1
Average Annual Death Rate in Married and Widowed Males Aged 25 to 35 Years (Rates/100k)[a]

Cause	Married	Widowed	Widowed and remarried
Tb	11.2	141.8	12.8
Inf/Pneu	2.6	20.1	7.7
ASHD	8.8	42.1	4.9
HBP	1.7	18.3	10.8

[a] Adapted from Kraus and Lillienfeld (1959).

of stress but can also have effects independent of the amount of stress. Kraus and Lillienfeld examined average annual death rates in married and widowed males, ages 25 to 35 years, from tuberculosis, pneumonia, heart disease, and hypertension (Kraus & Lillienfeld, 1959). As shown in Table 9-1, the average annual death rate sharply increased in widowed men as compared to married men, dropping almost back to base line in most cases in remarried men. Although the loss of a spouse is no doubt stressful, its effect on mortality has been thought to be based primarily on the loss of social support experienced by a man when his mate dies.

The effects of stress and family support on health appear to be mediated by neuroendocrine and immune mechanisms; that is, certain stressors cause the secretion of hormones, such as epinephrine, norepinephrine, and cortisol, which raise blood pressure, pulse rate, blood sugar levels, and cholesterol levels, blunt antibody responses, and decrease neutrophil functioning (Ader, 1981). These effects can result in exacerbations of many diseases, including hypertension, arteriosclerosis, diabetes mellitus, and infectious disease.

Thus, the socioepidemiologic model appears to have a great deal of validity in explaining how the family may affect health. However, despite its usefulness as a research construct, the socioepidemiologic model has not achieved widespread clinical use. One reason may be that within this model, disease is still seen as a disorder that exists entirely within the patient. Although many clinicians find this consistent with the biomedical model and thus are reasonably comfortable with it, many have found, for example, that treating an individual under a great deal of family stress with simple stress reduction techniques fails to address the underlying problem and is often just as unsuccessful as biomedical remedies that do not include the family within the treatment program. Thus, many physicians have turned to another model of the family's effect on health in an attempt to understand how the complexity of human relationships within the family can affect individual disease states in its members.

The Family System

The family system model grew out of general systems theory, which was first developed in the late 1940s by the biologist von Bertalanffy (1968). Von

Bertalanffy believed that science had become so reductionist by analyzing progressively smaller and smaller bits of a whole that the analyses were no longer meaningful to the behavior of the whole organism. In order to understand the whole, von Bertalanffy felt that one had to look at its behavior within the complex interaction of systems to which it belonged, rather than subjecting it to continued reductionistic analyses.

Von Bertalanffy defined a system as "a complex of elements standing in interaction." Systems occur at all levels throughout the biological spectrum from the biochemical and physiological systems in our body that regulate blood sugar to the human organizations of families, communities, and societies. Despite the diversity of biological systems, all systems have several characteristics in common.

First, the boundaries between the system and what occurs outside the system are either *opened* or *closed* depending on whether the system receives information from outside itself. One can often tell if the system is open or closed to certain information by observing whether the system responds and acts on information that it receives. If the system consistently never responds to certain information, then it is probably closed to that particular piece of information.

Second, biological systems always serve one or more biological *functions.* Those biological functions serve to justify the system's existence. Systems are arranged hierarchically based on the importance of their functions; the more important the function, the higher in the hierarchy (Fig. 9-1). This hierarchy is important to understand, as changes in one system, if those changes cause perturbations in a higher-level system, are likely to be resisted as the functioning of the higher-level system takes precedence.

Third, *feedback loops* (interaction patterns) within the system serve to regulate the behavior or functioning of the elements in the system. These feedback loops or interaction patterns are brought into play when a disturbance in individual functioning occurs. Their purpose is to restore the behavior of the individual elements to their previous level of functioning so that the entire system can fulfill its function. The tendency of a system to return individual elements to a stable level of functioning, maintaining systemic equilibrium, is termed **homeostasis.** Feedback loops and interaction patterns serve to maintain systemic homeostasis.

Fourth, systems are, therefore, *resistant to change,* because feedback loops continue to return the system to its previous level of functioning when it is perturbed. Because feedback loops also serve to maintain the functioning of individual elements of a system at a certain level, attempting to change the functioning of an individual element is very difficult, as feedback loops will attempt to restore the behavior of the individual element and thus the entire system to its previous equilibrium.

The physiological system within the human body that regulates blood sugar levels can be used as an example of these system principles (Fig. 9-2). The blood sugar regulatory system is primarily composed of two feedback loops. One loop involves pancreatic secretion of insulin in response to elevated blood sugar levels, and the other loop involves secretion of epinephrine, norepinephrine, cortisol, growth hormone, and glucagon in response to low blood sugar levels. These feedback loops serve to maintain blood sugar within a normal range, ensuring adequate functioning of the human brain and other organs that are dependent on blood sugar as a source of nutrition. In an attempt to fulfill this very important function, the system not only responds to *actual* blood sugar levels but also to other information, such as eating or exercise, that might in the future result in either elevation or reduction of blood sugar. This open boundary allows the system to prepare itself in advance of the activity that may have an effect on blood sugar.

Trying to change the level at which blood sugar is maintained by infusing a sugar solution into the vein of a human volunteer would, because of feedback loops designed to lower blood sugar, quickly result in restoration of blood sugar

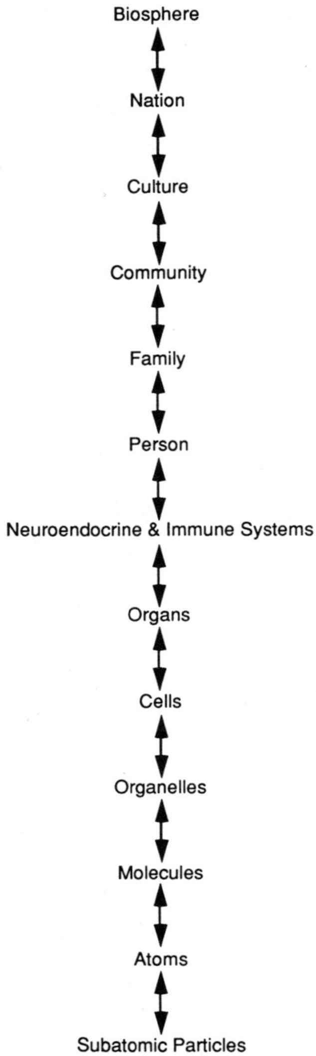

Figure 9-1. The hierarchy of natural systems. Adapted from Engel (1977).

levels to the normal range even if the infusion is increased to progressively higher and higher levels. Furthermore, if this primary system were exhausted and blood sugar rose above the normal range, secondary systems would come into play such as spillage of sugar in the urine, which would also attempt to restore blood sugar to normal.

Gregory Bateson was one of the first to apply systems principles to families (Bateson, 1972). He noted that, like the physiological system that regulates blood sugar within the human body, the family too develops feedback loops and interaction patterns that regulate the behavior of its individual members. Once these feedback loops or interaction patterns have been established, it becomes very difficult to change the behavior of a family member unless the feedback loops that maintain behavior are also changed.

Similarly, disease symptoms, illness behavior, and health behaviors can be stabilized by these feedback loops within the family. If illness behaviors, such as noncompliance, for example, are stabilized by the system, the clinician can become frustrated when repeated straightforward attempts to modify the illness-causing behavior are thwarted by the feedback loops within the family system.

Case 9-1 is a good example of systems principles. The disease state, diabetic ketoacidosis, should be fairly easily preventable with appropriate amounts of insulin injected by the diabetic adolescent. However, in this case the adolescent continues to have frequent attacks despite larger and larger doses of insulin. A family factor that could be maintaining this unhealthy situation is the fact that the patient has not been given the responsibility in her family to manage her IDDM. Because she is at a developmental stage in which independence is a critical issue, this fact could be causing her to rebel against her parents and her doctor's instructions by eating an excessive amount of foods high in sugar content in an attempt to establish independence from her parents. Her parents in turn may be responding to this by attempting to exert even more control over her IDDM by being very diligent in monitoring her blood sugar levels, causing her to rebel further and to become even more noncompliant with her diet. Such a feedback loop, consisting of the adolescent's IDDM becoming more out of control, resulting in more parental control, resulting in the patient's IDDM becoming more out of control, could explain the frequent attacks of diabetic ketoacidosis. Based on this theory, interventions can be designed to interfere with the feedback loop that is stabilizing the unhealthy behavior pattern.

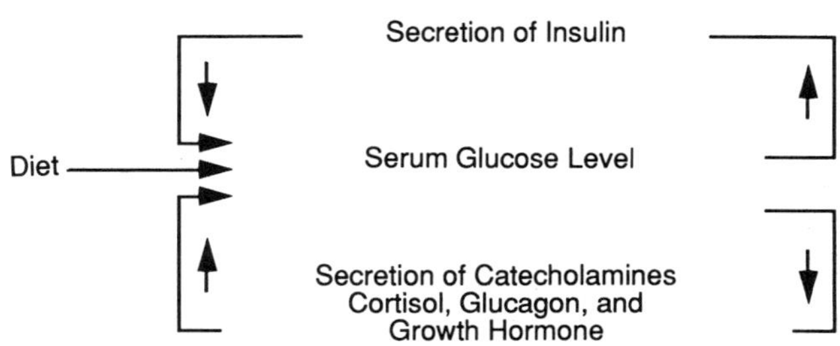

Figure 9-2. The physiological systems within humans that regulate blood sugar levels.

Because the family system model takes into account the rich complexity of relationships within the family, and because it ties in nicely with models of family therapy that enable clinicians to change systems and so improve their patient's health, it has achieved a slight dominance in the clinical setting over other models of how the family affects health. Because the family system model is more congruent with the biopsychosocial model of medical care, it is the model used in the rest of this chapter. Before preceding with more case examples and research studies, it is important to define some family system terms.

DEFINITION OF FAMILY SYSTEM TERMS

The first family systems term to be defined is family. Surprisingly, the definition of what constitutes a family is quite controversial. Structural definitions, such as "two or more people related by blood, marriage, or adoption who live in the same dwelling" are very common, yet they are to a certain degree too restrictive. For example, a heterosexual or homosexual couple who have lived together for 20 years would not constitute a family under the above definition. To compensate for the restrictive nature of structural definitions, functional definitions have been developed. For example, family can be defined as a handful of intimates who provide social support and to whom one turns in times of physical or emotional crises (Smilkstein, 1980). Given the remarkable changes in family structures that have occurred over the past two decades, it becomes important to maintain flexibility about what constitutes a family and, more importantly, to allow an individual the prerogative of defining his or her own family.

Family interaction patterns are stable, predictable, repetitive behaviors that regulate the behavior of family members. These patterns can be classified as normal or abnormal. Normal family interaction patterns are those that allow the family the best chance of fulfilling its functions. The most important function of the family is to encourage the growth and development of its members; however, other family functions are also important (Table 9-2). Normal family interaction patterns also change depending on the family's current developmental tasks. Therefore, it is particularly important to consider the family's developmental stage when assessing family interaction patterns (Table 9-3).

When looking at American middle-class families, Minuchin and Beavers have noted that the characteristics of normal family interaction patterns include the following: (1) the boundaries between the family and the outside environment are semipermeable in that information passes freely but selectively be-

Table 9-2
Family Functions

Individual growth and development
Provision of life-sustaining resources
Goal setting and problem solving
Sexual gratification of marital partners
Fulfillment of recreational needs

tween the family and the larger community; (2) the parents form a family subsystem in which adult needs are fulfilled, agreement on childrearing practices is mutual, both parents take an active and cooperative role in childrearing, and children are not involved in parental conflict; (3) children form a family subsystem in which they are not forced to behave inappropriately for their developmental stage and in which they receive an appropriate amount of parental support to ensure adequate growth and development; and (4) communication both among and within the subsystems is flexible, clear, and direct (Lewis, Beavers, & Gossett, 1976; Minuchin, 1974).

Abnormal family interaction patterns are those that prevent the normal growth and development of family members. Family therapists have described several types of interaction patterns that seem to be abnormal the great majority of time, particularly if they are rigid and do not yield easily to simple therapeutic interventions (Table 9-4).

The family in Case 9-1 illustrates an abnormal family interaction pattern. Clearly, from the brief presentation of this patient and her family, something appears to be wrong. First, the patient is not taking adequate responsibility for the management of her IDDM. Second, the parents seem overly close to her, knowing things about her, such as her blood sugar level, that even she does not know about herself and that are not verified by objective data. Third, the continued pattern of repeat hospitalizations for diabetic ketoacidosis suggests that this interaction pattern is rigid and unchanging.

The specific abnormal family interaction pattern that is exemplified by this case is called **enmeshment.** All members of the family are so close to one another emotionally that the patient cannot develop sufficiently as an individual to meet the demands of her IDDM. This parental response has been termed overprotectiveness. The combination of enmeshment, rigidity, parental overprotectiveness, and the apparent lack of conflict in this family are all characteristics of what Minuchin has called a "psychosomatic" family (Minuchin, Baker, Rosman, Liebman, Milman, & Todd, 1975).

Minuchin began studying diabetic adolescents from psychosomatic families when an endocrinologist named Baker came to him puzzled over a number of similar cases to the one described in Case 9-1. Minuchin studied them by subjecting both the patient and the family to a diagnostic interview while measuring free fatty acid levels via intravenous lines placed before the interview (Minuchin,

Table 9-3
Family Life Cycle Tasks

Stage	Tasks
Newly married	Negotiating roles/boundaries/ intimacy issues
Families with young children	Caretaking
Families with adolescents	Negotiating adolescent independence issues
Launching stage	Adapting to a smaller family
Older/retired families	Reemergence of couple issues

Rosman, & Baker, 1978). Minuchin's diagnostic interview with these families consisted of four phases: (1) accommodation, (2) parental conflict (induced by Minuchin) with the adolescent absent but watching through a one-way mirror, (3) parental conflict with the child present in the room with the parents, and (4) a resting phase. Minuchin and Baker hypothesized that these adolescents experienced frequent attacks of diabetic ketoacidosis because of increased secretion of catecholamines (reflected by increasing free fatty acid levels) resulting from abnormal interaction patterns within their families. Catecholamines are hormones whose actions are directly antagonistic to the effects of insulin, causing blood sugar levels to rise.

The results of the study were quite remarkable. Compared to a group of diabetic adolescents who were in good diabetic control, and a second group of diabetic adolescents who manifested noncompliant behavior, the adolescents from psychosomatic families had continued and sustained rises in their free fatty acid levels even during the resting phase. Free fatty acid levels in the other two groups of diabetic adolescents fell during phases 1 and 2, rising only during phase 3 when the diabetic adolescents were present during parental conflict and falling again during phase 4. In the psychosomatic family the parents' free fatty acid levels fell and continued to fall during phase four, while their child's free fatty acid levels continued to rise. Parents from families in which the diabetic adolescent was noncompliant showed continued elevation in their free fatty acid levels through phase 3, dropping in phase 4 back to base line, whereas parents from diabetic adolescents who were in good control showed little elevation of free fatty acids during any of the phases.

Minuchin felt that the rising free fatty acid levels of adolescents while free fatty acid levels of parents fell during phase 3 represented a "transfer of stress" in which the stress of the experimental situation was literally transferred to the adolescents in these psychosomatic families. In observing phase 3 interviews, Minuchin noted that parents from psychosomatic families did not continue their

Table 9-4
Abnormal Family Interaction Patterns[a]

Variable	Definition
Conflict	Emotional disagreement between members of the same system
Triangle	Triadic interaction pattern often characterized by an alliance between two members of a system against a third
Disengagement	Quality of a family in which members are emotionally distant
Enmeshment	Quality of a family system in which members are overly close emotionally
Complementary	Communication pattern in dyadic relationships in which differences between participants are maximized, for example, when one partner is overly assertive and the other is overly submissive
Symmetric	Communication pattern in dyadic relationships in which differences between participants are minimized; for example, communications among friends of the same peer group is often symmetrical
Rules/issues	Interaction patterns or behavioral laws that stabilize the family system, often manifestations of the ways families avoid open, active conflict

[a] Adapted from Mengel (1987c).

phase 2 arguments but instead focused on the adolescent, showing a great deal of concern for the adolescent. During phase 3 in the other two groups of families, parents continued their arguments, allowing the adolescent some input into the argument but not focusing on the adolescent as their sole concern.

As might be expected, Minuchin found that severe marital conflict existed between the spouses in these psychomsomatic families, which was buried beneath a show of concern and caring for their diabetic adolescent. Thus, the function of the frequent attacks of diabetic ketoacidosis that justified parental overprotectiveness was to keep the parents from fighting, keep the family together, and maintain the homeostasis of the family unit. Because the adolescent's IDDM being out of control served a function within these families, it was very difficult to bring these patients under better control through normal medical interventions. Fortunately, Minuchin discovered that structured family therapy enabled 80% of these families to return to a more normal existence, significantly decreasing the frequency of attacks of diabetic ketoacidosis in their adolescent children.

Case 9-2: Adolescent Abdominal Pain. A 12-year-old female presented to an emergency room late on a Saturday afternoon with complaints of bilateral lower abdominal pain. The physician was not able to see her until 1 h later. Because of that delay, when the physician eventually entered the room, the patient's father was very angry. After expressing his anger about the wait and hearing the physician's explanation, he sat back in his chair in a corner of the room, crossed his arms, and uttered little during the rest of the interview. Turning his attention to the child, the physician noted that she was on the verge of tears but gave an adequate description of her pain. Her pain was dull, achy in quality, had started 1 week ago, and was not associated with any other gastrointestinal or genitourinary symptoms. A physical examination revealed a temperature of 102°F and severe rebound tenderness in both lower quadrants of the abdomen.

After noting that the child was severely ill and noting that the father had not provided any information during the interview and examination of the patient, the physician asked the father specifically why he had not brought the daughter into the emergency room sooner. He replied that he felt that his daughter was always "faking" and so did not think that her pain was real. When the physician asked why he had finally brought his daughter to the emergency room if he thought that she was faking, the father stated that his wife, who was attending a baseball game with their son, had ordered him to bring her in. The physician then asked the father to leave the room and confirmed his suspicions of pelvic inflammatory disease by performing a pelvic exam (Mengel, 1987a).

The above case illustrates an abnormal family interaction pattern that occurred between the patient and her father. The almost total lack of emotional feeling or attachment between the father and daughter suggests *disengagement.* Most parents cannot resist to some degree interrupting their children when physicians are taking a history or performing a physical examination on their offspring. They usually demonstrate at least some measure of sympathy when their children are in pain. In this case, no expression of emotion was displayed by the father toward his daughter. Recognizing this disengagement helped the physician to make the proper diagnosis in this case, since many dysfunctional events can occur in a disengaged family without the knowledge of other family members. In this case, brother–sister incest was the cause of the patient's pelvic inflammatory disease resulting in her pain and her emergency room visit. When the father was confronted with this fact, he admitted that incest had occurred in the past between his daughter and her older brother, but he felt that he had put a stop to it. He reasoned that his son had committed this violation of his daughter because he had recently left the family to join the army. However, the father was able to get in touch with his son's drill sergeant, who ordered his son to submit to an examination that yielded a positive culture for *Neisseria gonorrhoeae*. The daughter's culture was also positive for *Neisseria gonorrhoeae*.

As the physician continued to care for members of this family, further information came to light that helped him to understand how disengagement had developed within this family. Fourteen years prior to the emergency room visit all four of the parents' natural children had perished in a house fire. The couple was visiting friends at the time. Even though the fire was in no way their fault, their grief and guilt over the death of their children must have been tremendous. A few years later, as they were unable to have more children, the couple began adopting children, actually replacing as best they could the children they had lost in the fire. They eventually adopted four children, all from different parents, actually mimicking the sex and closely mimicking the age distribution of their natural children from oldest to youngest.

Such attempts to replace lost loved ones rarely work and are usually a sign of a person's attempt, in this case the couple's attempt, to prevent working through a very painful grief response, accepting a loss, and moving on to future endeavors. The reason this replacement rarely works is that the physical presence of the surrogate loved ones continually reminds the person of their loss. In an attempt to prevent such a continual reminder, the family in this case became very disengaged. Thus, the disengagement in this family functioned to bury the couple's grief even further.

Unfortunately, the health cost of this disengagement was very high, in that adequate supervision of the children was not possible, resulting in the awful event that caused the daughter's illness. One could also hypothesize that the psychological development of these children was not optimal, as family disengagement prevented the necessary support the children needed to develop into mature adults.

Case 9-3: Family Obesity. Jennifer is a poor middle-aged female on food stamps who claims to eat less than is metabolically possible given her 260-lb weight. For the past month her physician has been asking Jennifer to record all that she eats; however, that record has not yielded any significant reason for her obesity. The physician then prescribes a diet for Jennifer; however, over the next month Jennifer makes little progress on that diet and, in fact, gains 5 lb. Instead of becoming frustrated with Jennifer's noncompliance, the physician tells Jennifer that she is trying too hard with her diet and that she is probably going a bit too fast. He suggests to Jennifer that she go more slowly, staying in control and maintaining her present weight, before she takes any steps toward further dieting. One week later Jennifer returns having lost 3 lb.

Why might this reverse psychology, called a "paradoxical intervention," work? To answer that question, an examination of Jennifer's family is necessary. Jennifer recently stopped living with her mother, on whom she was very dependent. Jennifer states that her mother was clearly "in charge" of their relationship, with Jennifer receiving many orders on how to behave and what to eat. Jennifer left because she was "fed up" with her mother's orders even though she had stopped following them years ago, wanting to be more in charge of her own life.

Jennifer and her mother were in a *complementary* interaction pattern in which the mother ordered and Jennifer obeyed or appeared to obey. Jennifer was never treated as an equal in her interactions with her mother. In fact, in this system the only area in which Jennifer appeared to have some control was in her eating behavior. Despite her mother's orders, Jennifer could control what food entered her mouth. Thus, although many might see Jennifer's inability or unwillingness to follow her mother's and doctor's dietary instructions as a subtle form of rebellion, it actually appears that this was also Jennifer's way of asserting independence.

Because of this period of her life when Jennifer was not able to assert her independence in a responsible manner, when confronted with parental figures such as doctors she follows previous complementary interaction patterns by receiving orders from authority figures but then not following them. Thus, when her physician prescribed a diet, the inevitable happened: she appeared to comply with the diet but actually rebelled by eating something not on the diet but not specifically forbidden either. The physician, noting the failure of standard dietary interventions, used Jennifer's comfort with complementary interaction patterns by ordering her not to diet but to stay in control. Jennifer accepted the order without questioning but then rebelled against the doctor, as she would her mother, by actually eating less. The physician continued this pattern of paradox by expressing shock and regret that Jennifer had lost so much weight when she came back for a follow-up visit. He sternly warned her that she was moving too fast and that she should slow down and stay in control or else something terrible might happen.

Paradoxical intervention is a difficult and powerful therapeutic technique and thus should not be done without great care. It is mentioned here not so much to illustrate the technique but to illustrate complementary interaction patterns. The key therapeutic point to determine is how Jennifer's eating behavior functions in her family system. As mentioned previously, Jennifer's eating behavior not only represented a way that she could assert herself, thus achieving individual growth and development within her family system, but in addition, it served as a behavior example that justified her mother's belief that Jennifer was incapable of caring for herself, thus needing continued maternal intervention. Thus, Jennifer's behavior served two critical functions within her family system. As long as Jennifer was obese, she could continue to assert her independence, and her mother felt needed.

By seeing how Jennifer's behavior fit in her family system, it is easier to understand Jennifer's rebelliousness. If Jennifer became thin too quickly, she would lose her only method of asserting her independence and enabling her mother to feel needed. The doctor's intervention took this into account by allowing Jennifer to assert her independence by losing weight rather than gaining it. One might hypothesize that since Jennifer's mother was not involved in this intervention, it too might eventually fail as Jennifer's dieting might suggest to the mother that she was no longer needed. The mother might then begin to covertly sabotage the doctor's efforts to encourage Jennifer to lose weight.

Recent research supports many of the above points. Brownell *et al.* studied obese adolescents treated in a 1-year intensive weight reduction program (Brownell, Kelman, & Stunkard, 1983). Adolescents were divided into three groups: (1) *mother involved,* in which the adolescent's mother was actively involved in the treatment program, (2) *mother present,* in which the adolescents' mothers met in their own separate groups apart from the adolescents' groups, and (3) *mother uninvolved,* in which the adolescent's mothers were not involved in the weight loss program whatsoever. Significant weight loss occurred only in the mother-present group. The adolescents in the mother-involved group and the adolescents in the mother-uninvolved group did not lose significant weight during the study period. Brownell *et al.* hypothesized that these findings resulted from the fact that the adolescent's problem-maintaining system, in this case, an obesity-maintaining system, was blocked by treating the mother and adolescent separately. An overinvolved complementary mother could no longer suppress the adolescent's desire for independence (and subsequent rebellion by overeating), as mothers were not directly involved in the adolescent's treatment and because the mother's separate treatment group blocked attempts by the mothers to interfere with their adolescent's treatment at home. Maternal interference was not blocked by the group in which the adolescent's mother was actively involved in treatment, and thus, the results were similar to those of the group in which the adolescent's mother was not involved at all.

Case 9-4: The Family Alcoholism Cycle. A 43-year-old male presented to his physician's office with a 2-week history of intermittent epigastric pain that was partially relieved by antacids. A physical exam did not reveal any abnormalities, but laboratory testing showed a megaloblastic anemia (decreased numbers of larger than normal red blood cells) and abnormal liver function tests. When the gentleman, a government executive, returned after a trial of cimetidine (an ulcer medication) had been only partially successful, the physician discussed the laboratory abnormalities with him. He asked specifically about his use of alcohol. The gentlemen replied, "Sure, I drink, but its under control. No, no, not much, just a couple of beers when I get home from work, maybe two highballs if I go out with the guys from work. No, I've had only two blackout spells, and no it doesn't affect my work. Now, just a minute, Doc, let's get off this alcohol stuff. What are you going to do about my stomach?"

The physician quickly recognized that this man was chemically dependent and guessed that his stomach pains were related to alcoholic gastritis. This man, in contrast to the overweight patient in the previous case, who at least recognized that there was a problem, denied any problem except for his pain. He stated that he could stop his drinking at any time without any trouble at all. He just wanted something done about his stomach pain—now.

When this patient's family was invited to the physician's office for a visit, they did not mention the patient's use of alcohol until the physician raised the issue. Everyone in the family expressed shock and surprise, particularly the patient's spouse, when the physician mentioned his hypothesis that the patient might be an alcoholic. In fact, the spouse stated almost exactly the same thing as the patient, saying, "No, no, Doc, you've got it all wrong. He's got his use of alcohol under control. It doesn't affect his job and it doesn't affect our relationship at all. Now, what are you going to do about his stomach pain?" The couple presented a very united front when it came to defending against the alcoholism hypothesis. The physician explored their family power structure in some detail and was struck by the almost rigid equality in their relationship. Further questioning by the physician confirmed the *symmetrical* nature of the interaction pattern that existed between the couple.

The symmetry of alcoholism is displayed in Fig. 9-3. Bateson has commented that symmetrical interaction patterns are characterized by positive feedback loops that maintain the problem behavior to such an extent that it can spiral out of control quite quickly (Bateson, 1972). Drinking behavior begins either because of a genetic disposition or as a learned social behavior. Most people who drink respond to societal checks that control drinking behavior so that it doesn't lead to irresponsible actions. Such checks are usually provided by spouses and employers who are willing to act in a complementary fashion to the alcoholic, suggesting or ordering that the alcoholic stop drinking. However, spouses and employers who act in a symmetric fashion and do not check the alcoholic's drinking behavior actually encourage that behavior. The failure to check the alcoholic's drinking behavior leads to irresponsible behavior on the part of the alcoholic and a poorer self-image, which predisposes to further drinking behavior.

The feedback loop on the right of Fig. 9-3 further reinforces the cycle of drinking behavior as spouses, employers, or even children overcompensate for the alcoholic's irresponsible behavior by performing tasks that the alcoholic

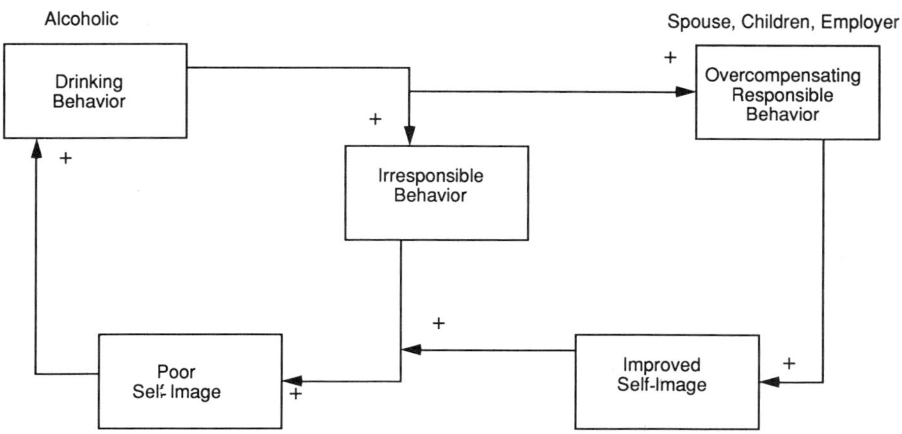

Figure 9-3. Symmetrical interaction patterns that maintain alcoholism.

should be performing, resulting in an improvement in their own self-image, which encourages more of the same. This behavior on the part of the alcoholic's significant others is called *enabling behavior* and is very important to take into account when treating alcoholism.

The treatment of alcoholism is most successful if a multimodality approach is utilized. In most cases, the alcoholic patient is referred to Alcoholics Anonymous, which attempt to improve the self-image of the alcoholic. Enabling behavior is treated through the use of Al-Anon or Alateen, organizations that encourage spouses and children of alcoholics to act complementary to the alcoholic when he or she is drinking in an attempt to discourage the drinking behavior. Likewise, employer assistance programs seek to present the alcoholic with employer sanctions if the alcoholic behavior does not improve. Use of this multimodality approach has resulted in greater than 60% 1-year abstinence rates if the alcoholic is treated at an early stage (Mendelson & Mello, 1985; Blum & Roman, 1986). Unfortunately, if the cycle is allowed to run for a long time, cure rates decrease substantially.

Unfortunately, in the case described above, the patient and his wife refused therapy and refused to see the physician further. However, the confrontation was not necessarily without value. It may require several confrontations, and even a personal or family crisis may be needed, to convince an alcoholic to seek treatment.

Case 9-5: Family Hair Loss. A 28-year-old woman presented to her physician's office with multiple circular patches of hair loss beginning a week before. The physician diagnosed alopecia areata and began treating her with monthly intralesional injections of a steroid medication, which were moderately successful in restoring her hair over the next 4 months. However, over the next 3 years she continued to develop outbreaks of alopecia areata approximately one to two times per year, sometimes accompanied by frequent headaches. Because of the recurrent nature of her alopecia areata in the absence of any systemic disease to account for the recurrences, a more detailed assessment of the family was undertaken.

The family assessment uncovered the following information. The patient married for the second time 4 years ago. Her first marriage had ended because her former spouse was both verbally and physically abusive. She had two children during her first marriage, none during her current marriage. She was concerned that her current husband might be "two-timing" her and might be drinking too much. When her level of anxiety about her husband's behavior peaked, arguments and sometimes physical fights developed between her and her spouse, fortunately with no significant injuries. An examination of the relationship between spousal conflict and her attacks of alopecia areata over the past 3 years revealed a pattern in which attacks of alopecia areata seemed to follow times of intense family conflict (Mengel, 1987b).

This case illustrates the profound effect family conflict can have on individual health. The physician in this case hypothesized that the patient's family conflict represented a stress to her immune system, resulting in the formation of or failure to control the actions of autoantibodies that attacked her hair follicles causing alopecia areata. Research linking attacks of herpes simplex to family stress also support this hypothesis (Katcher, Brightman, Luborsky, & Ship, 1973; Monjan & Collector, 1977).

This case also demonstrates the development of an *emotional triangle* that stabilized the patient's symptoms. When conflicts develop between two people who are close emotionally, a very natural human response is to seek an ally or friend who can provide support in the battle against a close adversary. If one is successful in seeking an ally but not successful in ending the conflict, a triangle is formed. Triangles or triads are important stabilizers in family systems. In this case, the triangle that stabilized the patient's family system consisted of her, her husband, and the health care provider. Her physician's support allowed her to withstand the marital conflict without having to fully resolve it. In fact, any verbal support from the physician for her position in the conflict was no doubt brought home and used as fuel for the fire.

The physician finally intervened in the family conflict by inviting the husband in for a visit. Instead of finding a "mean ogre," the physician found a soft-spoken, meek, almost "Casper Milquetoast" kind of man. During the interview, the patient was very strong in her criticism of her husband and almost verbally abusive. It seemed as if the patient, probably because she was an abused child herself, needed to see her husband as a victimizer and so did everything in her power short of buying him a gun to make him into one. The interview revealed that she not only taunted him and accused him of marital crimes he did not commit but withheld sex from him and did not allow him to participate in the raising of his two children. Being so treated, the husband did not get his emotional needs met and so responded, according to his past family of origin pattern, by drinking. The physician, recognizing the abnormal pattern that was maintaining the illness behavior, referred the couple to marital therapy, the wife into group therapy with other victims of abuse, and the husband into alcoholism treatment. This intervention met with moderate success such that at last report 1 year later, no attacks of alopecia areata had occurred.

The above cases serve to illustrate the point that the family is more than simply a collection of individuals. It is an organization in its own right with very important functions to fulfill. These functions are fulfilled by interaction patterns that regulate members' behaviors. When symptoms or disease states serve a stabilizing function within the family, they can be very difficult to treat. Recognizing abnormal interaction patterns associated with symptoms within a family can help the physician make a more accurate diagnosis (as in the case of pelvic inflammatory disease), understand chronic disease exacerbations (as in the IDDM case), and effectively treat resistant medical problems, such as obesity, alcoholism, and even alopecia areata.

FAMILY ASSESSMENT

Assessment of a patient's family is a clinical activity in which the physician attempts to determine if abnormal family interaction patterns are present and, if so, how those patterns may be contributing to the patient's illness. Like any clinical activity, family assessment should be carried out only when indicated, it should be directed by a clinical hypothesis, and it should be a search for objective evidence obtained from the patient and his or her family. Multiple tools are available to the physician who wishes to perform a family assessment, including direct observation, specific questions about the family system, and construction of a family genogram.

Most clinicians have found that family assessment proceeds best if it is conducted with the patient's family present, even though it can be done with the patient alone. Other family members often present the clinician with different and sometimes competing viewpoints, and thus, more information regarding family interaction patterns can be gained. Additionally, observing family interaction patterns during the family interview offers the clinician a rich source of data.

General indications for a family assessment have been developed by several authors and are listed in Table 9-5 (Sawa, 1988; Schmidt, 1978). Many clinicians also feel that a family assessment and interview are indicated at the time of the initial diagnosis of any chronic disease, not only to determine family resources that will aid the patient in his or her initial adjustment to the disease but also to allow the physician and patient to begin to mobilize those resources. Such an interview would obviously serve an educational function for the family as well.

After determining that a family assessment needs to be performed, the physician should formulate several hypotheses regarding family interaction patterns that might be contributing to the problem at hand. Formulation of these hypotheses should be based on the physician's knowledge of the state of the patient's disease, age, psychological development, cultural issues, and the specific indications for the family assessment. For example, a person with the new diagnosis of terminal cancer will adjust better to that disease if her family rallies around her and supports her adjustment efforts. A clinician who is unaware of this helpful family adaptation to the patient's terminal disease might in fact wrongly label the patient's family as enmeshed and attempt interventions.

Table 9-5
Indications for a Family Assessment

Frequent acute illnesses
Uncontrolled chronic disease
Frequent somatic complaints
Noncompliance
Mental illness
Drug and alcohol abuse
Obesity
Behavioral problems in children
Marital problems
Hospitalization
Terminal illness
Pregnancy
Genetic counseling
Overutilization of medical services

If specific hypotheses cannot be formulated from the patient's clinical situation, then a more general approach to family assessment has been advocated by Doherty and Baird (1983) in their book entitled *Family Therapy in Family Medicine.* Doherty and Baird recommend that clinicians assess sources of stress (both within the family and outside of the family), family adaptability, family cohesion, and family interaction patterns that may lead to chronic family dysfunction. Perhaps the simplest method of conducting a general family assessment is by watching the family members interact during a clinical interview. For example, in a family in which other members often answer for the identified patient and seem to exhibit a lot of anxiety about the identified patient's case, the possibility of family enmeshment should be entertained. Observing the interaction between spouses is often very fruitful in confirming a diagnosis of family conflict or triangulation, particularly if children become involved in parental conflicts.

If simple observation does not yield enough evidence to confirm or refute a suspected abnormal family interaction pattern, direct questioning about the patient's family system may be necessary. Recently, several family therapists have developed the technique of circular questioning, in which questions are asked of one member about a situation between two other members of the family. This technique has proven especially useful in elucidating family interaction patterns (Selvini, Boscola, Ceccin, & Prata, 1980). Sawa (1988) has grouped circular questions within three categories: triadic questions, interpersonal perception questions, and differences questions. Triadic questions are questions put to one family member about a relationship between two other family members. For example, the physician may ask a child in the family, "What does your father do when your mother attempts to discipline you?" The child is commenting on his observations of the relationship between the mother and father, and if the father's behavior tends to undermine maternal discipline, then a hypothesis of conflict between the spouses is strengthened. Similarly, a father may be asked, "What does your wife do when your child's IDDM becomes out of control?" If the father's response indicates overprotectiveness on the part of the mother, then a hypothesis of enmeshment is strengthened.

Interpersonal perception questions are questions designed to explore how one person perceives another's feelings about a certain event. For example, a child could be asked, "How do you think your mother feels when your father becomes drunk?" Such a question could be followed by asking the child how she herself feels. Although similar feelings do not necessarily indicate enmeshment, they at least raise the possibility. In addition, such questions will encourage the family to discuss their feelings toward one another, feelings often buried in dysfunctional families.

A third type of circular question has to do with family differences. These questions are designed to yield information about distinctions that family members draw in comparing relationships with other family members. They often disclose alliances and triangles within the family. For example, a child may be asked, "When you misbehave, which parent is more likely to discipline you; which parent is less likely to discipline you?" In families where discipline is consistent and agreed on by the parents, most children find it slightly difficult to answer that question. When a child readily answers that question with one parent's name, the possibility of family triangulation should be raised.

Perhaps the simplest and most useful technique developed in recent years to assess the family is the construction of a genogram. A genogram is a pictorial representation of the patient's family using predefined symbols (McGoldrick & Gerson, 1985). A basic or "skeletal" genogram consisting of family structure, dates of important events, and important medical diseases can be completed in a brief period of time by the physician, yielding a great deal of information about family structure, familial disease patterns, and family adaptability to major stressful events (Crouch & Davis, 1987). Additional information about family

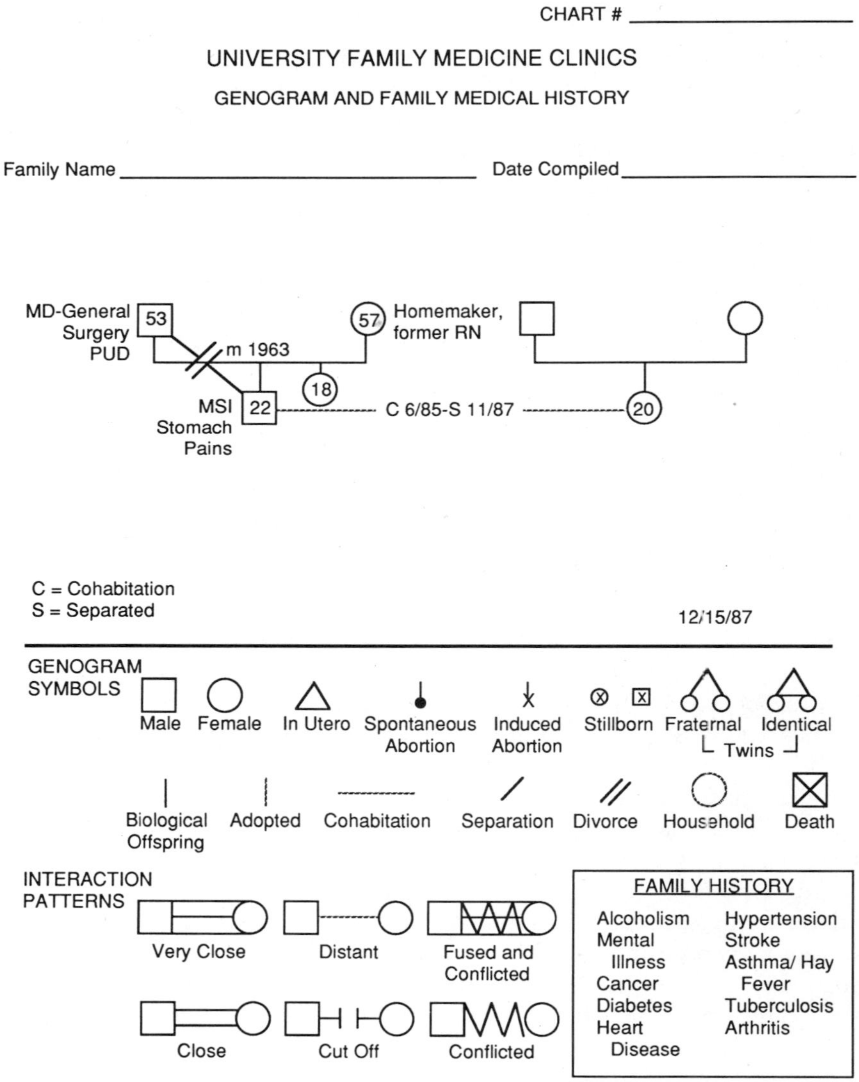

Figure 9-4. Family genogram for Case 9-6: the romantic stomach.

relationship patterns, repetitive family patterns across generations, and family imbalances in individual functioning or resource allocation can be added to the skeletal genogram as needed when the practitioner has more time.

Case 9-6: The Romantic Stomach. A 22-year-old first-year medical student presented to the student health service with complaints of stomach pains of 2 weeks' duration. The patient's description of the pains was consistent with stress-induced gastritis or peptic ulcer diseases. To investigate possible sources of stress, the physician constructed a genogram that showed that the patient had recently ended a long-term relationship at the request of his partner because he was studying too much and because his partner had found someone else (Fig. 9-4). The patient, however, wanted to resume the relationship and still saw her often as a friend, even though she was actively dating another. The patient believed that they might get back together, since his former girlfriend had never told him that reconciliation was impossible. The patient had a very close relationship with his mother, who "only wanted the best for her son" and urged him to "drop the hussy." He felt that he was very distant from his father, who worked long hours in his job as a surgeon and offered no opinion about his son's current predicament. The patient was also in the midst of final exams.

Recognizing the multiple sources of stress on this young man, the physician prescribed antiulcer medication and referred him for counseling to help him resolve his current relationship difficulties. Two months later the medication was stopped when the patient was able to formally end his relationship with his long-time partner by meeting with her and saying good-bye.

The above case illustrates the use of the genogram in assessing a patient's family. If after a family assessment is done utilizing tools of observation, questioning, and genogram construction, dysfunctional family dynamics are discovered that the clinician feels are contributing to the patient's illness, then the clinician has several intervention options depending on his or her level of comfort with family care and counseling. Doherty and Baird have recently developed five levels of physician involvement with families Table 9-6 (Doherty & Baird, 1987). No doubt most clinicians simply do not have the time to learn about and develop the skills necessary to practice family therapy (level 5 involvement), as was necessary in Case 9-6. However, many clinicians feel comfortable with

Table 9-6
Levels of Physician Involvement with Families[a]

Level	Involvement
1	Minimal emphasis on family
2	Ongoing medical information and advice
3	Exploring feelings and providing support
4	Systematic assessment and planned intervention
5	Family therapy

[a] Adapted from Doherty and Baird (1987).

level 2 and 3 involvement, for example, convening a family conference when the diagnosis of a serious or chronic disease is made in an effort to educate the family (level 2) and mobilize resources (level 3). Some clinicians enjoy level 4 work. The next case will illustrate family assessment and level 4 physician involvement.

Case 9-7: Family Hypertension. A 46-year-old female patient tells her physician that she is very worried about the health of her husband, who is an insurance executive. She states that several times during the past 2 to 3 years he has had his blood pressure taken, and it has been "borderline to high." She says that her husband is a heavy smoker, gets little regular exercise, and is overweight. She wonders if you could call him to come in for a physical exam.

At this point, the physician states that Mrs. C.'s concerns about her husband are valid and important and that he does indeed think that her husband should be examined. However, he says that he would feel uncomfortable asking Mr. C. to come in for a physical exam if he did not want to be examined. The physician does feel comfortable talking with Mr. C. on the phone and relaying Mrs. C.'s concerns to her husband. Additionally, if Mr. C. does choose to come in for an exam, he would like for Mrs. C. to come in as well. Mrs. C. asks the physician to call her husband, who after learning of his wife's concern does agree to come in for an examination. He also somewhat reluctantly agrees to have his wife accompany him.

During the meeting with the C.s, the physician begins by asking each of the partners why they have come. He learns that Mrs. C. is very concerned about her husband's health and that she has been expressing that concern by trying to get her husband to begin an exercise program, eat less, and stop smoking. She has also been asking Mr. C. to come to the physician for a physical examination almost daily during the past 2 months. From Mr. C. the physician learns that he is coming in to "get his wife off his back" and doesn't really feel that he has any health problems worth mentioning. The physician than asks Mr. C. if he is concerned about any of his wife's health problems and elicits the history that her menstrual irregularities do trouble him somewhat and he wishes that his wife would mention them. Mrs. C. simply states that she is going through menopause and doesn't feel her irregularities are important.

After eliciting these concerns, the physician mentions that it seems as though each partner is very concerned about the other's health but does not appear to share a similar concern about his or her own health. He asks them if both would be willing to submit to an examination in the next few weeks and then get back together again to hear his report.

During Mr. C.'s exam, the physician finds borderline hypertension, BP of 150/95, 20 lb of excess weight, a 60 pack-year smoking history, and a fasting cholesterol of 268 mg/dl (normal $<$ 200 mg/dl). During Mrs. C.'s exam he elicits a history of abnormal uterine bleeding occurring a year after her period ceased and a slightly enlarged uterus. He then asks the C.s to return for a joint appointment.

During the joint appointment, the physician frankly discusses the abnormalities that he found on each patient's exam. He then explains to Mr. C. that his continued sedentary life style, borderline hypertension, and smoking history will increase his risk of lung cancer, pulmonary disease, heart disease, and stroke. He explains to Mrs. C. that her abnormal uterine bleeding and her enlarged uterus raise the possibility of endometrial cancer. The physician then discusses some treatment options that each member of the pair might elect. He then asks each partner what they think about their own health conditions and options for improvement and what they think about the other partner's condition as well. Mrs. C. again states that she is very concerned about her husband's health and wishes he would adopt a healthier life style but is not worried at all about her own problem, saying that it will probably go away in a few months anyway. Mr. C. likewise states that he is "as healthy as a horse" but thinks that his wife should submit to a biopsy to ensure that she does not have endometrial cancer.

The physician then opens up a period of negotiation by stating that it again seems that both partners have significant health problems that may lead to even worse health if left untreated. He asks each spouse what he or she thinks the other could do to encourage her or him to be healthier. From Mr. C. he learns that he is tired of his wife's nagging, and if she would just "get off his back," he would have sought doctor's advice anyway. Likewise, from Mrs. C. the physician learns that she is tired of hearing of her husband's concern over her bleeding and wishes that he would spend more time at home. She is also very concerned about their only child, a son, who is going to college for his freshman year within the next several weeks. She wishes that Mr. C. would take more interest in their son so that she could feel that they are more like a family before he goes away.

After eliciting this information, he then asks each spouse if he or she would agree to discontinue the behavior that the other spouse dislikes and begin doing more of the behavior that the other spouse likes, so that each will be encouraged to take better care of him- or herself. The physician further suggests that he have separate meetings with each spouse to further discuss the options involved, since it appears that each spouse wishes that further involvement of the other in his or her health problems would stop. He obtains commitments from Mrs. C. that she will no longer "nag" her husband about his health problems and from Mr. C. that he will come home early at least twice a week to be with his family and take the family out at least once a week for an outing.

Subsequent follow-up visits with Mrs. C. reveal that she is pleased that her husband is spending more time at home. She submits to an endometrial biopsy, which does not reveal cancer. Likewise, Mr. C. is pleased that his wife is no longer nagging him about his health problems. He agrees to begin working on one of his risk factors at a time, choosing to stop smoking first by using a nicotine-containing chewing gum and enrolling in a stop-smoking group. Over the next 6 months he not only quits smoking but, without any further intervention from the clinician, lowers the amount of salt in his diet and begins an exercise program that results in a lowering of his blood pressure.

Physicians can have very powerful effects on their patients by utilizing their knowledge of family systems and being willing to attempt simple educational and supportive interventions after a process of negotiation with their patients. As illustrated by the above case, these straightforward family interventions can sometimes achieve a higher rate of success than more traditional biomedical ones. For example, if the physician in the above case had prematurely allied with the wife and requested her husband to come in for a physical exam without the husband being given a similar chance to express his concerns about his wife's health, then much of the physician's efforts to get the husband to change his behavior would have no doubt been resisted, since the husband would have perceived the physician to be an ally of his nagging wife. The physician's knowledge of systems theory helped him to free himself of that potential triangle and uncover the symmetrically conflicted relationship that existed between the spouses and the added stress of a member of the family leaving the household. By utilizing that information the physician was able to successfully negotiate an intervention with the couple. The key to this negotiated intervention was the fact that both spouses had concerns about the other's health; therefore, both would have to agree to exhibit more helpful behaviors toward the other spouse while at the same time agreeing to stop unhelpful behaviors. When an agreement was obtained from both spouses at the same time, the symmetry of the relationship was maintained, and a healthier outcome was possible.

Joint education is perhaps the easiest family intervention that a physician can undertake (level 2). The effect of family education has been shown to improve patient compliance and blood pressure control in a study by Morisky *et al.* of 400 ambulatory hypertensive outpatients over a 5-year period (Morisky, Levine, Grein, Shapiro, Russell, & Smith, 1983). Patients were randomized to receive either all or part of three educational interventions: (1) an exit interview to increase understanding of and compliance with prescribed medicine, (2) a home visit to encourage a family member to provide support for the patient's regimen, and (3) an invitation to attend a small group session to increase patient confidence and the ability to manage his or her problems. Patients who received any of the educational interventions increased their compliance, improved their blood pressure control, and decreased their overall hypertension-related mortality at 5 years when compared to the control groups that received none of the educational interventions. When examining the group of patients that received the home visit in which the spouse was educated about the patient's hypertension and encouraged to support the patient in controlling his or her blood pressure, Morisky *et al.* found that these people had even fewer missed appointments, even better blood pressure control, and experienced a further 57% decrease in hypertension-rated mortality when compared to those groups of patients who did not receive such a family intervention.

Doherty and Baird have recently developed an intervention that clinicians can utilize with noncompliant adult patients and their families (Doherty & Baird, 1984). The main facet of this approach is not only family education and support but negotiation of a contract with family members. The contract details very specific ways family members agree to support the patient as he or she attempts to adhere to the treatment regimen. Steps in this protocol are shown in Table 9-7. Actually establishing a family contract with frequent visits to monitor the effects of the contract may be necessary for some families resistant to simple educational or supportive family interventions.

Unfortunately, physicians often *underestimate* the degree to which patients do in fact want a family conference (Kushner & Meyer, 1989). Additionally, patients wanted their primary care physicians to provide *all* of Doherty and Baird's levels of physician–family involvement, including family therapy! Although this thought may be frightening to many physicians who already suffer under significant time constraints, these desires do indicate that patients often want the involvement of their families in their health care, and they want their physicians to coordinate such involvement.

Another study by Kushner, Meyer, and Hansen (1989) provides further support for the idea that patients want family conferences in certain situations. In a survey of family practice patients, these investigators showed that patients want family conferences for the following situations: hospitalization for serious illness (89%), new diagnosis of a serious illness (83%), depression (71%), marital relationship problems (48%), stress-related symptoms (49%), and frequent visits without improvement (37%). Recently, McDaniel, Campbell, and Seaburn developed a protocol for convening the family that attempts to alleviate patient and physician discomfort at the idea of family involvement (McDaniel, Campbell, & Seaburn, 1990).

If a family conference where education, attempts to increase family supportive behavior, negotiation, and contracting does not seem to have the desired effect on the health of the patient, then the physician should consider referring the patient and his or her family to a family therapist for a more thorough assessment and intervention. Likewise, physicians who are uncomfortable with even straightforward family interventions may wish to refer their patients to a family therapist earlier if traditional biomedical interventions fail to improve their patients' health.

Table 9-7
Steps in Doherty and Baird's Family Compliance Counseling Protocol[a]

Steps	Process
1	Assemble the family to talk about the patient's illness and its treatment
2	Discuss the medical problem with the family
3	Elicit questions from the family about the illness
4	Elicit family feelings and reactions to the illness
5	Formulate a supportive family contract centering around adherence by the patient to the treatment regimen
6	Hand out educational materials for the family to read
7	Schedule follow-up visits or referrals as needed

[a] Adapted from Doherty and Baird (1984).

Family therapists have developed a wide variety of theories and techniques that can be applied to the correction of dysfunctional aspects of patients' families. Minuchin developed structural family therapy, which has been very successful in correcting family enmeshment and conflicts centering around control issues (Minuchin, 1974). A brief goal-oriented approach has been developed by theorists at the Mental Research Institute that has been very helpful in changing rigid patterns of interactions (Fisch, Weakland, & Segal, 1982). Strategic family therapists have designed "paradoxical" interventions that have proven useful in changing rigid interaction patterns unresponsive to more straightforward methods (Madanes, 1981; Palazzoli, Boscolo, Cecchin, & Prata, 1978). Finally, experiential therapists such as Whittaker and Satir have utilized techniques that can resolve issues of family intimacy (Whittaker & Keith, 1981; Satir, 1972).

Finally, clinicians practicing from a systemic point of view should continually check to insure that they have not unsuspectingly become allied with a certain subsystem of the family to the exclusion of other subsystems (Mengel, 1987c). Dysfunctional families are often very good at embroiling unsuspecting physicians in their own conflicts. Such alliances unfortunately only serve to maintain the problem rather than encouraging a change in the system. Maintenance of an open, compassionate, neutral stance with all members of the family, and a commitment to negotiation over the goals and modalities of therapy are important, particularly when working with dysfunctional families.

CONCLUSIONS

The patient's family is one of, if not the, most important social systems to which a person belongs. Powerful interaction patterns within the family system often serve to maintain established patterns of behavior. These dynamics, when understood and rechanneled, can be used to improve the health of individual family members.

Viewing the patient's family from either the socioepidemiologic model or the systems model has great utility in determining if patients' families may be affecting disease states or illness behavior. The systems model of family functioning has enabled clinicians to assess patients' families to determine whether abnormal interaction patterns are occurring and then to tailor their therapeutic interventions based on those patterns.

Obtaining a genogram has emerged as the dominant family assessment technique in the clinical setting, although observation and questioning, particularly circular questioning if other family members are present, are also valuable assessment techniques. The genogram is a pictorial display in which standardized symbols represent family structure, important facts about the family, and family dynamics. Once enough information has been collected, the physician can formulate specific hypotheses of how the family is affecting the patient's health.

Physicians can choose the level of family intervention at which they would like to participate, referring patients to skilled family therapists when such patients don't respond to standard biomedical or straightforward family educational, supportive, or negotiated interventions. Improving dysfunctional family systems has great potential not only for improving family functioning but for favorably affecting the course of the patients' disease as well.

CASES FOR DISCUSSION

Case 1

A 27-year-old man presents to your office with complaints of palpitations. He is worried about his heart and specifically requests a stress test. A history reveals that he has no cardiac symptoms other than intermittent palpitations. His physical exam is normal. A resting ECG in your office reveals no abnormalities. At this point you explain to him that a stress test is very expensive, and since there is no medical indications for the test, his insurance will probably not cover it and he will have to pay for the test himself. The patients states "there is no problem," saying that his mother will pay for the cost of the test. At that point you take a more complete social history and learn that the patient was the youngest of five children. He is unmarried and lives with his mother. His father died 10 years ago of alcoholism. Although your patient does not admit to alcohol use, he does say that he uses cocaine intermittently, but emphatically denies that he is addicted.

1. Would you order the stress test on this patient?
2. Is there any evidence that abnormal family interaction patterns are present in this case?
3. What function could those abnormal family interaction patterns be serving?
4. If you suspect that your patient is a cocaine addict, what strategy would you use to encourage him to enroll in a treatment program, and why? (a) State flatly that you think he is a cocaine addict and then encourage him to enroll in an inpatient rehabilitation immediately. (b) Ask to meet with the patient, his mother, and any other family members who are in the area to discuss the patient's use of cocaine. (c) Order the stress test and, if that is normal, state to the patient that his use of cocaine does not appear to be affecting his heart and believe him when he says he only uses cocaine recreationally. (d) Not order the stress test, believe the patient when he says he is not addicted to cocaine, and ask him to return if he has any more problems.

Case 2

A 16-year-old girl with mild to moderate asthma presents to your office with an attack lasting 1 to 2 days. You have been following this patient for the past 5 months and have noticed that every time she comes in for an attack, almost monthly, her theophylline level is subtherapeutic even though you have asked her to take a regular dose of medication every day. You also note that her inhaler prescription is very old and has not been refilled recently. Her mother is present, and so you ask her about her child's medication. She states that she simply gives her daughter the money to get the medicines and doesn't know if she has obtained them or not. She states that her daughter's asthma is her responsibility, and she would just like you to "fix her up" so she can get back to work. Further social history reveals that she is a single mother who works not only a full-time job as a secretary but a part-time job as a waitress in order to support her three children. You further learn that your patient is not doing well in school, having been suspended twice during the past year. The mother states that she knows her daughter has a problem but she simply doesn't have the time to meet with the school to discuss it. In talking with the child you learn that she spends her medication money on snacks, does not feel she has any problem in school but that the teachers are against her, and she also just wants her asthma treated so she can go back to the mall where she spends her time with her friends after school.

1. Is there any evidence for abnormal family interaction patterns in this case?
2. What would be your strategy in attempting to improve this patient's compliance with her medication?
3. Do you think the mother should assume more responsibility in obtaining her child's prescriptions? How would you negotiate that?
4. If your interventions fail, do you think family therapy is indicated?

Case 3

A 23-year-old female who works as a social worker at a local hospital presents to your office having missed her last period. You diagnose an intrauterine pregnancy and invite her back 2 weeks later for her first prenatal visit. You also invite her husband. At that visit you learn that they have been married for a year and are happy that they are having a child. They ask a lot of questions about what they need to do to ensure a successful delivery. After answering their questions, you examine your patient and allow them to hear the baby's heartbeat. That substantially reassures them, and they appear happy with your demonstration that the baby is alive.

1. Is a family assessment indicated at this time?
2. If you were to obtain the genogram in Fig. 9-5, would you take any additional steps to ensure a successful pregnancy?
3. Do you feel that family therapy is indicated?

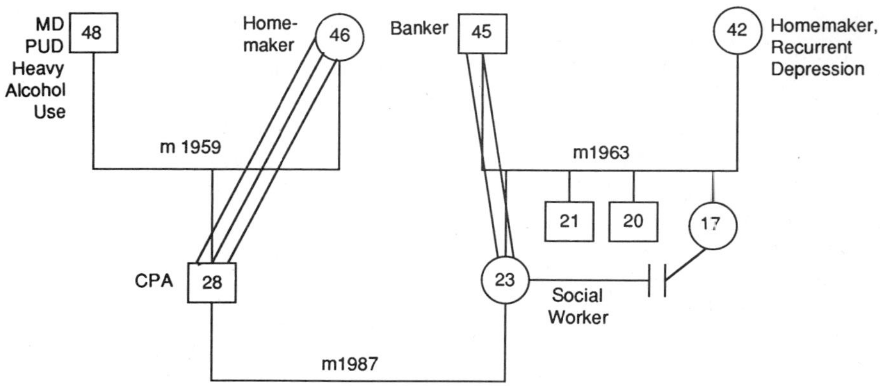

Figure 9-5. Family genogram for Case 3 for discussion.

Case 4

A 45-year-old woman presents to your office with complaints of migraine headaches. She has not had migraine headaches for 20 years, so it is quite surprising to her that they have started again. In examining her you note no abnormal physical findings and so treat her with ergotamine. One week later she comes back unimproved and wants something that will "really work" for her headaches.

1. Is a family assessment indicated?
2. If you obtain the genogram shown in Fig. 9-6, is there any evidence that family factors might have contributed to the onset of these headaches? If so what?
3. Given those factors, what would your strategy be in caring for this patient?
4. Is family therapy indicated?

Case 5

A 64-year-old white male with hypertension and diabetes sustained a stroke 2 weeks ago, leaving the left side of his body totally paralyzed. He was recently transferred to a local rehabilitation hospital where you are the attending physician. In examining the patient you note that he has a very dense left-sided hemiparesis. He doesn't seem very motivated for rehabilitation, but you feel that he at least deserves an evaluation by the physical and occupational therapists at your center. His wife then enters the room and asks you many questions about her husband's condition. You are perplexed by these questions since you assume that she has been adequately informed by her family physician on the nature of the stroke and what deficiencies to expect. The wife then asks you if she can stay in her husband's room to "help him out." She is very concerned that if she does not stay in his room something awful might happen to him. You look at the husband and he agrees with his wife by passively nodding his head.

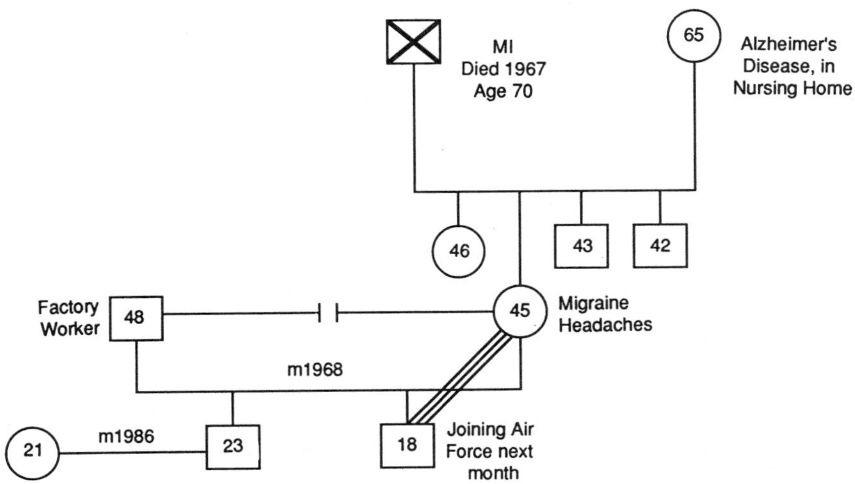

Figure 9-6. Family genogram for Case 4 for discussion.

1. Would you grant the wife's request to stay in the hospital room with her husband?
2. Is there any evidence of abnormal family interaction pattern. If so, what patterns. If so, how will that affect your decision?
3. How might the abnormal family interaction pattern you suspect affect the patient's rehabilitation?
4. You eventually decide that the wife cannot stay with her husband. Over the next several weeks the husband makes poor progress in rehabilitation. The wife is constantly complaining to you and the hospital administrators that she is not pleased with her husband's progress. What would be your strategy?

EXERCISES FOR PRACTICE

The best way to learn family assessment through genogram construction as described in this chapter is to practice it on either real or simulated patients. If real or simulated patients are not available, then role-playing an encounter can be equally effective.

During the role-play, one student should play the patient and one the physician. The patient can either "make up" an appropriate family or use his own family. The physician then interviews the patient, obtaining a social history and constructing a genogram. The genogram should include at least three generations of the patient's family, ages and health status of members, dates of important family events, and important relationship patterns. The genogram symbols displayed on Fig. 9-4 should be used. After the interview, the patient can provide feedback to the physician on his interview style and the completeness of the social history and genogram construction. The roles then change, and the process is repeated.

RECOMMENDED READINGS

Crouch, M. A., & Roberts, L. (1987). *The family in medical practice: A family systems primer.* New York: Springer-Verlag.

A short text describing all aspects of a family systems approach to medical care, focusing not only on the patient's family but on the physician's family and the doctor–patient relationship itself as well.

Doherty, W. J., & Baird, M. A. (1983). *Family therapy and family medicine.* New York: Guilford Press.

The book unites two sister disciplines by successfully demonstrating how family systems concepts may be applied to the medical setting. It is practical, clearly written, and still remarkably up to date even though it was published in the early 1980s.

McDaniel, S., Campbell, T. L., & Seaburn, D. B. (1990). *Family-oriented primary care: A manual for medical providers.* New York: Springer-Verlag.

The text advances the field of family systems medicine by providing practical ways busy physicians can integrate these concepts into their daily practice. Case examples and protocols at the end of each chapter help illustrate key points and summarize information into a useful clinical method.

McGoldrick, M., & Gerson, R. (1985). *Genograms in family assessment.* New York: W. W. Norton.

The classic text on not only the use of genograms to conduct a family assessment but their interpretation as well. Genograms of famous historical figures and entertainers illustrate key points.

CHAPTER 10

The Cultural World of the Patient

Howard F. Stein

Case 10-1. A primary care resident complained to the author after seeing a 23-year-old Navaho patient in the clinic exam room: "He didn't once look me in the eye. I couldn't tell whether he really understood what I was saying or whether he'll take the medication I prescribed." [Among traditional Navahos, aversion of gaze, avoidance of direct eye contact, is a sign of respect toward and deference to another.]

Case 10-2. A post-myocardial-infarction 63-year-old white patient on the cardiac rehabilitation unit suddenly stopped eating, refusing any food or drink for a day. The nurse carefully noted this in the patient's chart; the attending physician, wanting to rule out depression, asked for a liaison psychiatry consult. [The psychiatrist quickly learned that the "refusal to eat" occurred on a religious fast day, Yom Kippur, the Day of Atonement, and that the patient was an Orthodox Jew.]

Case 10-3. A 38-year-old wife of a successful executive tearfully said to her family doctor: "I never see him any more. I feel abandoned to raise the kids and make a home all by myself. When he's not working late into the night at corporate headquarters, he's spending hours jogging around the neighborhood and working out at the corporate club. He's become obsessed with his body, keeping it in shape. What shape does that leave our marriage in?" [The wellness and fitness movements that emerged in the late 1970s among popular American culture, and widely endorsed by professionals in clinical medicine and public health alike, embody a core of meanings that are rarely addressed by those mostly concerned with cardiac fitness: among them, dread of aging and death, atonement for earlier forbidden pleasures, search for an elusive "high" in life, fear of personal intimacy, image enhancement under professional peer pressure, sense of loss of control over the larger environment, fear of nuclear war.]

INTRODUCTION

People live in groups, from small, nuclear to large, extended family groups, from face-to-face villages to complex, urban, national societies cemented by electronic communications media. Even in small, bounded societies such as aboriginal hunting–gathering bands, people are never members of only a single group; even there, they move in and out of several microcultures, although the differences between them are not as dramatic as those in our industrial society. It is in such groups that people become ill, are defined as ill, receive treatment, recover or decline, and eventually die.

Unlike small-scale, face-to-face, closed, kin-based preliterate societies, in our complex, secularized, urbanized, and pluralistic society, practitioner and patient often come from different cultural groups. Their values, beliefs, rules, roles, attitudes, expectations, and world views thus may markedly differ. Added to this is the fact that the clinician will have undergone years of training in a professional culture that is supposed to supersede all those earlier ones from childhood that bear the mark of being "lay."

This chapter explores the cultural world of the patient and its consequences for sickness and treatment. Following a number of conceptual topics, four types of cultural settings are discussed: ethnic or nation of ancestry, religious, occupational, and popular. The reader should understand, however, that such a classification is at some level heuristic and arbitrary, that all of these overlap, and that culture is a fluid, not a static, process.

APPROACHES TO THE CONCEPT OF CULTURE

Culture may be understood conceptually in a number of ways.

1. As a "design for living," culture is a normative system, with both prescriptive and proscriptive rules, values, attitudes, roles, expectations, and the like (Parry, 1984; Spiegel, 1971). It is full of "Thou shalts" and "Thou shalt nots."

2. Culture likewise consists of the description of actual patterns of living, patterns that reveal their own rules, values, and roles that might markedly depart from the official design. Elsewhere (Stein & Hill, 1977), the distinction is proposed between "ideological" and "behavioral" ethnicity, that is, what people say versus what people do.

3. Culture is an abstraction constructed by outside observers and interpreters, an inference about group norms and behavior made from observations of many individuals, an abstraction that may be welcomed or unwelcomed by the "natives"; in this sense, culture is a composite drawing made from numerous observers' individual drawings.

4. Culture is the unit to which the sense of belonging and loyalty are attached, the unit associated with one's social boundary. That is, to say, "This is

who and what I am. This is who and what we are. This is what we do." Or, "That is not who and what I am. That is what we do not do." Cultural content here serves to define what is "me" and what is "not me." For example, many male members of the "cowboy culture" of the North American Great Plains consider cowboy boots to be an intrinsic part of the self and of one's masculinity. Other forms of footwear are viewed as alien, feminine, if not downright wrong. For such persons with temporary foot-related orthopedic problems, the prospect of not being able to wear cowboy boots is experienced as a threat to the self. Of course, group boundaries are permeable, and one can have multiple "group" identities and affiliations.

5. Culture can be regarded as patterned, preferred solutions to common problems, solutions that lead to often standardized, stereotyped responses to these problems. For instance, the Irish Catholic lively sense of sin and guilt may sensibly lead the patient from that background to believe that if a medicine is really beneficial, then it should be expected to taste bad or to hurt when applied to the body.

6. Culture is transmitted between generations or via socialization to newcomers. Although conventionally, the "unit" of culture studied and defined has been that beyond the family (e.g., hunter–gatherer bands, nomadic tribes, peasant villages, sedentary kingdoms, nation-states), the fact of family-boundedness as a culture unit was recognized and described nearly four decades ago by Roberts (1951) in his classic, *Three Navaho Households.*

7. Cultural content changes as its ability to fulfill human functions diminishes. Culture is not static or immutable. For instance, Native Americans' hunting and raiding by foot on the Great Plains was succeeded and replaced by equestrian hunting and warfare. One need only think of the revolutionary movements associated over history with such names as Buddha, Moses, Jesus, St. Paul, Martin Luther, John Calvin, Thomas Jefferson, Napoleon Bonaparte, Vladimir Lenin, Adolf Hitler, Isaac Newton, Albert Einstein, Louis Pasteur, Alexander Fleming, or Jonas Salk to realize how cultural ideas to which people are passionately committed do change.

8. Culture can be described statistically, in terms of population characteristics, and then interpreted. For example, at one family medicine residency clinic, "like clockwork" in the middle of March there will be several three- and four-wheeler vehicle (ATV, all-terrain vehicle) accident victims, mostly teenagers, in the hospital. With the first sign of a break in the winter weather, young people will take their restless energy to daredevil courses on the clay mounds and in the fields.

9. All cultures have some degree of intracultural variation. It is more pronounced and more tolerated in complex, secularized, urban society. In complex society, people move in and out of numerous subcultures, whereas in more primitive, small-scale society, these tend to merge or at least greatly overlap. The more complex the society, the less homogeneity, and the more heterogeneity. For instance, in a hunting–gathering band, one's kin group is also one's occupational group and one's religious congregation.

10. All cultures have their stereotypes about themselves and about others (Henry, 1963). Such stereotypes "feel" and "ring" true because they perform vital functions of preserving self-esteem and cohesiveness. But their price is that

they distort reality. Groups cannot learn when they feel that they cannot afford to perceive the world differently. For instance, cultural groups rife with suspicion and mistrust, and abounding in malevolent supernatural beings who inflict disease and death, will be unlikely candidates for easy acceptance of the more neutral and impersonal biomedical disease model.

To say that culture is a *system*, and not a mere collection of elements or traits, is to say that culture is an *organizing principle* of people's lives. This can be taken too far as much as it can be overlooked. Physicians, mental health practitioners, social scientists, and public policy makers frequently use cultural formulations to "pigeonhole" people, to adopt cultural profiles as cookbooks, to turn description, inquiry, and interpretation into stereotypes that oversimplify and distort rather than illumine. Especially in complex, pluralistic society, statements about people's ancestral ethnicity, a label about their personal or parental religion, a classification of their job, or a statement that they largely self-medicate based on popular American folk culture should not be construed to be the whole story.

For many patients, socioeconomic status, education, and sheer access or lack of access to the mainstream biomedical health care system are powerful facilitating or limiting factors in their lives. Such factors are likely to be overlooked by explaining away people's health behavior exclusively in terms of one or more cultural systems. Indeed, social class, education, and other "access" issues may be masked by looking solely at culture.

There can be no substitute for the painstaking and time-consuming elicitation of the patient's story, including the patient's family and wider intimate network, a fact that is no less true in the era of corporate medicine than it was in the prior era of fee-for-service practice (Stein & Apprey, 1987). To know that a person is Vietnamese, Afro-American, Southern Baptist, Ashkenazic Jewish, Latin Rite Catholic, Mennonite German, Great Plains wheat farmer, physician, or avid reader of *Reader's Digest* and *The National Enquirer* as sources for medical advice is rightfully to generate a set of hypotheses to be questioned in order to understand and culturally calibrate the individual better. At its worst, most excessive, and fallacious, cultural extrapolation from a mere label (Polish, Baptist, carpenter, vitamin taker) is an indulgence that reveals more the projections of the observer than the cultural worlds inhabited by the one ostensibly under observation.

PATIENTS' INFORMAL CARE NETWORKS, ROLES, AND TREATMENT CHOICE

Most people's sickness episodes are cared for outside the formal health care system. Even when this latter system becomes involved, it is usually after a number of assessments and interventions by the *patient's own personal network*. Indeed, it is helpful for the physician to see the act of "going to the doctor" as an act of including the physician's world within the patient's expanding cultural world and to ask "What is the patient seeking in doing so?" Christman (1977) has identified five steps that characterize the health-seeking process: (1) symptom definition, (2) illness-related shifts in role behavior, (3) lay consultation and referral, (4) treatment actions, and (5) adherence.

People consult with and seek treatment from a variety of others in the popular (lay), folk (e.g., root-worker, medicine man, chiropractor), and professional sectors (Foster & Anderson, 1978). This can be sequential or concurrent. For instance, a person might consult an aunt, a local pharmacist, a chiropractor, and a physician for different facets of the same illness episode. Or the person might seek help from them in some sequence as a result of the progression or nonresolution of symptoms. Johnson and Kleinman (1984) note that

> most illness episodes are dealt with in the context of the family, regardless of ethnic background. This may involve special diets, foods, herbs, massage, exercise, religious treatment, and prescribed or nonprescribed medications. Ethnic patients also may consult with folk practitioners such as *curanderos* among Hispanics, root-workers and spiritualist ministers among blacks, herb doctors and acupuncturists among East Asians, voodoo specialists among Haitians, and medicine men among Native Americans. It is common for patients to engage in lay healing practices and to consult traditional practitioners while simultaneously seeking health care from physicians (pp. 279–280).

A decade ago, Kleinman (1978) introduced a useful conceptual distinction between disease and illness, defining "disease" as "malfunctioning and maladaptation of biological and/or psychological processes" and defining "illness" as "the personal and social significance of and life problems created by the experience of perceived disease" (p. 428). Disease is the conceptual domain and chief interest of the medical professional, whereas illness is the conceptual domain and chief interest of the patient. The degree of congruence between the physician's (professional and other cultural) and patient's (ethnic, religious, occupational, popular, lay) cultural models of the illness episode and expectations for treatment deeply affects the clinical relationship (Christman & Maretzki, 1982; Eisenberg & Kleinman, 1981).

Johnson and Kleinman (1984) begin their chapter on "Cultural concerns in consultation psychiatry" with the observation that

> People are taught by their culture how to interpret and communicate about symptoms, from whom to seek care, how to explain illness etiology and pathophysiology, how serious and long-lasting the problem is, and what to expect from treatment.
>
> An appreciation of the differences in styles of communication and codes of etiquette for physician–patient interaction is important in working with culturally diverse patients (p. 275).

Based on Kleinman, Eisenberg, and Good (1978) and Kleinman (1980), Johnson and Kleinman (1984) suggest a series of questions that the physician might use to elicit the patient's culturally based and shared "explanatory model" of the illness episode:

1. What do you call your problem?
2. What do you think has caused your problem(s)?
3. Why do you think it started when it did?
4. What does this sickness do to you? How does it work?
5. How serious is this illness? How long will it last?
6. What kind of treatment is best for this illness?
7. What results do you expect from treatment?
8. What are the chief problems your illness has caused you?
9. What worries you most about being sick? (p. 282).

Sickness and healer roles, together with the definition of what qualifies as legitimate illness, are inseparably bound up with shared notions about the self and its boundaries. This collective self-image, together with the range of deviation allowed within the cultural category of "normal," is not only a social fact but an important value. In the United States, for instance, disease conceptualization and treatment are embedded in the value system of self-reliance, rugged individualism, independence, pragmatism, empiricism, atomism, privatism, emotional minimalism, and a mechanistic conception of the body and its "repair" (Kluckhohn & Strodtbeck, 1961; Ohnuki-Tierney, 1984). The horror of dependency (the conscious expression of a repudiated wish) is a powerful fuel that influences and confers authority on the biomedical conceptual, diagnostic, and treatment system. Hocking (1987) writes that

> Because the sick are dependent, sickness is seen as deviant behavior, undesirable, and only to be legitimated on certain terms ([Talcott] Parsons' sick role concept). Legitimation of sickness has become the prerogative of the medical profession which uses the biomedical concept of disease as its yardstick (p. 526).

In American culture, the biomedical conceptualization and treatment of disease has been welcomed and widely adopted precisely because it fits so well with the image of the self as a physical thing that could be broken and repaired.

ILLNESS-RELATED WORDS AND THEIR MEANINGS

Language is a common area of misunderstanding and ill will between physician and patient (Dirckx, 1982). Physicians often discount irrational-seeming patient folk expressions. However, some of the worst impasses occur when the words doctors and patients say *seem* to be the same but carry divergent meanings. Many black patients, for example, visualize illness in terms of blood imbalance. Physicians talk about high and low blood *pressure,* where many lower-class blacks talk about high and low blood (and parallel terms thick/thin and sweet/bitter blood) (Snow, 1974, 1983; Hill & Mathews, 1981).

The terms "high" and "low" blood

> may refer to either the amount of blood in the body or a shift in its location, that is, "high blood" may be too *much* blood or it may be that a normal amount of blood is present in the body but has suddenly shot up into the head. Changes in blood volume and shifts in location can result from improper dietary practices or emotional shock or both (Snow, 1983, p. 824).

Foods included in the etiology of "high blood" include red meat (especially pork), beets, red wine, carrots, grape juice, and other foods that are regarded as too rich or red in color. Blackouts, especially in males, are often regarded as a symptom of high blood. Low blood

> is associated with lack of energy, fainting spells, and constipation. Treatment for both of these illnesses involves diet modification, family counseling to deal with interpersonal relations related to stress, and herbal remedies (Hill & Mathews, 1981, p. 316).

Typical remedies for high, sweet, thick blood are substances believed to help thin down the blood: bitter herbs, epsom salts, vinegar, garlic, peach leaf, horehound, snake root, pickle juice (Hill & Mathews, 1981, p. 317), many of which increase the patient's sodium intake and are thus anathema from a biomedical viewpoint. In lowering "high blood," the goal is to try to sweat the excess out through the pores, to try to eliminate it through the bowels, or, in women, through menstruation (Snow, 1983, p. 824). In part, conditions of "high" and "low" blood are related to gravity. Elderly black patients who diagnose themselves as suffering from "high blood" might drink pickle brine to dilute their blood and sleep sitting upright in bed (propped up with boxes and pillows) so that their thinned blood could run down from their head and redistribute itself in the rest of the body.

Among many whites and other mainstream Americans, Blumhagen (1982) notes that in popular culture, many Americans believe the diagnosis "hypertension" to mean that they are hypertense, anxious, nervous, irritable, highstrung, and that the logical cure is relaxation. In such a scheme, drastic diet management, exercise, and medication for life often make little sense. When the medical diagnosis of "essential hypertension" is made, many hear "hypertension." Also, within American popular culture, the heart is a deeply metaphoric subject; one has only to think of its association with Valentine's Day (love, intimacy), sadness and depression (having "a heavy heart"), pride ("a stout heart"), etc. Americans are attentive to cardiovascular imagery akin to the French and Latin focus on the liver, the Japanese on the stomach (*hara*), etc. This may prepare fertile ground for misunderstanding between physician and patient, since physicians are often looking for a mechanical malfunction, whereas patients might be referring to a different, personal meaning.

For another example, mainstream, acculturated Americans might feel emotionally "close" to their families and friends, maintaining contact by telephone and travel, yet actually live thousands of miles from them. Mexican Americans, studied by Keefe (1984), feel deeply close to their families, but such closeness has a markedly different meaning. It is not that Anglos are less familistic than Mexican Americans, but that the meaning of familism and closeness is different. "Mexican Americans value the physical presence of family members while Anglo-Americans are satisfied with intermittent meetings with kin supplemented by telephone calls and letters" (Keefe, 1984, p. 68). For Mexican Americans, close familism is associated with geographic stability, whereas for Anglos, it is associated with considerable social and geographic mobility. Keefe (1984) concludes that

> Urban Mexican Americans live in kin-based communities while Anglo Americans do not. By community, I do not mean a place-community or neighborhood [similar to ethnic "ghettos" early in the 20th century around or near urban factories], but rather a personal network made up of people living within a limited geographic area in which face-to-face interaction can occur frequently . . . (p. 69).

When patients use familiar-sounding words, it is useful if not necessary to find out from them their own meanings. By doing so, say, with respect to the word "close" family, the physician can assess the extent to which closeness corresponds to his or her expectation or is functional or pathological (as, for instance, in "enmeshed" families). Such inquiry can clarify the extent to which the family can realistically function as support system and which member(s) the physician can rely on or contact during a sickness episode if it were necessary.

Consider, further, the range of cultural meanings of the seemingly self-evident word "togetherness" and of the clinical misunderstandings between patient (or family) and physician when the physician assumes that his or her meaning is the same as that of the patient or family. From clinical experience and research, Nguyen Nga (1988), a psychiatrist, has discovered that whereas "Caucasian," highly acculturated, mainstream Americans associate "family togetherness" with the notion of spending the weekend together at the lake or going on a picnic, the Vietnamese-American meaning is that of "us versus them," "our family united against other families and against the world." The American connotation is inclusive and expansive, whereas the Vietnamese connotation is exclusive and encapsulating. An American clinician would miss crucial information if he or she did not elicit the boundary aspect of Vietnamese family togetherness.

A further distinction lies in the fact that when mainstream Americans speak of togetherness, they mean a collection of distinct selves, each with a personal identity. Traditional Vietnamese, on the other hand, more regard themselves in terms of a shared "family identity" from which each member sees himself or herself as inseparable. This family identity encompasses deceased ancestors for whom the living must perform rites so that their souls do not wander aimlessly forever. Thus, something as seemingly elemental and universal as the definition and the experience of the *self* is influenced by the culture in which one grows up and in which one participates.

In Japan, Korea, and traditional China, the family is also experienced as identical and coextensive with the self. In Confucianism, whose "moral principles . . . supported the legitimacy of [the Japanese] family and state" (De Vos 1980, p. 121), there is

> no place for individualisitic concepts of the person. There are no individuals as such—only family members whose roles change through the life cycle. At no time is the person regarded as separate from his family and social roles, and maturation is a deepening of understanding of one's ultimate psychological security, is to be found in family or group continuity, not in the continuity of the self. . . . Tensions experienced through a conflict of occupational expectations or family role versus disruptive private feelings are most frequently resolved in Japan by directing the individual back toward the family. The goals of attempts to alleviate psychiatric problems are therefore defined in terms of family or occupational integration. (De Vos 1980, pp. 121–122)

In such families, duty to the family and wider cultural unit predominates over duty to an individual self, a value organization that may make it difficult for the patient from such cultures to "follow doctor's orders" when they conflict with obligations to one's family role. Obligations to one's kinship network often supersede obligations to strangers such as the physician. American individualism and the tightly bounded doctor–patient relationship might differ markedly from the value system and expectations of such patients. As Parry(1984) notes,

> seeking help for oneself may be a threat in cultures in which the family or other social networks are more important than the individuals. A set of behaviors that threatens to change a role in a family would be viewed as displaying selfishness, disloyalty, or even hostility (p. 930).

Thus, for Americans and a number of families of Far Eastern heritage, to speak of birth, adolescence, marriage, and death as "family events" may carry vastly different cultural meanings and burdens.

ETHNICITY AND HEALTH BEHAVIOR

Within the United States, the terms "ethnic" and "ethnicity" denote a major social typology according to which people are classified by others and classify themselves in terms of nation or tribe of origin: for instance, Poles, Irish, Slovaks, English, German, Navahos, Hispanics, Iroquois, Jews, and so forth. As has been discussed at length elsewhere, the term "ethnicity" is complex (see Committee on International Relations, 1987; De Vos & Romanucci-Ross, 1975; Glazer & Moynihan, 1975; Stein, 1987d; Stein & Hill, 1977). Jews, for example, are sometimes regarded, and sometimes regard themselves, as a nation, as an ethnic group, as a race, and as a religion.

Until the civil rights and Black Power movements of the 1960s, large numbers of American blacks regarded themselves, and were regarded by the larger society, as a race (and anthropologists were quick to point out that the American folk notions about "race" should not be confused with the concept as is used in scientific biology). Since the mid-1960s, many blacks have renounced the racial classification and have strongly identified themselves as Afro-Americans, that is, in terms of their continent of origin. Not only has the black/white/yellow/red American "racial" classification distorted the deep cultural diversity *within* each ostensibly homogeneous racial category, but "race" has often been used as an "ethnic" category. Moreover, groups that now qualify as whites, e.g., Serbians, Poles, Ukrainians, Italians, Spaniards, Greeks, were, earlier in the 20th century, regarded as inferior, darker races by those "whites" who feared that the largely north European, Protestant culture of their United States would be defiled! In this section, ethnicity is an American cultural system of categorizing social diversity.

The important point to keep in mind in all aspects of medical care is that *anything* can have group-shared, symbolic significance that bears consequences for clinical outcome. Consider food, whose symbolic weight is at least as great as its objective, nutritional value. One immigrant Italian American male in his 60s was recovering postsurgically in the hospital. His physicians and nursing staff were becoming alarmed that he was hardly eating anything from his well-stocked hospital tray. Finally, an Italian-speaking social worker was brought in to find out what was wrong. It turned out that the soft-spoken patient objected to the *way* the food was served: it was so unappetizing that he could not bring himself to eat it. Yet to regain strength from the surgery, he had to eat. He protested: "Couldn't they make the same meat into a nice patty or meat ball and put some garlic and spicy tomato sauce on it?"

For another example: In a largely Protestant and Catholic small town lived a retired Jewish widower in his 80s. He contacted the local hospital-based "Meals on Wheels" organization to bring his lunch and dinner meals 5 days per week. Although he was unable to keep a strictly kosher diet (that is, one in complete accord with Orthodox Jewish dietary law), he was able to arrange that the Meals on Wheels kitchen send him sandwiches and hot meals without pork products (the meat of the pig was perhaps the most forbidden). Through this arrangement, Meals on Wheels could provide him with nutritionally high-quality food that at the same time met his sense of religious obligations as well.

The *form,* rather than the *substance,* of prescribed medication may become a source of conflict. Many Hispanic-Americans prefer to have their medicine in the form of a "shot" (which is more masculine) than in the form of a "pill" (which is more sissifying). One Irish-Catholic male in his early 70s staunchly believed that "Good medicine tastes bad. If it don't hurt going down, it mustn't be very strong." For him and many of his religious/ethnic culture, "taking your medicine" is as much a form of punishment as it is a form of treatment. To soothe the conscience as well as to perform its biomedical function, medicine that is acceptable must inflict a little physical pain.

Many traditional Hispanic-American patients (Mexican American, Puerto Rican) adhere to the Hippocratic, humoral-theory-derived "hot–cold" (*caliente–frio*) model of disease (Harwood, 1971, 1981). According to this system, certain diseases are classified as hot, cold, and "cool" (an intermediate category). "Cold-classified illnesses are treated with hot medication and foods, while hot illnesses are treated with cool substances" (Harwood, 1971, pp. 1153–1154). Hispanic women on diuretics might discontinue such doctor-prescribed potassium sources as bananas, oranges, or raisins during menstruation (a cold condition, and these foods are likewise regarded as cold or cool). The physician could prescribe potassium in the culturally acceptable form of vitamins (which are "hot"), together with such "hot" foods as coffee and cocoa, which are rich in potassium (Harwood, 1971, p. 1155). Or, consider pregnancy, a "hot" condition during which

> many women will not take hot iron supplements or vitamins. These patients might be encouraged to take these prescriptions with fruit juice or an herb tea [both of which are cool] to "neutralize" them (Harwood, 1971, p. 1157).

East European Jews tend to be as concerned about the meaning of pains as with their immediate alleviation through analgesics. Although American physicians of various ethnicities perceive Jews and Italians both to be vociferous about their pains, they often fail to perceive that the purpose or function of the complaint differs between the groups. Anglo-American ("WASP") patients, like Jews, tend to be health-conscious but attach very different significance to the search for health. Jews have been depicted as generally worried that something profoundly terrible might be wrong, whereas Anglo-Americans may be presented as viewing the body in a machine-like utilitarian way: when something seems broken, one is obligated to take care of oneself and bring one's body to the doctor to be fixed (Zborowski, 1969). Jews may see in the most minor symptom the harbinger or symbol of tragedy; Italians may primarily want to feel better and place less emphasis on the entire prescribed medical regimen; Irish patients might ignore their symptoms as long as possible, report only a few, and avoid the sense of sin that goes with too much preoccupation with the body; and WASP patients believe that rationality, hard work, control, and "pulling yourself up by your bootstraps" should suffice in the treatment of disease as with the rest of life.

The following brief case illustrates the importance of taking into account the acceptable cultural *form* of a recommended biomedical substance or procedure.

Case 10-4. A behavioral scientist was working with a married female family medicine resident who was irate about a pregnant Chinese American woman. This patient refused to take the prescribed iron-enriched vitamins and seemed otherwise noncompliant and uninterested in her own pregnancy. The patient had evidently not wanted to become pregnant and wanted to have her baby and be done with it (abortion was out of the question). A consultant was brought in to mediate the conflict. The consultant spoke with the patient in Chinese and learned that in her culture, pregnant women do *not* take vitamins because it was felt they would throw the body out of balance. The consultant discovered, however, that *within* the patient's framework, seaweed figured prominently in her diet. Then the consultant and the resident successfully reached agreement with the patient to increase her intake of seaweed to give her the necessary iron supplement. The resident was relieved that her patient was getting the iron, albeit in a culturally acceptable form.

Internist and family doctor Robert E. Pieroni reported the following case of hypokalemia in a pregnant black patient:

Case 10-5. I was recently asked to evaluate a 42-year-old black female with a dangerously low serum potassium level. She was 8 months pregnant and had been admitted to the hospital because of weakness and marked hypertension. She denied any significant vomiting, diarrhea, or use of drugs, which could have contributed to her considerable loss of potassium. I then questioned her about pica (an abnormal craving), which we frequently find in this area [the deep South]. She denied eating starch, dirt, or clay but on direct questioning did admit to chewing tobacco to ease her morning sickness. Such a practice is not uncommon in this region and has probably been handed down from generation to generation. Many brands of chewing tobacco, including the brand my patient was using, contain licorice, which can not only deplete the body of potassium but can also cause marked hypertension, weakness, and swelling. Fortunately, we were able to correct her potassium before further harm was done, and she went on to deliver a healthy baby. She is now spreading the word that chewing tobacco is not a panacea for morning sickness (Pieroni, 1981, p. 7).

All patients have a rationale for their medical actions. This rationale might not be organized into an Aristotelian explanatory system, nor might it follow the same rules of evidence that biomedical decision making at least officially strives to follow. Although many ethnomedical practices might contain irrational elements or aspects (Boyer, 1983), it is prejudicial to infer automatically that simply because a practice is different from one's own, or from one's official medical model, it is *ipso facto* inferior, wrong, crazy, or dangerous. On the other hand, it is dangerous to romanticize folk or popular medical practices. Pieroni's above example illustrates the importance of becoming intimately familiar with patients' various cultures, so that one might know what types of questions to ask the patient (e.g., regarding licorice, chewing tobacco ingestion).

Case 10-6. The Vietnamese American parents of a 4-year-old boy brought him to a primary care physician for persistent cough, sore throat, fever, diarrhea, upper respiratory distress, and poor appetite that had lasted a week. On physical exam, the physician found six symmetrical ovoid bruises (ecchymoses) on the boy's back and two on the front of his neck. He immediately suspected child abuse, especially since the child seemed so quiet, docile, and compliant. He wanted immediately to contact child protective services and have a social worker begin an investigation of the boy's home situation.

Consultation with a behavioral science faculty and subsequent inquiry of the parents revealed a different picture, however. The parents practiced an ethnomedical treatment regimen that they widely shared with coastal Vietnamese peoples. Many diseases are believed to be caused by "bad winds" that enter the body and cause an imbalance. "Winds" are believed to be one among the major elements of the universe. This Vietnamese theory of disease is a local variant on a balance theory widespread throughout the Buddhist/Confucian-influenced Orient. For the boy to recover, the parents resorted to custom to try to help restore the body's natural balance. They took a highly polished coin and rubbed it with an ointment (lubricant) at several places on their son's back and neck until these polaces bruised, thereby creating openings for the "bad winds" to escape from entrapment in the body, thus enabling the boy's body to restore its natural balance. This procedure is called *Cao gio* ("scratch away the wind": *cao* = scratch away, *gio* = wind) (Primosch & Young, 1980).

The boy and his parents alike described the practice as soothing, a little like a massage, that the warm ointment felt good being rubbed. The boy insisted that "it didn't hurt." The parents became concerned when their efforts did not result in the boy's rapid return to health. With this explanation, the physician was persuaded that with this family situation, he did not need to pursue child abuse investigation. It turned out that the boy had an especially virulent form of the flu, one that typically lasted around 10 days; the parents likewise felt reassured on hearing this.

As the physician became more familiar with the family over time, he learned that the parents' grave concern for this boy's welfare stemmed from the fact that he was their eldest son. They wished him particularly to carry on the family tradition, this in their new homeland, America. After being in the United States for 7 years, they still felt guilty for abandoning their ancestral home.

Not long ago I presented this same case to a group of family medicine residents; the topic was patients' and physicians' explanatory models. Their response was far from enthusiastic; one resident said monotonously, "We saw this kind of stuff at the Mecca (teaching hospital)." I then sought to draw a parallel between this "exotic" and "alien" cultural presentation and something perhaps more within their orbit. I said that the Vietnamese model is one among many "balance" theories of sickness, treatment, and health. I continued:

> Many of us in this room probably grew up with some degree of humoral folk medicine. Did your mother ever tell you that, when you finish a hot shower or bath, to be sure to run some cold water on yourself to be sure your pores closed? Otherwise, if you went outside or walked on the cold floor, you could catch a draft and get the flu or a cold.

The group brightened, joking about some of the stories they remembered from their childhoods 20 years earlier. Suddenly, the Vietnamese theory of ill winds gained some experiential plausibility. It was not simply silly, prescientific, and foreign. Rather, they (we) found aspects of their (our) own lives that could be used to identify with those of a different culture.

In a study of diabetes and diabetes management on the Devil's Lake Sioux Reservation, Lang (1985) found that "Food preferences, expense, and lack of time in a large household were the most frequently given reasons for lack of compliance" with the diabetes program. "In general, Dakota people today associate bigness and heaviness with a sense of well-being and health" (p. 252). Three widespread Dakota perceptions about diabetes are that (1) diabetes afflicts the Dakota because their way of life is out of balance; (2) diabetes is the most recent among diseases spread by the white man to destroy Indian society; (3) because few medicine men have the power to treat it, diabetes may not necessarily be treated by traditional Dakota means. There is "high regard for traditional foods and medicinal plants, and . . . the importance of the role of eating and food in marking social occasions" (Lang, 1985, p. 255). Moreover, "Diabetes is perceived as another imposition on Indian people by Europeans or 'whites,' and dietary regimens are perceived as telling people how to live their lives." Thus, not only are there cultural and religious aspects to food and diabetes, but *political* ones as well.

In a paper on physicians' "cultural blind spots" with regard to patients, Lin (1983), a Western-trained Chinese physician, challenges the popular assumption that similarities in cultural background between patient and physician invariably enhance clinical communication and outcomes. A common cultural heritage does not rule out intraethnic variation influenced by age, sex, personality, political orientation, socioeconomic class, rural/urban background, region of origin, dialect spoken, religion, occupation, education, family structure, or extent of acculturation (e.g., Americanization). Especially when the physician identifies himself or herself as belonging to the same ethnic group as the patient, "cultural stereotyping results in superficial generalizations that are often misleading in the case of individual patients (Lin, 1983, p. 92)." Lin's caution extends beyond ethnicity or nationality of origin to religion, occupation, and common popular cultural participation. The clinical error in all of these is the assumption that "You are the same as I," a psychological merging that prevents the physician from taking notice of potentially important differences between himself or herself and the patient. The reverse is also possible, where the patient tries to persuade the physician that they are the same. Both of these can be seen to be a variation on physician countertransference/patient transference issues. When one wants to see the patient as the same as oneself, the question to ask is: "What am I trying not to see in the patient?" (Devereux, 1980; Stein & Apprey, 1985).

RELIGION AND HEALTH BEHAVIOR

Religion is the domain of human life that concerns the belief in, and the experience of, spiritual beings and supernatural forces as well as the consequences of these beliefs for the conduct of life. In simpler, preliterate societies, and in earlier historical epochs in the West, religious life was inseparably interwoven with "ethnic," "occupational," and "popular" aspects of life. Early German Lutheran, Dutch Reformed, and Hasidic Jewish religions are instances of this fusion. It is only in more secularized, urbanized, industrialized, cosmopolitan settings that the pluralistic separation of religion and nation ("church" and "state") has occurred.

In any event, the physician would do well to keep in mind that patients' and families' religious beliefs, meanings, and practices may well influence any and all aspects of health-related decision making. Even where patients might accept the naturalistic, mechanistic, entity-oriented biomedical model for certain aspects of their disease and its treatment, they may well harbor more personalistic (Foster, 1976) ideas of why they are sick *now,* why *they* have fallen ill and not another, *what* they might have done in their relations with other people or with God that might have resulted in their "susceptibility" to disease or accident, and what to do about it now. Often patients, families, and physicians come to an impasse over how and whether to talk about these issues. Patients and doctors often think that the other only wants to talk about the "strictly medical" matters; or patients may feel afraid to bring up religious beliefs for fear of looking foolish or superstitious in the physician's eyes. On the other hand, patients may compartmentalize their medical care, allocating the corporeal "why" and biomedical treatment to the doctor while allocating the spiritual or psychological "why" and its restoration to their pastor. The following case illustrates the consequences for health behavior of one patient's religious beliefs.

Case 10-7. Some years ago I conducted lengthy counseling of a woman, Carol, who had suffered a spinal cord injury in an automobile accident. She had some loss of function in her right hand and leg. (The full description of the case is discussed elsewhere; see Stein, 1987f). In work with her, I learned of the intimate connection between her sense of self, her Southern Baptist religion (as belief system, as network of community relationships), and expectations she had of herself for full recovery of function. The auto accident and its aftermath stretched her values to the breaking point. These values then exacted from her more than she could physically give.

In Carol's Southern Baptist world of the rural Great Plains small town, self-control was prized. If she had lost it through the automobile accident (in which she had been a passenger), she expected to regain it—by herself. It was a test. If she regained complete use of her hand, arm, and leg, it would be proof that she was worthy in the eyes of God. If she failed, it would show to all that she was a failure. She severely reproached herself for not being able to restore herself to perfection (e.g., through exercise, physical therapy, etc.), to walk well, to carry even the heaviest casserole, to be a good enough wife, mother, and Christian.

Carol felt very much alone in her attempts at recovery and in her attempts at differentiating between what were realistic goals and what were magical ones. Her fear of failure and shame dominated much of the therapy. In her personal, family, and religious world, everything was a matter of either/or, black/white. Much of the counseling dealt with her haunting questing of how she could be a good woman and a good Christian if and when she could not make her body return to its condition of health prior to the accident.

In conversations related to this case, a Southern Baptist family physician colleague, who had counseled many ministerial couples and served as their family doctor, told me of one Baptist minister's wife's symptoms. He had treated her for multiple physical complaints, none of which could be attributed to an organic disease process. When he offered to her the interpretation that the symptoms might be stress related, she adamantly replied: "I am a Christian. I *can't* have stress," a statement that the physician, I believe accurately, construed as meaning that as she expected herself and her marriage to be perfect; any flaw in that perfection must be denied. In Carol's case, her self-blame and its association with evangelical Protestant religious values were not idiosyncratic or isolated but characterized the expectations of many born-again Christians and those seeking or awaiting spiritual rebirth.

In keeping with the mind–body dualism that has dominated Western religious and philosophical thought since the late Renaissance, it is acceptable for the body to be sick, though symptoms may have highly symbolic meanings. It is not acceptable, however, for the mind or soul to be sick; nor may the "soul" be permitted to have an influence on the "body." The split must be absolute for moral, religious reasons. Physicians and other therapists who harbor "psychosomatic" or "family-somatic" diagnostic models (that is, investigating family influences on disease etiology, severity, persistence, and remission) often encounter difficult communication processes when working with such patients for whom the somatic is the only personally and religiously acceptable idiom in which to be ill. Somatization also functions as a complex compromise, for through it one can demand to be cared for, one may be punished for making such demands, one may indirectly punish others through one's symptoms, and one may preserve the personal and family belief or myth that one remains good and Christian.

OCCUPATIONAL CULTURE AND HEALTH BEHAVIOR

The culture of the workplace is yet another source of health-behavior-related norms. These are often learned not via intergenerational socialization of the young (as is more characteristic of long-term ethnic and religious cultures) but through learning as a participant in one's work culture. (An exception, discussed below, is the culture of family farming.) One is subject to similar external stresses and expectations. One negotiates common meanings and interpretations of events from day-to-day interaction with superiors, co-workers, and subordinates.

Although the family farm, the family grocery store, the hospital, and the corporation, for instance, can all be labeled "occupational cultures," one must keep in mind that they differ markedly in the process of recruitment. Family farms and family businesses recruit from within, through procreation and socialization of the next, succeeding generation. However, "organizations [such as hospitals and corporations] are not *self-renewing* but must replace their memberships from the outside society" (Grieco, 1988, p. 85). Those recruited from without are already culture bearers, albeit those whose values are congruent with those of the organization and who are most easily socialized.

For 6 years I coordinated the behavioral science teaching at the family medicine residency program in Shawnee, Oklahoma, a clinic in which many workers from Tinker Air Force Base sought their primary care. Over the years, residents came to formulate what they somewhat humorously called the "Tinker syndrome." They described it as follows. Many workers did not find their job fulfilling; many did not feel productive. Many did not put in a great deal of effort during most of the year. They felt they just put in their hours and collected their paycheck. Many come to the clinic intermittently through the year, acknowledging depression or with multiple organic complaints. Toward early spring (March, April), the family medicine residents noticed that many of these workers would come into the clinic with symptoms they would relate to stress (anxiety, can't sleep, nervousness).

Early spring was the time of an annual site visit and major review of the Air Force base, when supervisors were expected to show how efficient and productive they were and units were to be evaluated for their performance. Suddenly, the base became self-consciously more active and busy. The physicians surmised that many of their patients were situationally anxious or suffering from vague guilt and fear of being judged and found inadequate, which they expressed in a wide spectrum of physical symptoms. During this "Tinker syndrome" influx, there were biomedically *bona fide* physical complaints as well. Some workers would literally strain themselves by trying to cram 12 months of physical labor into 2 to 3 weeks prior to the annual site visit. Unaccustomed to regular strenuous physical labor, some workers injured themselves when they attempted to perform intensive physical labor on their jobs.

Apart from this latter group, a visit to the doctor usually resulted in reassurance that no severe disease process was taking place. The workers were able to ventilate about their variously frustrating and bureaucratic governmental jobs and confess some anxiety, guilt, and shame for their lack of enthusiasm at an unrewarding job. Through their symptoms they received some degree of punishment for their lackluster attitude toward work and received assurance that neither their body nor their spirit was in such terrible shape, only to return to the base to commence the cycle anew. It required rather sophisticated cultural thinking on the part of these residents to (1) recognize an epidemiologic pattern rather than think exclusively of patients on a one-by-one basis and (2) learn to interpret a plethora of physical complaints as a metaphor for a disorder related to the culture of the workplace. (Gratitude is expressed to J. M. Pontious, M.D., for his collaboration on this case.)

A major element in the health care process is timing: when does the patient (often in league with relatives, co-workers, drinking partners, etc.) decide to come in for medical care? Physician and patient often become embroiled in conflict from the start because the physician's sense of timing does not correspond to that of the patient. Consider this issue from the viewpoint of the culture of Great Plains wheat-farming families, a regional cultural group congealed over the generations from immigrants and their descendants from western and central Europe, Great Britain, and Ireland. Often a farmer's presenting complaint at the emergency room or in the clinic is a variation on the following:

> My wife made me come. She's been on my back for 2 weeks now. I've had just a little pain in my chest, nothing that working out in the yard or on the tractor won't cure in time. But the only way I could get her off my back is to come in and prove it's nothing.

Moreover, it is often difficult if not impossible to elicit a "complete history" from the taciturn, terse farmer (who keeps words to a minimum, wants to avoid stirring a fuss over nothing, and serves up plenty of "Yup"s and "Nope"s); therefore, it becomes the role of the wife to provide the history of the symptoms. She is the person from whom the explanatory model can often be elicited. As described elsewhere in detail (Stein, 1987a,b), the preharvest months and harvest proper are times when only a seriously ill infant or child will be brought to the doctor; similarly, during holiday times of family togetherness (Thanksgiving, Christmas), trips to the doctor will be postponed.

The following case describes a physician's frustration when the patient gives higher priority to the wheat harvest than to his own health.

Case 10-8. "What a dirtball!" fumed an irate family medicine resident at a mortality and morbidity conference. "I told him 4 months ago that he'd better have that abnormal ECG followed up. So now his wife brings him in the ambulance with a massive MI. We couldn't even stabilize him in the CCU. All I can say is we could have saved him if he'd listened to me." It was now early July. The patient's abnormal ECG had been discovered in early April. The patient, a 58-year-old Oklahoma wheat farmer, had jokingly laughed off his physician's urging for follow-up.

"I didn't feel nothing different than before your test," the patient had protested. "Besides," he continued pithily. "I've got a lot on my mind to look out for first. There's all my machinery to get ready for harvest. I'll be lucky if we have everything ready for the big push in June or early July, when we're waiting for the weather to be just right so we can go cutting. It can't be too bad since I can still do all my work."

The physician said incredulously, sarcastically: "He left with a smile on his face. 'I'll see you after harvest. Then you can have my ticker checked out all you want.' We'll see who's smiling now."

A cultural chasm separated the physician and patient. For the physician, "health" was not only an abstraction about physical and mental status but the highest value in life. One's personal health came first; it should have a higher priority over all other values. For the wheat farmer, to assure the success of this year's crop, and thereby his one and only annual "paycheck," had highest priority. "Family" and "farm" came far before "self." Moreover, for him and countless others in the farmer/cowboy culture of the North American Great Plains, health is measured by the ability to work: "If I can do a good day's work, I'm not sick enough to go to a doctor," is the motto of many.

Work, too, is closely bound up with one's masculine identity. One does not go to the doctor until virtually at death's door; to do otherwise is to incur fear that one is, and will be seen as, a "wimp" or a "sissy." In sum, an overriding cultural feature of this case is the disparity in the sense of timing between patient and physician; a disparity that the physician can attempt to bridge but that he or she often can do little to alter. All cultures have their consequences; all cultures take their toll from their priorities and values.

A final case illustrates the discrepancy between biomedical practitioner cultural values and priorities and those that characterize many "white," Euro-American patients in the "cowboy culture" of the Great Plains (see Stein, 1987a,b).

Case 10-9. A 57-year-old wheat farmer from the Oklahoma panhandle was brought to the nearest minor emergency clinic in March by his concerned wife. He had been much more bent over than usual, and they both had suffered many restless, sleepless nights because he could not find a position in bed that did not give him pain. "She made me come in," was his presenting complaint to the physician. As the physician was taking a history and doing a physical exam, and ordering few tests in order to keep the farmer's expenses down, the farmer said, as if to minimize the situation: "It's just my arthritis acting up a little. Nuthin' that the sun and hard work won't straighten up. But she couldn't wait," he joked.

The family physician diagnosed muscle spasm in the lumbar spine. For treatment, he gave the patient a prescription for several days' muscle relaxants and urged him to try to avoid a lot of bending over and twisting, to try to "take it easy" for about a week, and then the back would probably settle down. The farmer, a quiet, respectful fellow, thanked the doctor, and left for the waiting room. His wife took the prescription and had it filled, over her husband's hapless protests.

He took two pills and refused to take any more. They relaxed him, but too much. He became drowsy, couldn't think straight. "It put me out of commission," he told her. It was calving season and time to repair all the farm machinery as the first days of spring heralded the push toward harvest in June. "The treatment is worse than the pain." Several days later, with his "arthritis" unchanged, he drove his pickup truck to his local chiropractor, over his wife's remonstrations, saying as he left the house, "He's straightened me out before, and he can do it again. I don't need them sissy pills."

Scheper-Hughes and Lock (1987, p. 18) write that:

> once an organ captures the imagination of people, there appears to be no end to the metaphorical uses to which it may be put. Among "old stock" American Midwestern farmers, for example, the backbone has great cultural and ethnomedical significance. When illness strikes at these industrious and "upright" people, being forced off their feet comes as a grave blow to the ego. Even among the elderly and infirm, well-being is defined as the ability to "get around," to be on one's feet. Obviously, the ability to stay "upright" . . . has two connotations to Americans: the first, to stand up, to be on one's feet; and the second, a moral implication "not to stoop to anything, to be honest and just, to be true to friends in danger, to stand by one's convictions." Among rural Midwesterners laziness is a most serious moral failing, and "spinelessness" is as reviled as godlessness. It is little wonder that a therapy concerned with adjusting perceived malalignments of the spine—chiropractic medicine—would have its origins in middle America (Cobb, 1958).

Thus, clinicians of all backgrounds may also bring and often unwittingly enact their ethnic-derived assumptions about how a good doctor or patient ought to act, what a good outcome ought to be, what degree of emotionality/impersonality is appropriate, and so forth (Abel, Metraux, & Roll, 1987). For example, many physicians drawn from and practicing among the farming/cowboy culture of the American Great Plains are intolerant of patients, especially males, who are more expressive than silently stoic about their pain or who take on the patient role for "minor" symptoms. In these physicians' stories, such patients do bear the labels of "wimps," "sissies," or "pussies."

POPULAR CULTURE AND HEALTH BEHAVIOR

Powerful folk medical currents exist among mainstream United States *popular* national culture, currents that flow into official professional culture as well. As the reader will discover throughout this chapter, the designation of cultures as "popular," "ethnic," "occupations," etc. is ultimately contextual if not arbitrary. Consider, for instance a person who grew up into mainstream American culture but who became, say, a business executive or oilfield worker in a Middle Eastern country. That person's familiar "popular" culture would be redefined elsewhere as his or her "ethnonational" popular culture, one that would differ markedly from the professional and popular medical cultures of the Middle East host nation. That is, what one calls culture depends in part on where one is!

We take for granted elements of American popular medical culture, although they become evident as soon as they are pointed out. Over-the-counter patent medicines available at pharmacies and supermarkets are part of this popular, folk-American culture. The wide-swinging deification and villification of doctors (who can do nothing wrong and who can do nothing right) is intrinsic to popular culture. The common preference for medication in pill (oral) form, together with the search for a pill for every ailment, "magic bullets," are popular ethnomedicine. Similarly, much of the impetus for high-technology solutions to human suffering come from this cultural "grass roots." Television commercials (from prime time to "soap operas"), newspaper and magazine ads, and articles in the popular press are rich treasure troves of fantasies and ideologies and practices within American popular medicine.

A strong theme within this popular culture is that of *germ phobia,* a long-term preoccupation of Americans and one into which AIDS fits grimly well. In popular culture, much of the painstaking, scientific method that at least officially characterizes the ideal self-image of biomedicine is replaced by abundant magical thinking, of which supernaturalized, menacing "germs" are the result. The popular medical cult of cleanliness, inside the body and outside, from laxatives through laundry detergents, is obsessed with the ritual purification of the body, to make it as in the Ivory Snow commercial, "99 and 44/100% pure." The popular image of the doctor, conqueror, warrior, doer, teacher, wise caretaker, and master of high technology holds that the physician is the one in whom the hope rests for the secularized purification of the body for life here on earth.

The deep embeddedness of biomedicine in the American imagination is immediately attested to by the consistent popularity of medical programs on television, e.g., "Marcus Welby, M.D."; "Ben Casey"; "Medical Center"; "MASH"; "After-MASH"; "Trapper John, M.D."; the daytime soap operas such as "General Hospital," and countless local call-in physician talk shows. Moreover, medical "miracles" and "breakthroughs" are featured on local and national "news" on radio and television, in the newspaper, and in national magazines. To be so worthy of prominence in the genres of "news" and "entertainment," medicine must tap deeply into the dominant meanings and fantasies of our time.

Professional culture is never far removed from popular American culture. An example is the prevalence of "management" imagery, language, and organization within biomedicine. In the 1920s, the movement led by Frederick Winslow Taylor introduced principles of scientific management into industry and organizational settings. Three decades later, Peter Drucker's (1954) rationalist approach called "management by objective" became widely accepted throughout American business culture. Work was conceived to be a strictly and narrowly linear enterprise, having expected outcomes and precise ways of reaching them and measuring productivity along the path toward that outcome. One might say that this managerial world view was a decontextualized one or rather one in which the only contexts to be considered were those regarded by the managers as important (e.g., specifically, variables that were supposed to be incentives for greater worker productivity).

This management ethos rapidly diffused throughout various cultural institutions, medicine among them. Common expressions are "medical management," "case management," "management conference," "It is a clinical management problem," and so forth. Not only the language but the way of *imaging* or *conceptualizing* medical problems, the way of treating them, and the way of relating to other medical colleagues in the treatment process are all consequences of the popular culturally managerial style of thinking. Clinically and elsewhere in life, people act toward themselves and toward others in terms of how and what they think of themselves. In medicine as in life, metaphors often become destinies.

In a powerful interpretive passage, Scheper-Hughes and Lock (1987) show how professional and medical cultures collude in the production of the obsession with anorexic fitness and ascetic wellness. In a sinister way, hypochondriasis is transformed from disease into cure!

> In our own increasingly "healthist" and body-conscious culture, the politically correct body for both sexes is the lean, strong, androgynous, and physically "fit" form through which the core cultural values of autonomy, toughness, competitiveness, youth, and self-control are readily manifest (Pollitt, 1982). Health is increasingly viewed in the United States as an achieved rather than an ascribed status, and each individual is expected to "work hard" at being strong, fit, and healthy. Conversely, ill health is no longer viewed as accidental, a mere quirk of nature, but rather is attributed to the individual's failure to live right, to eat well, to exercise, etc. We might ask what it is our society "wants" from this kind of body. DeMause (1984) has speculated that the fitness/toughness craze is a reflection of an international preparation for war. A hardening and toughening of the national fiber corresponds to a toughening of individual bodies. In attitude and ideology the self-help and fitness movements articulate both a militarist and a social Darwinist ethos: the fast and fit win; the fat and flabby lose and drop out of the human race (Scheper-Hughes & Stein, 1987). Crawford (1980, 1985),

> however, has suggested that the fitness movement may reflect, instead, a pathetic and individualized (also wholly inadequate) defense against the threat of nuclear holocaust. . . . Crawford (1985) has interpreted the eating disorders and distortions in body image expressed in obsessional jogging, anorexia, and bulimia as a symbolic mediation of the contradictory demands of postindustrial American society. The double-binding injunction to be self-controlled, fit, and productive workers and to be at the same time self-indulgent, pleasure-seeking consumers is especially destructive to the self-image of the "modern," "liberated" American woman. Expected to be fun-loving and sensual, she must also remain thin, lovely, and self-disciplined. Since one cannot be hedonistic and controlled simultaneously, one can alternate phases of binge eating, drinking, and drugging with phases of jogging, purging, and vomiting. Out of this cyclical resolution of the injunction to consume and to conserve is born, according to Crawford, the current epidemic of eating disorders (especially bulimia) among young women, some of whom literally eat and diet to death (Scheper-Hughes & Lock, 1987, pp. 25–26).

Linking professional biomedical and popular national American culture is the fact that "illness somatization has become a dominant metaphor for expressing individual and social complaint" (Scheper-Hughes & Lock, 1987, p. 27). Physician, health care system, third-party payers, patients, families, and society jointly collude in the diversion of attention from affect (emotion), conscious and unconscious meaning, and the experience of social injustice. Paradoxically, by defining virtually all problems and issues somatically, patients and families inadvertently surrender to physician control much of the autonomy and self-responsibility for which the medical consumerist movement of the 1970s fought so strenuously. Scheper-Hughes and Lock (1987) ironically point to "the usefulness to the body politic of filtering more and more human unrest, dissatisfaction, longing, and protest into the idiom of sickness, which can then be safely managed by doctor agents (p. 27)."

Consider the following case that illustrates one model of alcoholism in popular culture.

Case 10-10. A 47-year-old male was brought by ambulance to the emergency room following a fight that broke out at a New Year's Eve party. His wife accompanied him to the hospital. He had become severely intoxicated after drinking a number of mixed "hard liquor" beverages. He then got into an argument with another person and got into a fistfight that ended with abrasions, contusions, and a broken right femur. At the ER, his wife said with a mixture of embarrassment and naivete: "He's just not himself when he drinks. He's really a quiet man, always considerate of other people. He's a supervisor down at the plant, and he never lets anything get him ruffled. People admire him for being able to handle anything. He's a wonderful guy when he's sober. I just don't know what gets into him when he's been drinking."

The next day, the patient said to the physician: "I'm just a different person when I drink." His wife confided to the physician later on that: "When he's sober, he's all business. I guess that's the way he's got to be, taking charge of so much responsibility at the plant. He's not much fun. But when he drinks is about the only time we have good sex any more. I don't know what comes over him, but it's not the same person he is the rest of the time. When he drinks, I don't know whether to look forward to what happens or to dread it."

An implicit popular cultural theory of "possession" underlies the official professional pharmacological biomedical theory of alcoholism and drug abuse in America (Stein, 1982, 1985a, 1987c). In this folk model, alcoholism and chemical dependency constitute a form of *secular possession*. In imbibing the spirits, one incorporates the impersonal anima or "spirit" that has been bottled or canned and is soon possessed by it. Just as religious knowledge is said to come from the outside in, by divine "inspiration" or "revelation," likewise do drunkenness or drug-induced highs. All one need do to confirm this is to consult our cultural semantics, vividly illustrated by the above clinical example.

We say one becomes "intoxicated" after consuming alcoholic beverages. We speak of someone being "under the influence" of alcohol or "driving under the influence" (or "while intoxicated"). Alcohol is thereby associated with the profane, with badness, with poison that enters the body and does its evil work (e.g., "demon rum"). The initial part of our cultural ritual cure for alcoholics is, not unexpectedly, a form of exorcism: *detoxification* to expunge the poisons (toxins) from the body, often performed in special inpatient hospital wards or mental health units. Since possession by the debasing, alien agent caused the intoxication in the first place, detoxification will expel the noxious substance from the body. But expulsion is never complete ("Once an alcoholic, always an alcoholic"). Alcoholics, even after the exorcism (similar to drug abusers following chemical detoxification), remain vulnerable to being possessed once again by the vile but fascinating substance.

Although Americans proudly scorn the notion of spirit possession within other contexts as being "mere" superstition, scientific theory is often in fact only veiled supernatural, animistic possession theory in an acceptable form. Such cultural models, when applied to biomedicine in the designation of alcoholism as a disease, may be used to divert the attention of patient, family, physician, health care institution, and the wider culture away from the system of meanings, conscious and unconscious, of which alcoholism or drug abuse are only "the tip of the iceberg."

CONCLUSIONS

This chapter has introduced the reader to the cultural world of the patient, and perhaps has *re*introduced the reader to the cultural worlds he or she inhabits. In all clinical communication, the practitioner gains access to realms of the patient's experience, values, beliefs, expectations, explanations, feelings, meanings, and conflicts by having free access to those realms within himself or herself. The self of the clinician remains one of the finest instruments of observation, assessment, and treatment available. Physicians, no less than patients, are creators and bearers of culture, and suffer the consequences from unexamined assumptions about others' cultures.

In this chapter, after several approaches to the concept of culture were discussed, two aspects of culture were portrayed: (1) patients' informal care networks and (2) illness-related words and concepts, together with their meanings. Four cultural domains that affect patients' health behavior were explored: ethnicity, religion, occupation, and popular American culture. It is tempting for the practitioner to memorize lists of cultural traits, just as in medical school the student must memorize thousands of anatomic parts, biochemical terms, physiological processes, and pharmacological actions. The result, however, would be less an intimate understanding of a real other person and family than the imposition of a stereotype and the mistaking of that stereotype for the patient's reality. It is admittedly more difficult, yet at the same time more rewarding, for the physician (or other health care provider) to take an interest in the patient as a person, an interest that will quite naturally lead to inquiry into the universes of meaning the patient inhabits and in turn to a more satisfactory, productive clinical relationship.

CASES FOR DISCUSSION

Case 1

Work-culture pathologies occur not only in individuals but in groups. The astute clinician, by knowing the organizational culture, can know *what* is "infectious," and its timing as well. In a pioneering paper on "Anthropologic aspects of occupational illness epidemics," Hocking (1987) offers the following case:

> Macquire [1978] reported two outbreaks of skin disorders in English workplaces. One in a ceramics factory is described here. Eight female employees who worked in one room and two male porters were affected. One woman was (subsequently) found to have angioneurotic edema with cholinergic urticaria with impetigo complicating self-inflicted excoriation. The other seven women described how their difficulties began after seeing this woman, and they developed transient rashes on their exposed surfaces. The two men had a winter eczema. An extensive investigation was undertaken, the plant was temporarily closed, frank reassurance was given, and the rashes disappeared. Macquire notes that only the first employee sought medical help. "It was clearly evident from the consensus among the employees that the factory management was directly responsible for their illnesses, so it must cure them without anyone else's help." She also notes of the workplace "that there was no longer a sense of individuality, only units in a system of groups of varying sizes," Macquire does not term her cases MPI [Mass Psychogenic Illness], but "psychic possession" (Hocking, 1987, p. 527).

Hocking (1987) draws attention to "structural factors and grievances in the work force . . . industrial solutions by themselves should not be seen as adequate. The distress of the individual and the group must not be overlooked by physicians or social scientists" (p. 529). Hocking (1987) defines mass psychogenic illness as "the collective occurrence of physical [somatic] symptoms and related beliefs among two or more persons in the absence of an identifiable pathogen" (p. 527). He continues:

> MPI in the workplace is held to have certain features in that it largely involves females who are relatively uneducated and are performing routine repetitive work; it has an explosive onset and rapid remission but with relapses; and clusters are found without apparent cause. . . . The fact that these epidemics tend to involve women in certain work situations may reflect their powerlessness as well as the need for the group to define itself. This social function of illness is much removed from the biomedical definition of disease and not surprisingly perplexing to most physicians (Hocking, 1987, pp. 527–528).

Mass somatization in the workplace ironically occurs by the same mental mechanisms through which a cohesive work culture forms: the process of identification. The "infectiousness" of mass psychogenic or sociogenic illnesses can likewise be interpreted in terms of the dynamics of the psychiatric "*folie-à-deux*" to the *n*th degree.

1. As a physician in a community or corporate group, how do you learn to think in terms of epidemiologic or cultural patterns in addition to thinking clinically, one patient at a time?
2. As the physician for a corporation or plant, for whom do you work (that is, individual employee, the employee's supervisor, the management, the union, etc.)? What role conflicts might you expect in the setting of an industrial or corporate culture?
3. Discuss this case in terms of Kleinman's distinction between "disease" and "illness."
4. If somaticizing responses are corporately and culturally safe, how would you help employees to discuss feelings and grievances if these could be construed by management as threat or rebellion?
5. How would you clinically or administratively deal with the issues of female employees' low pay and relative powerlessness?

Case 2

John Deer is a 60-year-old white male who farms on the southern Plains (from Stein & Pontious, 1985, pp. 181–183). He works 14–16 h daily and is upset when unable to work. His farming activities consist mainly of large-scale pork production and several sections of wheat land that he and his son-in-law actively farm.

Over the last several years, John Deer was having increased difficulty with his right knee, especially when he bent down to work on feeders or was getting into a tractor cab. He visited several physicians to alleviate the pain. Although medication—when he would take it—somewhat decreased the pain, Mr. Deer continued to have an intermittent effusion over the knee and experienced a marked loss in his range of motion. As the more active seasons (spring and early summer) in his farming operation came about, the knee pain became worse, but Mr. Deer protested to the family that during these periods he had little time to take care of it. He would wait until November, December, or January to have it checked, for winter was the time he felt the farm needed the least attention. Mr. Deer postponed having anything major done about the knee for fear that it would restrict his activities and that he might come out of it worse than when he went in. His family physician son-in-law observed that: "For him not to have harvest is like a death notice." Mr. Deer relied on his family for medical advice and health care prior to and while utilizing medical facilities.

In October 1980, Mr. Deer consulted an orthopedic surgeon for evaluation in a city 30 miles from home. He was told that he had severe degenerative arthritis of the knee. The orthopedic surgeon recommended a total knee prosthesis. Mr. Deer informed the physician that he would consider surgery but needed time to think about it.

Mr. Deer returned home and asked the advice of his family physician son-in-law. The latter discussed with Mr. Deer the pros and cons of joint replacement and what he might expect in terms of outcome and length of convalescence. Mr. Deer continued to have difficulty in making a decision. At the suggestion of the son-in-law, he obtained a second opinion from a physician at a regional medical center some 100 miles from Mr. Deer's home. The second orthopedist concurred with the initial assessment and recommended a total knee replacement.

Mr. Deer subsequently developed low back pain, which his original orthopedic surgeon felt was secondary to his gait (which had changed because of the pain he initially had in the right knee). The back pain persisted, motivating Mr. Deer to consult a local chiropractor who had a reputation in the community of being able to improve resistant cases of back pain. Mr. Deer expected an instant cure (an assumption shared by many, that when one is treated by a chiropractor, one will feel better immediately; treatment by physicians, on the other hand, takes time, and its outcome is often uncertain). The chiropractor took a series of x rays and pointed out that indeed it was his back that was causing his pain and that to operate would be futile, since it was the back that was the difficulty and would respond to "manipulation."

After the treatment by the chiropractor had failed to reduce his pain, Mr. Deer tarried another 2 months prior to making his decision to undergo the knee surgery. In February 1981, he decided to have the surgery done. The cultural logic that the son-in-law employed to convince his father-in-law to undergo surgery in late winter was that, all things being equal, Mr. Deer should be mobile enough by late May to participate fully in the wheat harvest.

In early March 1981, a total knee prosthesis was performed. There were no intra- or postoperative complications. Mr. Deer was discharged in mid-March. At that time he had but 60° range of motion in his right knee, and it was painful to ambulate. His orthopedic surgeon informed him that his restriction was entirely "within normal limits" and that he would gradually be able to increase his range of motion. His physical therapist, one of his daughters, worked consistently with him over the ensuing weeks to improve the range of motion. Mr. Deer was markedly dissatisfied with his progress. With the wheat harvest rapidly approaching, he was anxious that he would be in "no condition" to oversee the harvesting of his crops.

Knee immobility played a role in his investment in new equipment, specifically a combine "with a cab large enough" to accommodate a leg in the extended position. This purchase enabled him to harvest his crops as he had done for 40 years. Five months later, Mr. Deer had full range of motion of his right knee and was contemplating having a prosthesis done on the left knee.

1. What occupationally related difficulties was Mr. Deer having that led him to seek medical consultation?
2. Why did Mr. Deer postpone for so long having "anything major" (surgery) performed on his right knee?
3. What was Mr. Deer's rationale in seeking the services of a chiropractor?
4. What is the "right time" for surgery according to the cultural rules of farmer John Deer? According to those of his physicians?
5. Describe the *sequence* of family, folk, and biomedical personnel whom Mr. Deer consulted and explain how this sequence "makes sense" within Mr. Deer's rural, agricultural world.

Case 3

Mary Tinsley, a woman in her mid-60s presents at the office of her family physician with a complaint of mid- and low-back pain (from Stein, 1987a, pp. 170–171). It is late September, and her annual visits are like clockwork. Her ritual has been going on for some 30 years. She alleges that years ago she had some back injury, but no vertebral fractures or compressions can be detected. Recent workups confirm the present physician's conviction that the problem is psychosomatic. The present physician is one in a distinguished line of family physicians, general practitioners, and orthopedic surgeons, all of whom were able to "find nothing."

Every year during the September planting season, John Tinsley, her husband, a man in his late 60s, spends nearly 2 weeks away from the house, working in the field. Mary feels isolated, abandoned. She felt this way even when their young children were living with them, when they lived in a house on the farm. She feels the same now that she and her husband have moved from the farm to a nearby town. Thirty years ago, her back pain was so bad that she had to move about in a wheel chair, and her irate husband and children had to take care of *her.* Over the years, she had admirably run the household and reared the children. During the rest of the year, she is not sick a day. But come September and planting, her low-back pain is as predictable as is the change of season. The annual onset of symptoms coincides with John's departure. By the time plowing is finished, she has become a veritable cripple (while continuing to perform domestic duties to a fault) and seeks medical relief. The physician prescribes meperidine HCl (a narcotic pain medicine) or flurazepam HCl (a tranquilizer) to alleviate the pain.

Mary reports that her husband berates her as "excess baggage," accusing her of not holding her own in her responsibilities about the house. As they both have grown older, Mary has apparently "aged" more than John—who even now cannot seem to work enough. John wants the freedom to work his farm, to come and go as he pleases, to be accountable to no one, and to not be tied to home or wife. Over time John's expectations have not at all diminished, whereas Mary resents being saddled with these expectations, feeling unappreciated for her role and abandoned and ridiculed as "excess baggage."

1. Explain the timing of the wife's symptoms.
2. Speculate on the role of her symptoms in her marriage.
3. How would you as a physician go about inquiring into the meaning and function of her physical symptoms?
4. How would you avoid the temptation to do a "million-dollar workup" on a patient of this kind—who is "presenting" somatically?
5. How would you introduce "psychosocial" issues to a patient whose familial–cultural–religious beliefs militate against such an interpretation?

Case 4

A farmer in his early 50s was scheduled for gallbladder surgery (from Stein, 1985b, pp. 87–88). Hospitalized, he was being prepped for surgery, his family gathering in the waiting area. As the anesthesiologist approached the patient, he developed supraventricular tachycardia, whereupon she stepped back and waited for him to calm down. She tried this unsuccessfully several times. Finally, she decided to postpone the surgery until a later time—one in which the patient would presumably be less nervous.

In the waiting area, the family wondered why it took so long for him to be readied for surgery. First, the anesthesiologist attempted to explain the problem by saying that the patient had developed supraventricular tachycardia; she explained anatomically all that was involved; she even drew an elementary diagram. The family didn't understand, standing around puzzled, wondering whether something undiscovered was wrong. The surgeon then attempted to redeem the situation, going basically through the same explanation as had the anesthesiologist—with similar success.

Down the hall walked a family physician who overheard the vain attempts to explain to the family through recourse to anatomy and physiology. He put his arm around the shoulder of one of the members of the family, and said: "Your father's heart is shimmying like the front end of an old Chevy." The family said, with one voice, "Oh!"—finally feeling that they understood what was wrong. Satisfied, they were ready to leave until the next attempt could be made.

1. How would you have tried to explain the patient's cardiac reaction to the patient and family?
2. How do you think you would have responded (feeling, behavior) to the patient's and family's incomprehension of an accurate, elegant biomedical explanation you had just offered to them?
3. What cues would "tell" you that you need to talk with them in a different language?
4. Why do you think the family practitioner's explanation succeeded, since a heart is not the same as the front end of a pick-up truck?
5. Had this been an emergency situation, how would you have proceeded medically?

Case 5

Mrs. S. was a 27-year-old Native American female with a 6-year history of systemic lupus erythematosis and treatment with [cortico]steroids [cortisone] who was referred to the University Hospital in Seattle [pregnant] at 30 weeks' gestation with symptoms of preeclampsia (from Kleinman, 1982, p. 95). The patient had had four previous miscarriages in the last 6 years at early stages of gestation. She had one daughter, age 8, and strongly desired another child.

Because of severe preeclampsia, labor was induced during her second hospital day, and a nonviable premature infant was delivered. Psychiatric consultation was obtained 3 days later for "psychotic depression with hallucinations."

The following history was obtained from the patient. She was mourning the death of her baby and had "heard the baby cry" 2 days after the death. She stated that it was normal in her American Indian culture for loved ones to talk with close family members after death to try to bring relatives with them into the hereafter. Although she had no prior experience with this custom, many of her friends had spoken of their experiences with loved ones after death. The staff reacted with anxiety and alarm on hearing that Mrs. S. had heard her baby cry after it had been dead for 2 days and never bothered to elicit her cultural explanation. Thus, a psychiatric consultation was requested.

After talking with the patient and the staff, we recommended that the staff help the patient ventilate her feelings about the death of the baby and also enable her to perform any cultural ceremony that she and her husband would normally go through at home. During the next 7 days of the hospitalization the patient "heard her baby cry" daily, but with the help of the staff and her husband this became less alarming to the patient. She and her husband went through their indigenous rite of destroying all traces of the baby's existence, including blankets, baby clothes, and an echogram picture. The patient made an uneventful recovery both physically and emotionally (Katon & Kleinman, 1981, pp. 259–260). Reports of similar culturally constituted acute grief reactions can be found in the ethnographic literature on Native Americans.

1. Describe how you would go about distinguishing between behavior that is cultural from behavior that might be labeled "psychotic depression." (Moreover, can cultural behavior also be psychotic or depressive?)
2. Describe the differences between the cultural accounts of the medical staff and the Native American woman with respect to hearing the deceased baby cry.
3. What are some differences between Judeo-Christian and Native American religious beliefs and practices that affect how the patient and the staff respond to the birth of a premature infant? (There are, admittedly, enormous *intra*-group differences.)
4. If you were working clinically with this woman and her family, how would you assist in the grieving process?
5. What is your personal reaction to this case, and how do you think your response affects how, when, or even whether you would elicit her explanation for her reaction?

RECOMMENDED READINGS

Abel, T. M., Metraux, R., & Roll, S. (1987). *Psychotherapy and culture.* Albuquerque, NM: University of New Mexico.

Abel, Metraux, and Roll offer a view of the therapeutic process based on a psychodynamic model of human relationships and meanings.

Christman, N. J., & Maretzki, T. W. (Eds.). (1982). *Clinically applied anthropology.* Dordrecht, Holland: D. Reidel.

This edited volume describes the clinical contributions of applied anthropologists who conduct research and teach in health science settings.

Harwood, A. (Ed.). (1981). *Ethnicity and medical care.* Cambridge, MA: Harvard University Press.

This edited volume offers rich accounts of the role of cultural values, attitudes, expectations, language, and beliefs in a wide array of ethnic groups' members' health behaviors.

Henry, J. (1963). *Culture against man.* New York: Random House.

Henry critically examines family, education, values, political ideologies, attitudes toward aging, and much more in this classic work on American culture.

Stein, H. F., & Apprey, M. (1987). *From metaphor to meaning: Papers in psychoanalytic anthropology.* Charlottesville, VA: University Press of Virginia.

Stein and Apprey offer interpretations of the intrapsychic story that is simultaneously represented and veiled by culture. They demonstrate how deceptively simple personal, familial, clinical, and larger cultural symbols condense complex ideas and feelings.

CHAPTER 11

The Health Care System

James W. Mold*

Case 11-1. Dr. S. had become increasingly active on the staff of a comprehensive rehabilitation hospital. He was particularly interested in geriatric rehabilitation, becoming the most frequent admitter of older patients to the facility. With the encouragement of the Chief of Staff and the administrator of the hospital, he began having meetings with the staff to discuss ways to improve the care of older rehabilitation patients. One of the ideas he presented to the group, which was made up of physicians, nurses, speech–language pathologists, occupational therapists, physical therapists, recreational therapists, social workers, case managers, and dieticians, was to have providers document their portions of the initial assessment in a single unified section of the chart and to put all progress notes within another single unified section using a goal-oriented, rather than a problem-oriented (SOAP), format.

Dr. S. was surprised at the amount of resistance to his idea. The other physicians in the group did not want other providers writing in the physicians' progress notes section of the chart and felt that a problem-oriented format was more appropriate than a goal-oriented system. The nursing staff was using a separate chart altogether, had put a great deal of effort into developing it, and saw no reason to change their system. Many of the therapists were enthusiastic about the idea but felt that differences in terminology and approach might make communication difficult even within a unified chart. They were also concerned about who would be involved in constructing the goals list, specifically wondering whether the physicians would control the process.

*With the assistance of **Kevin T. Avery,** D.M.D., **Julia Eyer,** Ph.D., CCC-SP, **Martha J. Ferretti,** M.P.H., P.T., **Marjorie Greer,** LPT, **Don Lanquist,** RRT, **Carol McCoy,** Ph.D., MT (ASCP), CLS, **Earl Schmitt,** O.D., Ed.D., **Roberta Warner,** R.D./L.D., **Terry Pace,** Ph.D., **Linda E. Reed,** P.A.-C., M.Ed., **Bob Shahan,** R.T., **Carole A. Sullivan,** M.Ed., R.T.(R)T, FASRT, **Sheila Tiarks,** M.S.W., **Shirley Wunder,** R.N.

INTRODUCTION

Although physicians are typically considered to be the principal providers of health care in this country, in actuality they represent one of a large number of disciplines that make up the health care system. Many of the other disciplines are comparatively new, reflecting the increasing complexity of modern health care. Table 11-1 is a partial list of health care providers.

For such a large and complex system to be most effective and efficient in its mission to improve the quantity and quality of life of individual patients, a certain amount of teamwork is required. Unfortunately, the training received by providers in each discipline is usually discipline specific, taught by members of that discipline, with surprisingly little integration among training programs. For example, physicians are rarely taught by nurses except informally on the hospital wards, and social workers learn very little about physical therapists until they are forced to work with them later in the workplace. As a result, approaches to health care and even the terminologies used by providers from different disciplines often differ considerably. In addition, because of differences in responsibilities and rewards as well as some overlap of competencies, there is a natural tendency for the various groups to be suspicious and sometimes envious of each other, a tendency that, at its worst, leads to what is commonly called "turfism" (protecting one's turf), as illustrated in Case 11-1.

When the barriers between disciplines can be overcome, the health care system can function in a truly interdisciplinary way. Such cooperation results in better coordination of health care with less duplication of efforts. More overall energy can be applied to patient care, since less is spent on "turf" battles.

The goals of this chapter are to introduce the major health care providers including information about roles, practice settings, training, and certification. The consultation and referral process is described. The interdisciplinary team approach to health care is introduced and described as desirable even if it is often difficult to achieve. Some of the obstacles to implementation of a team approach are discussed, and suggestions are made regarding ways to overcome those obstacles.

Table 11-1
Partial List of Health Care Providers

Dentistry	Pharmacy
Dietetics	Physical therapy
Clinical laboratory science	Podiatry
Family therapy	Psychology
Medical records	Radiologic technology
Medicine	Recreational therapy
Nursing	Social work
Occupational therapy	Speech–language pathology
Optometry	

Case 11-2. Mrs. B.F. was a 68-year-old woman who had coronary artery bypass surgery 6 years earlier and now was experiencing recurrent symptoms related to her severe coronary artery disease, uncontrolled by medications. Her physician, Dr. J., requested a cardiologist's opinion regarding the risks and benefits to Mrs. F. of another coronary artery bypass operation. The cardiologist, after evaluating Mrs. F., agreed that surgery was a possible option and requested the additional input of a cardiothoracic surgeon. The surgeon, after reviewing the cardiac catheterization results, recommended against surgery because of the high operative risk for this particular patient.

However, Dr. J. felt that his questions had not been properly answered. He already knew that the risk associated with a second cardiac surgery would be high, but he felt that his patient might be willing to take a substantial risk considering that she was unable to do anything without experiencing chest pain and had tried all other available treatments without benefit. What Dr. J. really needed to know were the probability of benefit and the probabilities of the various possible adverse outcomes associated with surgery for his patient so that he could intelligently assist Mrs. F. to make the best possible decision taking into account her own values and preferences.

In 1986 there were 569,160 physicians in the United States. Of these, 462,126 were involved in patient care activities. There were 230 physicians per 100,000 population in 1986 compared to 142 per 100,000 in 1960. The number of physicians increased $3^1/_2$ times more rapidly than the population as a whole over that period of time, leading some authorities to speculate that an oversupply of physicians now exists (see Chapter 14). Approximately 40% of physicians in 1986 were classified as primary care physicians (family physicians, general practitioners, general internists, and pediatricians). Fifteen percent are women, up from 7% in 1967 (AMA, 1987).

Physicians have traditionally been male, whereas most of the other health care disciplines are predominantly female. Differentials in average income undoubtedly reflect not only differences in training and responsibility but also a measure of sexism. As more women become physicians and more men become nurses and allied health professionals, these differences may become less significant.

Because of their extensive training as well as their highly revered position in society, physicians have tended to occupy the highest leadership roles in the health care delivery systems. Physicians are often the chairmen of hospital committees. They are frequently the directors of peer review organizations (PROs) and often hold important positions within health insurance companies. Hospital medical staffs have a great deal of control over hospital administrators. State and national physician organizations such as state medical societies and the American Medical Association exert a powerful influence on legislators. Although administrators are now taking away some of the authority and responsibility that has traditionally belonged to physicians, among health care providers it is still physicians who most frequently give orders that other providers are expected to follow and physicians who bear the greatest liability when something goes wrong. Many physicians believe strongly that other health care professionals are, or should be, under their direct control and should only be involved in patient care by direct order of a physician.

Because of the current dominance of the biomedical model of health, physicians, as the most highly trained applied scientists, are the most respected members of the health care team. Other health professionals are often forced, then, to function in supporting roles. There is some reason to believe, however, that the current biomedical model may soon be transformed into a new approach that will also transform the traditional hierarchy to some degree. The pressure for such a paradigm shift is coming as a result of changes in both the content and definition of health care and from consumers who have become increasingly dissatisfied with the current biotechnical, physician-dominated approach, which is viewed as too impersonal, mechanistic, and expensive (Freymann, 1989).

Interactions among Physicians

As the field of medicine has become more and more complex, physicians themselves have become increasingly fragmented into groups defined by specialization and subspecialization. Table 11-2 lists the major medical and surgical specialties. The same sorts of turf struggles that occur between health care disciplines occur between specialties of medicine for similar reasons. Interestingly, more specialized physicians tend to have greater status and higher incomes than generalists. This trend is in stark contrast to the situation that exists in most modern corporations, for instance, in which individuals with the most specialized training are the heads of divisions, whereas the corporate leaders are of necessity generalists. Part of the income differential between specialists and generalists is the result of third party reimbursement practices, which have tended to favor procedures over cognitive activities (see Chapter 14).

Despite their higher incomes and status, specialists are dependent on generalists for consultations and referral of patients. Thus, there is some pressure on

Table 11-2
Major Medical and Surgical Specialties[a]

Allergy and immunology	Otolaryngology
Anesthesiology	Pathology
Colon and rectal surgery	Pediatrics
Dermatology	Physical medicine and rehabilitation
Emergency medicine	Plastic surgery
Family practice	Preventive medicine
Internal medicine	Psychiatry and neurology
Neurological surgery	Radiology
Nuclear medicine	Surgery
Obstetrics and gynecology	Thoracic surgery
Ophthalmology	Urology
Orthopedic surgery	

[a] *American Board of Medical Specialties Compendium of Certified Medical Specialists,* (American Board of Medical Specialties, 1986).

specialists to be gracious and to return referred patients to the referring physicians as promptly as possible. This graciousness unfortunately often evaporates within medical centers and other larger organizations in which, for one reason or another, specialists are less dependent on, or are less aware of their dependency on, primary care physician referrals, as in Case 11-2.

Patients interested in obtaining the best possible health care are faced with the confusing choice of either seeing the appropriate specialists for each of their health problems or of seeing a generalist (family physician, internist, or pediatrician), whom they must trust to refer them to specialists when appropriate. Studies indicate that family physicians can skillfully manage 85% to 95% of the health care problems that their patients present to them (Geyman, Brown, & Rivers, 1976; Brock, 1977). Because of their familiarity with specialist colleagues and with the health care system in general, primary care (generalist) physicians are often in an ideal position to advise their patients when consultation with other providers is necessary and which specialists would provide the best service in specific situations.

Generalists can also serve as health care coordinators and patient advocates when problems are multiple or complex. Most physicians would agree that a critical requirement for good patient care is that one physician or other health care professional must take a primary decision-making and coordinating role in the care of each patient. When this does not occur, the patient is in danger of becoming overtested, overmedicated, frustrated, and confused. The modern health care system is complex enough that most individuals at some point need the services of a personal advocate. Lately this coordinating role is being referred to as "primary medical care" when it is assumed by a physician or as "case management" when it is assumed by a nonphysician.

Generalists are less likely to recognize and diagnose unusual problems as quickly and accurately as specialists can within their areas of expertise. They are therefore susceptible to *errors of omission*. Specialists, on the other hand, are less able to view health problems in context, are expected not to make errors of omission, and have more technology at their fingertips, making them more susceptible to *errors of commission* (doing too much). Errors of omission are often more obvious than errors of commission but are not necessarily more harmful. Increasingly aggressive attempts, through testing and other interventions, to reduce uncertainty and the anxiety that accompanies it at times may result in an avalanche of unwanted consequences. This phenomenon has been called the "cascade effect" (Mold & Stein, 1986). Clinical cascades may be catastrophic and obvious, but they are more often indolent and unrecognized.

Integral to the professional relationship between physicians is the consultative process (McWhinney, 1989). Classically, a physician asks, on behalf of his patient, a particular specialist for expert advice regarding the diagnosis or treatment of a particular health problem. The request may be communicated by phone, letter, or by the patient directly. The more effectively the request is communicated, the more likely the consultant is to be helpful by providing the answers to the referring physician's questions. Once the specialist has reached an opinion, he communicates it to the patient and to the referring physician in one or more of the same ways and returns the patient to the care of the referring physician unless requested to do otherwise. Obviously, good communication between physicians is essential to the consultative process, but for several reasons, including time restraints, fear of disclosure of incompetence, and lack of training in the consultative process, it may not always occur.

A proper request for consultation should include the specific questions that are being asked of the consultant and specific directives as to the extent of involvement requested of the consultant in the evaluation and management of the patient. The physician requesting the consultation may, for example, request that the consultant render an opinion regarding diagnosis or treatment but not assume responsibility for implementation of the recommended treatment or for ongoing care.

Although the opinion of the consultant should obviously be given a great deal of consideration, it is in no way binding. Neither the physician requesting the consultation nor the patient is under any ethical or legal obligation to follow the advice of the consultant. It should be remembered that although the consultant brings specialized knowledge and skills to bear on the problem in question, the referring physician and patient have equally important information that must be considered before a final decision can be made. Under no circumstances should a consultant send the patient to a second consultant without the authorization and approval of the primary physician, as was done in Case 11-2 (McWhinney, 1989). Unfortunately, even when the request for a consultation is communicated effectively, the consultation does not always prove helpful. In such a situation, the physicians involved may need to communicate the request again directly, or it may be necessary for the primary physician to consult a different physician.

At times it is necessary and appropriate for one physician to refer a patient to another physician for ongoing management of one or more problems. This process, which is called referral, requires the same careful communication as described for the consultative process.

Osteopathic Physicians

There have been as many as four different physician groups in the United States. However, at the present time there are two distinct groups of physicians in this country, allopathic and osteopathic. Allopathic physicians, M.D.s who rely primarily on drug or surgical cures, have been described in the previous section. Osteopathic physicians, D.O.s, are described next.

Osteopathy was founded in 1874 by Dr. Andrew Still. It was based on the following principles, which apparently were sufficiently distinct from those of allopathic physicians at that time (Jones, 1978):

1. The body is an integral unit, a whole. The structure of the body and its functions work together, interdependently.
2. The body systems have built-in repair processes, which are self-regulating and self-healing in the face of disease.
3. The circulatory system or distributing channels of the body, along with the nervous system, provide the integrating functions for the rest of the body.

4. The contribution of the musculoskeletal system to a person's health is much more than providing framework and support.
5. While disease may be manifested in specific parts of the body, other body parts may contribute to a restoration or correction of the disease.

Dr. Still had become fascinated with the musculoskeletal system, spending large amounts of time studying it in great detail. At the same time he was opposed to many of the medicinal remedies that were in vogue at the time and was therefore interested in nonpharmacological treatments for disease that could enhance the body's natural repair mechanisms. He became convinced that manipulation of the musculoskeletal system could effect beneficial changes in all other systems, particularly the circulatory and nervous systems, which he felt were critical to the body's natural reparative mechanisms.

Although osteopathic manipulation is a relatively small part of the training and practice of osteopathic physicians today, it has never been accepted by allopathic medicine as a valid approach and has been singled out and magnified as part of a historically aggressive and persistent, though weakening, campaign by allopaths to discredit and ostracize osteopaths. It has only been within the last two decades that osteopaths have been allowed to be members of the medical staffs at predominantly allopathic hospitals. It is still difficult for osteopaths to obtain malpractice insurance.

The number of osteopathic physicians in the United States increased from 14,300 in 1970 to 24,000 in 1985. The ratio of allopaths to osteopaths in 1985 was approximately 23 to 1. Currently osteopathic physicians receive essentially the same quantity and quality of training as allopathic physicians, with only minor differences in philosophy and emphasis. Although barriers and philosophical distinctions between the two physician groups are diminishing, there are no obvious signs that they intend to unite in the near future.

For a variety of reasons including the basic principles of the discipline, osteopaths have always been trained as generalists first and foremost, and although specialty training is available in all of the traditional areas, a larger percentage of osteopaths end up in general practice compared to allopathic physicians. Osteopathic physicians have also been more likely to practice in rural settings than their allopathic counterparts, a fact that has not gone unnoticed by state legislatures, resulting in substantial political power for osteopaths.

PHYSICIAN ASSOCIATES

Physician associates (PA) are well-recognized health care professionals who provide services to patients under the supervision of physicians. In order to assist in extending medical services, physician associates take medical histories, perform physical examinations, and order laboratory tests. Under the direct or indirect supervision of either an allopathic or osteopathic physician they make diagnoses and initiate treatment plans. Patient education and counseling are also performed by PAs.

In 1989 there were 17,379 Certified Physician Associates in the United

States. The majority (78%) were practicing in either hospitals or medical clinics (American Academy of Physician Assistants' Survey, 1988). Specifically, PAs can be found in private practices, health maintenance organizations, nursing homes, student health services, urban and rural clinics, correctional institutions, and industry. In addition, physician associates may decide to enter the fields of medical education, health administration, or research.

Physician associates graduate from programs accredited by the Committee on Allied Health Education and Accreditation (CAHEA), which is sponsored by the American Medical Association. The training required to become a PA involves basic prerequisite college-level courses followed by a 24-month training program consisting of two phases. The first phase includes classroom and laboratory instruction in the basic medical sciences. The second phase consists of structured clinical rotations providing the students with direct patient contact. These rotations are intensive hands-on learning experiences in private and institutional medical settings that emphasize training in primary care (family practice, internal medicine, and pediatrics) but also include experience in obstetrics and gynecology, surgery, and emergency medicine.

Degrees awarded on completion of a program vary, depending on the institution offering the program and the educational background of the student. Most programs offer a baccalaureate degree on graduation. A few master-level and residency programs are available either within the core PA curriculums or for postgraduate specialization in such areas as occupational medicine, surgery, and pediatrics.

Physician associates, working with other members of the health care team, promote better distribution of health care services and improve accessibility to care in rural areas and underserved communities. They also increase the efficiency of ambulatory care practices, reduce patient waiting time, and allow physicians more time for difficult cases. Ultimately, PAs may help to decrease the escalating cost of health care through the reduction of costly hospitalizations by stressing preventive health maintenance as well as increasing the practice productivity of their supervising physicians or their respective medical institutions.

DENTISTS

Case 11-3. A 40-year-old insulin-dependent diabetic, E.W., who had previously achieved excellent diabetic control, had recently begun to have blood glucose levels in the 200–300 mg/dl range for reasons that were unclear to him. His physician seemed equally puzzled. Because of some gum swelling and irritation, he saw his dentist. The dentist discovered an abscess under one of E.W.'s teeth, which he treated with antibiotics and surgical drainage. One week later, E.W.'s diabetes again came under good control. No communication occurred between the two health professionals involved in this case.

There are approximately 145,000 dental practitioners in the United States (DDSs and DMDs). Eighty-five percent of dentists are generalists. Eight dental specialties are recognized by the American Dental Association: orthodontics, oral surgery, oral pathology, endodontics, pediatric dentistry, dental public health, periodontics, and prosthodontics.

The majority of dentists practice on a full-time basis. Ninety-three percent share in the ownership of their practice, most as sole proprietors. Only a small number of women are represented in the profession, although enrollment in dental school is now 33% female. Nine out of ten dentists employ a chairside dental assistant, and more than half employ a full- or part-time dental hygienist (American Dental Association Bureau of Economic and Behavioral Research, 1988).

Most applicants to dental school complete an undergraduate degree. However, it is possible to apply to most dental schools after 2 years (60 h) of college credits. On completion of the 4-year curriculum, graduates are eligible for licensure. Only one state (Delaware) requires a year of residency training. National Board examinations are required by most states. Practical clinical examinations are also conducted in most jurisdictions. In some areas, regional clinical board examinations have been organized.

Dentists provide a wide variety of services, which include the prevention, diagnosis, and treatment of dental caries, gingival and periodontal disease, malocclusion, temporomandibular joint dysharmony, soft tissue pathology, and various cosmetic problems. The dental caries rate in the U.S. population has been substantially reduced as a result of water fluoridation. Subsequently, the rate of edentulism is much lower, and many more people are at risk for periodontal disease. The profile of services that dentists provide has therefore shifted to include fewer fillings and extractions and more endodontics, periodontics, and cosmetic restorations (Ring, 1985). Part of this shift is also related to new technology and to patient expectations. People now expect to keep their natural teeth over a lifetime and are demanding treatment in order to do so. In 1988 the U.S. population spent more than 37 billion dollars on dental care. Half of that amount came directly from patients, almost half from third parties, and very little from the government.

Physicians and dentists need to work together to educate their patients, identify problems early, and make appropriate referrals, in contrast to what often happens as illustrated in Case 11-3. Most dental diseases are preventable or much easier and less costly to treat in the incipient stages. Pediatricians, obstetricians, and physicians working in geriatrics should be especially conscious of the oral health of their patients.

NURSES

Case 11-4. Mrs. R., a 60-year-old debilitated white female, was admitted for pneumonia and dehydration. Her regular physician, Dr. P., was on vacation. His associate did not know Mrs. R., nor did he have access to her chart in the emergency room. The doctor's orders at admission included a regular diet, an intravenous infusion of 5% dextrose and normal saline, and penicillin to be given intravenously.

During the admission assessment by a registered nurse, Mrs. R.'s daughter arrived. Prior to instituting the doctor's orders, the nurse interviewed the daughter and found out that Mrs. R. had insulin-dependent diabetes mellitus and had not eaten or taken her insulin in the last 24 h. She also discovered that Mrs. R. was allergic to penicillin. The nurse placed a call to the doctor and, while waiting for his return call, started an intravenous infusion with just normal saline, withholding dextrose until appropriate insulin and diet orders could be given. The nurse then called the pharmacy and put a hold on the penicillin order and clearly marked the chart so that the penicillin would not be given inadvertently by another nurse.

Nursing is the largest single health profession. In 1985 there were 1,531,200 practicing nurses in the United States. This represented 533 nurses per 100,000 population, up from 425 in 1978. Only about 3% of nurses are men. Ten percent are from racial or ethnic minority groups. Sixty-six percent work in hospital settings.

Nursing education is extremely heterogeneous. For example, registered nurses (R.N.s) may receive their training in a 2-year community college program, 3-year hospital diploma program, or a 4-year baccalaureate degree program in a college or university. Licensed practical nurses (L.P.N.s) generally receive 1 year of training in trade, technical, or vocational schools, community colleges, or hospitals. Nearly 7% of nurses hold master's or doctoral degrees.

The American Nurses' Association has recommended standardization of nursing education. The primary goal is to require a baccalaureate degree for registered professional nurses, a 2-year associate degree for registered associate nurses, and a 1-year training program for licensed practical nurses. This will undoubtedly take a number of years to accomplish, since state laws govern nurse practice.

Nursing, like medicine, has begun to develop a specialty structure, which will allow nurses to develop greater expertise in more limited areas and should result in increased status, income, and decision-making responsibility. Nursing clinical specialties have for the most part been organized around medical specialties, but with a clearer differentiation between ambulatory and hospital-based practice. Specialty-trained, master's degree nurses in hospital practice are called clinical nurse specialists, whereas those in ambulatory settings are more often educationally prepared as nurse practitioners or as nurse midwives (Mechanic, 1983).

Florence Nightingale, in 1859, described a nurse's role as "putting the patient in the best condition for nature to act upon him." In 1980, the American Nurses Association redefined nursing as "the diagnosis and treatment of human responses to actual or potential health problems," reflecting a somewhat more expansive concept of the involvement of nurses in patient care. In most clinical settings, nurses spend a greater amount of time working directly with patients than any of the other health care professionals. Their impact on outcomes is often underestimated. For example, studies of postoperative mortality rates between hospitals have consistently pointed to the experience and qualifications of the nursing staff as one of the major variables determining outcome. Case 11-4 is another example of good nursing care that could easily be inadequately recognized and rewarded by other members of the health care team.

Collaboration between physicians and nurses, though vitally important for optimal patient care, is too often suboptimal. Physicians frequently regard nurses as subordinates whose major responsibility is to carry out their orders. Nurses, on the other hand, consider themselves to be health care professionals with roles that are equally important to and in many ways distinct from those of physicians. Although nurse practice acts vary from state to state, several legal opinions have held nurses responsible for failing to take timely and responsive action, such as failing to communicate patient condition changes to the physician and failure to discover conditions not found by the physician.

Mechanic (1983) described the tension between nurses and physicians regarding clinical decision-making responsibilities as follows:

> Clinical decision making is the major source of continuing tension between nurses and physicians in the hospital context. Nurses have been cast in roles where they frequently must make clinical decisions, some of critical life-and-death significance, but they work under institutional rules that recognize only physicians as having authority to make independent professional decisions about patients. . . . Much of the continuing conflict between nurses and physicians could be reduced if better agreements regarding decision making could be achieved which appropriately recognized nurses' levels of expertise and their particular responsibilities for seriously ill patients.

OPTOMETRISTS

Optometrists are concerned with maximization of optimal visual performance through the evaluation and care of their patients' ocular health. Binocular and refractive conditions, along with accommodative and convergence relationships that can influence reading, learning, and other visual tasks, are major professional concerns. At the same time, optometrists evaluate, diagnose, and manage a variety of ocular pathological conditions. As is the case with other primary health care professions, the scope of optometric practice is governed by individual state laws. Optometrists may employ topical diagnostic pharmaceuticals throughout the nation and may administer a wider selection of appropriate therapeutic agents in half the states.

The professional optometric curriculum consists of a 4-year academic program. Although admission to an optometric institution occasionally may be gained after 3 years of postsecondary undergraduate preparation, the majority of current applicants hold baccalaureate degrees. Preadmission undergraduate requirements are parallel to those of other major health professions and include basic science courses such as biology, physics, advanced mathematics, organic chemistry, and microbiology.

Whether they are independent or affiliated with major universities, optometric schools and colleges are accredited by independent national regional agencies for higher education. Further evaluation is made by the Council on Optometric Education, a subsidiary of the American Optometric Association. The Council particularly is concerned with clinical aspects of an optometric curriculum and also accredits the many postdoctoral optometric residency programs that are maintained throughout the country.

In order to deliver professional care, the optometric graduate must pass a board examination administered by the state in which he would practice.

Demarcations are sometimes indistinct between the professional roles of optometry and ophthalmology. Matters of serious ocular pathology and invasive surgical intervention are clearly within the realm of the ophthalmologist. Likewise, systemic therapy, as might be suitable to remedy ocular pathologies and related disorders at a secondary or tertiary level of referral, usually require the level of skill and training of an ophthalmologist. Otherwise, in primary ophthalmic health care, the clinical activities of the two professions are very similar. Optometrists are employed as members of HMOs, in group practices, as industrial and sports vision consultants, in research capacities by ophthalmic companies, and in academic institutions.

ALLIED HEALTH PROFESSIONALS

Case 11-5. O.L. was a 79-year-old man admitted to the hospital because of intractable pain and resultant disability from a vertebral compression fracture. His physician pursued a diagnostic evaluation and ordered narcotics for the pain. He also consulted a physical therapist for advice regarding pain management and mobilization. The physical therapist fitted O.L. with a thoracolumbar extension brace and taught him to use a transcutaneous nerve stimulation unit. She taught him bed exercises and provided him with a walker for trips to the bathroom.

Although he was much more comfortable, O.L. felt that he would be benefited by a short nursing home stay before returning to his home to fend for himself. The hospital social worker helped him make the necessary arrangements and discussed home care options in case he should need them once he returned home. He also mentioned to O.L. that an occupational therapist might be able to suggest some home modifications and adaptive equipment that might allow O.L. to return home more quickly.

The major allied health professions are listed in Table 11-3. During this century, the rise of the allied health disciplines has been one of the most dramat-

Table 11-3
Allied Health Professionals

Audiologists
Dietitians
Laboratory professionals
Medical technologists
Medical laboratory technicians
Cytotechnologists
Histological technicians
Occupational therapists and OT assistants
Physical therapists
Radiologic technologists
Recreational therapists
Respiratory therapists
Social workers
Speech pathologists and audiologists

ic developments in the health care delivery system, reflecting both the increasing complexity of patient care and the increasing use of technology for diagnosis and treatment.

The relationships among the various allied health professional associations, the American Medical Association, and the certifying and licensing bodies governing each discipline are somewhat complicated, at times strained, and subject to fairly frequent modifications. An additional complicating factor in recent years has been the tension between the federal government (Medicare, Medicaid), state governments (Medicaid), and the private sector created by efforts to contain costs while assuring quality (Mechanic, 1983).

Clinical Dietitians

A patient's nutritional status is obviously very important to his overall health and well-being. The evaluation of current nutritional status, determination of adjustments needed to achieve nutritional well-being, development and implementation of a plan to meet those goals, and education of the patient and other care givers are all important and expected responsibilities of the health care professional providing nutritional services.

Most accredited hospitals and rehabilitation facilities require that nutrition support be provided by a registered or licensed dietitian. These titles denote a level of expertise acquired through an American Dietetics Association (ADA)-regulated combination of didactic and clinical learning. A dietitian must have a Bachelor of Science degree in Foods and Nutrition or a comparable major from an accredited university and an additional 900 hours in preplanned and ADA-approved clinical experience. In addition, many facilities require ADA registration, which requires passage of a professional examination and monitored maintenance of continuing education hours in compliance with ADA regulations. Some states have also implemented a licensing procedure through state medical licensure boards, which protects the consumer from persons practicing under false credentials and guards against inappropriate practice behavior of its members. The initials R.D. or L.D. will appear with the person's signature if these higher levels of certification have been achieved.

The term "nutritionist" has been used by many to imply professional expertise in the area of human nutrition. However, this title is not protected from misuse by persons with questionable educational background and possible unethical presentation of information to the consumer. Persons using this title should be able and willing to provide information to verify their level of professional qualification.

Medical Technologists/Cytotechnologists

Case 11-6. A.R. was an 8-year-old girl brought to the emergency room by her parents for evaluation of recurrent leg pains occurring at night, preventing her from sleeping. The episodes had been occurring occasionally for 4 months but had been getting more frequent and severe for the past 2 weeks.

Dr. Y. was covering the emergency room on the night that A.R. presented. His examination of her was completely unremarkable. However, he ordered a complete blood count (CBC) with a differential count and an erythrocyte sedimentation rate (ESR) as a precaution. The machine-run CBC results showed normal parameters. Review of the differential by the medical technologist revealed the presence of immature white blood cells. To confirm the diagnosis of acute leukemia, a bone marrow biopsy was performed. After results of the special stains performed by the medical technologist and review of the bone marrow aspirate by the pathologist, the diagnosis was confirmed. A.R. was thought to have a good prognosis because her disease was diagnosed at such an early stage.

Laboratory professionals represent the single largest group of allied health professionals. This reflects the heavy reliance of modern patient care on analytical laboratory testing and procedures for the diagnosis, treatment, and monitoring of patient care. There are several categories of laboratory professionals. Educational requirements differ based on the scope of practice.

Medical technologists represent the largest group. Their education requires extensive coursework in chemistry and the biological sciences. A baccalaureate degree, usually in medical technology or a related science, is the prerequisite for the national certifying exam. Their professional education also includes 1 year in a hospital laboratory. Both hospital-based and university-based programs utilize the clinical setting in hospital laboratories for this part of the educational experience. All programs integrate theory with analytical testing performed in the clinical laboratory.

The medical technologist performs analytical testing, evaluates the validity of the results, and reports the results to the physician who requested the test, as illustrated in Case 11-6. If there is a question regarding the clinical correlation of the results and the patient's condition, a clinical pathologist provides the consultation.

Medical technologists are able to work in any of the clinical laboratory specialties, i.e., blood bank, chemistry, toxicology, microbiology, and hematology. They are employed in hospital and independent laboratories as well as medical and industrial research laboratories. Some obtain specialty certifications after the medical technology certification. Many supervisors and managers hold master's degrees.

The *medical laboratory technician* works in the clinical laboratory under the supervision of a medical technologist. Accrediting agencies will not allow them to work in a setting that does not also employ medical technologists. Most medical laboratory technicians possess an associate degree in which their didactic and clinical education is integrated. There are a few certificate programs in which technicians complete a 12-month training program. Either program will allow them to take the certification exam. Medical laboratory technicians perform many of the same procedures as medical technologists; however, they do not engage in the problem-solving activities of the technologist.

A *cytotechnologist* now must earn a degree as a prerequisite for the certification exam. Their education has less emphasis on chemistry but a stronger emphasis on anatomy than that of the medical technologist. Cytotechnologists screen slides for the presence of cancer and other disease states. Any diagnosis of malignancy is confirmed by an anatomic pathologist. The largest portion of the work performed by a cytotechnologist is in the screening of pap smears. They also screen many nongynecological specimens such as bronchial washing and fine-needle aspirations of masses for the presence of cancer cells. Some cytotechnologists take additional training and are employed in cytogenetics laboratories.

Histological technicians have completed either a 2-year associate degree program or a 1-year, on-the-job training program. Either route will allow them to take the certification exam. They prepare tissue specimens for viewing by a pathologist. The histology laboratory has recently expanded its diagnostic capabilities via special types of stains, e.g., immunochemistry.

There are other employees in laboratories who have not completed college-level course work. *Phlebotomists* are usually trained on the job, to obtain blood specimens for laboratory testing. A certification exam and special curriculum have just been developed for phlebotomists. Some laboratories use *lab assistants* to process the blood and body fluids that are analyzed by the medical technologists. Lab assistants are also trained on the job (American Society of Clinical Pathologists Board of Registry, 1989).

Occupational Therapists

Occupational therapists use selected educational, vocational, and rehabilitative activities to help individuals reach the highest functional levels possible, become self-reliant, and build a balanced life style of work and leisure. In partnership with their clients, they frequently work with other members of a health care team and with community agencies not only to treat patients with various disabilities but to attempt to prevent injury from occurring. Whereas physical therapists focus on mobility, strength, and endurance, occupational therapists deal more frequently with activities of daily living such as bathing, dressing, cooking, and driving (See Case 11-5).

Occupational therapists may work in hospitals, clinics, schools, rehabilitation centers, home care programs, private practice, community health centers, nursing homes, day care centers, or psychiatric facilities. A registered occupational therapist (OTR) carries professional and administrative responsibilities for occupational therapy programs and services and is responsible for evaluating clients, deciding on program goals, working with clients to implement goals, and evaluating progress. In addition, OTRs educate students entering the field and may be involved in research. The certified occupational therapy assistant (COTA), working under the supervision of an OTR, assists clients in carrying out program goals, participates in client evaluation, and assists the OTR in evaluating progress and program effectiveness.

As college graduates, OTRs have completed either a baccalaureate degree in occupational therapy after 4 years in an accredited program, 2 years at a liberal arts college and 2 years in an occupational therapy program, or a master's degree in occupational therapy following a bachelor's degree in a related field of science or liberal arts. Each of these programs includes 6 to 9 months of field work. After the successful completion of all requirements, an applicant must pass a national certification examination.

Certified occupational therapy assistants (COTAs) are high school graduates or the equivalent who complete an associate degree program in an accredited university or community college or a 1-year certificate program in an accredited educational institution. A minimum of 2 months of supervised field work is also included. Graduates are eligible for certification as a COTA on passage of a national certification examination.

A career ladder program for the experienced COTA is available. Credentialing as an OTR is possible by meeting criteria for admission to the certification examination, which must be passed. The criteria for admission include 4 years of work experience as a COTA. Currently there are 33,000 OTRs and 7700 COTAs working in the United States; 45.3% of OTRs and 35.8% of COTAs are working in hospital settings.

Physical Therapists

The United States Bureau of Labor Statistics reports that there are an estimated 70,000 licensed physical therapists in the United States currently. Physical therapists practice in a variety of settings, providing inpatient, outpatient, and community-based services. Unique settings include community health centers, public schools, private practices, athletic centers, and specialty medical clinics as well as hospitals and rehabilitation centers

The academic preparation required to become a licensed physical therapist can be obtained through one of two routes. Students may complete 2 years of undergraduate college prerequisite coursework, apply to a professional program in physical therapy, and, if accepted, complete 2½ years in a physical therapy curriculum achieving a baccalaureate degree. Alternatively, they may finish an undergraduate degree in a related area and apply to an "entry-level" graduate program in physical therapy.

Opportunities for specialization following entry-level education are increasing. The American Physical Therapy Association (APTA)-sponsored American Board of Physical Therapy Specialties presently offers board certification in six specialty areas: pediatric physical therapy, orthopedic physical therapy, sports physical therapy, clinical electrophysiology physical therapy, cardiopulmonary physical therapy, and neurological physical therapy.

Physical therapists provide direct patient care services by first completing a comprehensive assessment, on which an appropriate therapeutic program is based. Assessment includes but is not limited to determination of motion, strength, and endurance abilities of the patient; evaluation of balance, coordination, and postural (static and dynamic) abilities; establishment of quantitative and qualitative profiles of movement abilities; development of a profile of the cardiopulmonary abilities of the patient; and definition of electrophysiological responses to various electrical modalities. Therapeutic regimens consist of a wide range of interventions from the application of specific modalities to exercise, musculoskeletal rehabilitation, and the reeducation of various functions.

Additionally, physical therapists provide a wide range of consulting services in areas such as health promotion and fitness, prevention of athletic injuries, and the prevention of work-related injuries and trauma. Research activities of physical therapists reflect the diversity of the profession.

Radiologic Technologists

Radiologic technologists can be subdivided into four major groups: radiographers, nuclear medicine technologists, radiation therapy technologists (to be changed to radiation therapists once the subgroup of radiologists using that name change the name of their discipline to radiation oncology), and diagnostic medical sonographers. Members of the first three groups, who are involved in the use of radiation of various types for either diagnostic or therapeutic purposes, are different in several other ways from diagnostic medical ultrasonographers, who are involved in the use of high-frequency sound waves. Their training must include at least 24 months of didactic and clinical training. In fact, nuclear medicine technologists and radiation therapy technologists have often completed an additional 24 months of training in their chosen field. Currently, diagnostic medical sonographers must complete a 12-month training program only. In addition, diagnostic medical sonographers are credentialed by the American Registry of Medical Sonographers, whereas the others receive their credentialing through the American Registry of Radiologic Technologists.

Radiologic technologists may receive their training in 24-month certificate programs generally offered by hospitals and vocational technology schools, associate degree programs offered by community and junior colleges, or in baccalaureate programs offered by colleges and universities.

Radiographers [R.T.(R)s] are responsible for obtaining high-quality radiographs (x-ray pictures) as requested by a physician to be interpreted by a radiologist. This involves working closely with patients and with a variety of sophisticated kinds of equipment. They must know how properly to position the patient, set the proper radiation exposure levels, protect the patient from unnecessary radiation exposure, and determine whether adequate images have been obtained. In addition to routine radiographs of the chest, extremities, etc., radiographers make sophisticated images such as computerized axial tomographic (CAT) scans and magnetic resonance imaging (MRI) pictures.

Nuclear medicine technologists [R.T.(N)s] administer radiopharmaceuticals to patients and operate a variety of scanning equipment that produces radiographic images of various parts of the body for diagnostic purposes. Brain, bone, liver, and thyroid scans as well as dynamic cardiac and pulmonary scans are examples of the kinds of tests they routinely perform.

Radiation therapy technologists are involved in the administration of ionizing radiation primarily to cancer patients for therapeutic purposes. Because of the nature of cancer, and since treatments are generally given repetitively over a period of time, radiation therapy technologists often develop close relationships with patients and their families and are often called on to function as members of interdisciplinary teams.

Although most radiologic technologists frequently work in hospital settings or in large clinics, *diagnostic medical ultrasonographers* work in a wide variety of settings. Cardiologists, obstetricians and gynecologists, and even general surgeons and primary care physicians may employ ultrasonographers to assist them in the evaluation of common problems such as valvular heart disease and congestive heart failure, pelvic masses, pregnancy dating, gallstones, and peripheral vascular diseases.

Recreational Therapists

Recreational therapists constitute a fairly diverse group of professionals with regard to their areas of interest and activity. Some of the distinct areas of interest and expertise are (1) self-esteem/confidence building, (2) independent living/self-reliance building, (3) self-expression/enrichment of life, (4) group acceptance/development of interpersonal skills, (5) hospital and play therapy/fear reduction, (6) art and music therapy/self-expression and fulfillment, and (7) physical activities/physical conditioning and stress reduction. They are employed in a variety of settings including hospitals, rehabilitation centers, nursing homes, mental health centers, community parks and recreation departments, schools, sheltered workshops, and correctional centers.

To become a recreational therapist one must complete an approved baccalaureate program in recreation, recreational therapy, or physical education. Masters and doctorate degree programs are also available. Recreational therapy assistants must complete an approved associate's degree program. Certification is awarded by The National Council for Therapeutic Recreational Certification after satisfactory completion of a certifying examination. Licensure or registration is also required in many states, often through the state's Board of Medical Examiners.

The responsibilities of a recreational therapist include (1) evaluation of needs, interests, and capabilities of individuals regarding their participation in recreational activities; (2) education and encouragement regarding appropriate use of therapeutic recreational modalities; (3) development of a therapeutic plan to meet the needs of each individual including individual goals and objectives; (4) organization and direction of therapeutic recreational activities; and (5) documentation of activities and progress toward achievement of goals (National Therapeutic Recreation Society, 1989).

Respiratory Therapists

Respiratory therapists must complete a 2- to 4-year hospital- or college-affiliated, American Medical Association-approved program designed to prepare them to qualify for the registry examination of the National Board for Respiratory Therapy (NBRT). Once they pass the examination, they become registered respiratory therapists (RRT). Certified respiratory therapy technicians (CRTT) have completed a 1-year hospital-affiliated program and have passed an NBRT certifying examination. There were approximately 34,000 RRTs and 48,400 CRTTs in the United States in 1989.

Under the direction of a physician, respiratory therapists are responsible for the administration of therapeutic gases (oxygen, carbon dioxide–oxygen mixtures, etc.), aerosols and humidity (bronchodilators, corticosteroids, aerosolized water, etc.), assisted ventilation (respirators, etc.), positive airway pressure, and chest physical therapy (to mobilize secretions and stimulate cough, breathing exercises, etc.). They perform blood gas sampling and pulmonary function testing, and they provide individualized patient education and follow-up.

Social Workers

Social work practice focuses on the relationship between individuals and their environment and is directed toward defining and resolving problems that develop in this relationship. Social workers are therefore trained to evaluate the psychosocial aspects of an individual's situation. They are often able to provide supportive psychological counseling to individuals and families and act as advocates in situations where environmental changes would be helpful, as in Case 11-5. They are especially well trained to locate community resources that may enhance the quality of life of an individual or family (Mechanic, 1983).

The specific activities of a social worker depend somewhat on the occupational setting in which the social worker practices as well as the amount and type of training she or he has received. Common practice settings include medical and psychiatric hospitals and clinics, schools, nursing homes, special shelters, government agencies, the workplace, family service agencies, churches, and private practice.

Social workers may achieve a bachelor's degree, master's degree, or doctoral degree in social work from programs accredited by the Council on Social Work Education. Special training for social workers is also available in mental health services such as individual or family therapy. Individuals who have received such training are often called psychiatric social workers.

Speech–Language Pathologists and Audiologists

Speech–language pathologists and audiologists are health professionals who have either a master's degree or a doctorate and have completed at least 60 semester hours of prescribed academic credit dealing with the normal and developmental aspects of human communication, communication disorders, and clinical techniques for evaluation and management of these disorders. In addition, they have completed at least 300 hours of supervised clinical experience and 9 months of full-time professional experience, termed a clinical fellowship (American Speech–Language–Hearing Association, 1989).

To receive the Certificate of Clinical Competence in speech–language pathology and/or audiology (CCC-SP, CCC-A, or CCC-SP/A), they must pass the National Examination in Speech–Language Pathology or the National Examination in Audiology or both. Most states require state licensure as well.

In 1988 there were 52,600 active members of The American Speech–Language–Hearing Association, the national association of speech pathologists and audiologists (*ASHA Membership Directory 1989–90*). In a variety of settings, including hospitals, rehabilitation facilities, and public and private outpatient settings, these professionals identify, evaluate, and provide treatment for individuals with communication disorders of all types. They often work closely with otorhinolaryngologists, neurologists, physiatrists, dentists, and plastic surgeons. Much of their work involves children (congenital and developmental disorders) and the elderly (acquired disabilities such as deafness and aphasia). Audiologists are responsible for diagnosis and remediation of hearing loss. Responsibilities include prescription and fitting of amplification and provision of auditory and speechreading training. Speech–language pathologists diagnose and remediate speech disorders (e.g., problems of fluency, voice, and articulation) and language disorders (e.g., aphasia, reading disorders, and delayed language development). Some speech–language pathologists are also involved in the evaluation and treatment of eating and swallowing problems, augmentative communication devices, and alternate forms of communication such as sign language and esophageal speech.

PHARMACISTS

There are currently approximately 164,000 pharmacists in the United States (72 pharmacists per 100,000 people), making pharmacy the third largest health profession after registered nurses and physicians. There are over 1.5 billion prescription orders dispensed annually from community and hospital pharmacies in the United States (Smith & Knapp, 1987). In addition to prescription medications, pharmacists are involved in the dispensing of nonprescription (over the counter or OTC) medications.

Almost 90% of active pharmacists are practicing in clinical settings. Another 10% are involved in the development, production, or distribution of drugs, teaching, research, legal and regulatory activities regarding pharmaceutical practice, public health activities, association work, and journalism. The clinical work of pharmacists includes community pharmacy, hospital pharmacy, drug information centers, poison control centers, and supervision of dispensing practices in long-term care facilities such as nursing homes. Although pharmacy has traditionally been a male-oriented profession, the number of female pharmacy graduates has increased from 12% in 1960 to 48% in 1984 (Penna & Sherman, 1985).

Since 1960 the entry-level degree for pharmacists has been a 5-year baccalaureate degree. However, there has been an increasing trend toward requirement of a 6-year doctor of pharmacy degree as the entry-level degree. The number of doctor of pharmacy (Pharm.D.) degrees granted annually almost tripled between 1974 and 1984 (Penna & Sherman, 1985). In addition to academic coursework, pharmacists are required to have 100 to 2000 hours of professional experience to qualify for state licensure. This professional experience is usually incorporated into the 5- or 6-year academic program. Master of science and doctor of philosophy degrees are also available for pharmacists interested in pursing an academic, administrative, or industrial career. An increasing number of residencies and fellowships are also available for both academic and clinical pharmacists in specialized areas such as psychiatry, geriatrics, internal medicine, pediatrics, pharmacokinetics, family medicine, and others.

The many clinical activities in which pharmacists are involved include verification of prescriptions for accuracy, legality, and physical and chemical compatibility; advice to patients and other health care providers regarding proper administration, potential side effects, and potential drug–drug and drug–nutrient interactions of prescription drugs; advice to patients and other health care providers regarding proper use and choice of over-the-counter medications; advice to patients regarding personal health habits (smoking, drug abuse, etc.); referral of patients to other health professionals; instruction of patients and other health care providers regarding proper use of medical or surgical appliances (inhalers, colostomy bags, splints, and bandages); participation in mass screening programs (stool occult blood testing, hypertension screening, etc.); and participation in utilization review, medical audits, and other medical care evaluations in hospitals, nursing homes, etc. (Rosenfeld & Thornton, 1978. Other services of a more innovative and advanced nature include pharmacokinetic and nutrition consultations and primary care of patients with special emphasis on hypertension, diabetes, hyperlipidemia, etc. Additionally, advanced trained pharmacists are now able to conduct drug research with human subjects provided that a physician is part of the study team.

Pharmacists may be the nation's most accessible health care professionals. However, in retail community pharmacy practice, a significant factor limiting the ability of pharmacists to provide good care is their lack of access to complete patient-related information. Pharmacists, more than any other health care professionals, are usually relatively isolated from other professionals. Some pharmacists have difficulty dealing with physicians on an equal basis and find it hard, for example, to confront physicians about possible prescribing errors. Patients would benefit greatly from efforts to improve communication between physicians and pharmacists.

THE MENTAL HEALTH PROFESSIONS

As in other health care professions, the decades since World War II have seen dramatic developments within the mental health and clinical behavioral science professions. These developments have been spurred by the maturing and professionalization of these relatively young disciplines. The emergence of new theoretical perspectives on mental health, an accumulating empirical data base, demonstrations of effective and generalizable clinical procedures and programs, and broader social acceptance of mental health concerns have all contributed to the growth of the mental health professions (Richardson, 1988). The development of the biopsychosocial (Engel, 1977) and multisystem (Tapp & Warner, 1985) theories of health and illness along with theories of stress and coping (Lazarus, 1966; Selye, 1976) have blurred the distinctions between physical and mental health and resulted in the development of the fields of behavioral medicine (Schwartz & Weiss, 1978) and health psychology (Millon, Green, & Meagher, 1982). Mental health professionals have been increasingly integrated into medical settings.

These developments have resulted in a diverse array of distinct yet overlapping clinical mental health professions. The primary mental health professions include psychiatry, psychology, counseling and marital and family therapy, social work, and psychiatric nursing. In sorting out these disciplines there are several guidelines that may be used by the physician or consumer. Despite much overlap, these professions are heterogeneous regarding type and level of training, roles and practice settings, and licensure or certification for independent clinical practice.

Psychiatrists are physicians who specialize by completing a 3-year psychiatric residency during which they receive training and experience in the diagnosis and treatment of major mental illness. They may further subspecialize in order to work primarily with adults, children, or other identified groups.

There are two major schools of philosophy and training regarding American psychiatry (Richardson, 1988). The traditional approach emphasizes the biological aspects of psychiatric illness. A second approach is primarily social and emphasizes environmental aspects of psychiatric illness. Most contemporary American psychiatrists have a strong biological orientation and are highly trained in the diagnosis and pharmacological treatment of major mental illness. Depending on training and interest, psychiatrists may also be skilled in psychotherapy and other forms of psychosocial treatment. As physicians, psychiatrists are licensed to practice medicine by each state and, after completion of an approved residency and comprehensive examination, are certified by the American Board of Psychiatry.

Often confused with psychiatrists, psychologists are doctoral-level behavioral scientists, typically holding doctor of philosophy (Ph.D.) degrees. Some psychologists hold doctor of psychology (Psy.D.) or doctor of education (Ed.D.) degrees. Psychologists typically complete a bachelor's degree in psychology or a related area and may complete a master's degree along the way to the doctoral degree. Total graduate school education typically requires between 4 and 6 years of full-time study.

Not all psychologists are professionally trained as clinical practitioners. Many are academic and research specialists in different areas of psychological science. The American Psychological Association recognizes four professional specialties within psychology: clinical psychology, counseling psychology, school psychology, and industrial–organizational psychology (American Psychological Association, 1981). There are three additional professional specialty areas that are emerging with distinct identities but are not yet fully recognized: neuropsychology, health psychology, and forensic psychology. The highest credentialing for a professional psychologist in one of these specialty areas (except for health psychology, which is not yet certified by the board) is Diplomate status granted by the American Board of Professional Psychology, which requires at least 4 years of postdoctoral experience in the specialty area, a written examination, and direct peer review of clinical skills.

Professional psychologists are licensed for independent practice by all states. A major distinction between psychologists and other mental health professionals is that licensed psychologists are the only mental health specialists, except for psychiatrists, who are always trained at the doctoral level. Also, psychologists are primarily behavioral scientists before they become clinical practitioners and are the only professionals with special training and qualifications in the administration and interpretation of the more complex psychological tests and in the application of cognitive–behavioral learning principles to behavioral modification (Richardson, 1988).

Clinical and counseling psychologists are the most broadly trained psychological specialists in regard to clinical behavioral science and mental health services. Both are required to complete basic studies in all the major areas of scientific psychology, including physiological, cognitive–behavioral, educational, personality, developmental, social, organizational, and multicultural psychology. The emphasis in this basic training is on scientific theory, methodology, and empirical knowledge bases. In addition, clinical and counseling psychologists complete a sequence of educational experiences in basic scientific methodology with a focus on research design and statistical analysis. Both receive training in psychological evaluation, assessment, and diagnosis with special focus on the use of psychometric testing in clinical settings. Finally, both complete a sequence of clinical courses and practicums focusing on basic counseling and psychotherapy skills with a diversity of psychological disorders and problems, with a focus on broad skill development and in-depth understanding of the theoretical and empirical literature regarding psychological problems and interventions. The culmination of doctoral training for the clinical or counseling psychologist is a 1-year full-time American Psychological Association-accredited clinical internship in a medical or mental health setting and the completion of an independent dissertation research project. Both clinical and counseling psychologists may specialize via focused studies and clinical training in any number of areas but are initially trained as scientifically oriented general mental health practitioners.

Clinical and counseling psychology have evolved out of different historical contexts (Tipton, 1983; Whitley, 1984). Clinical psychology has traditionally had a greater emphasis on the diagnosis and treatment of children, severe psychopathology in all ages, and services delivered in inpatient mental health settings, whereas counseling psychology has had a greater focus on assessment and treatment in rehabilitation settings, vocational, educational, and family counseling agencies, and with persons experiencing adjustment problems and other less severe forms of psychopathology. Despite these differences, it has been estimated that these two specialties have 80% to 90% overlap in training, skills, work settings, and professional roles (Watkins, Lopez, Campbell, & Himmell, 1986). Clinical and counseling psychologists are employed in many settings, including private practice, medical schools, hospitals, universities, mental health centers, other human service agencies, and research foundations.

School psychologists specialize in the learning and mental health needs of children in educational settings. School psychologists are usually employed in school systems or academic research institutions. Industrial–organizational psychologists specialize in the study and design of organizational settings with regard to human performance and interpersonal relationships and are usually employed by large corporations and public institutions or in academic research settings. Neuropsychologists are typically clinical or counseling psychologists who complete special pre- and postdoctoral training in neuropsychology. Neuropsychologists conduct neuropsychological evaluations and contribute to diagnosis and treatment planning of patients with a variety of neurological injuries and rehabilitation concerns. They are typically employed in medical and rehabilitation settings but may also work with school systems and in academic research capacities. Health psychologists are also trained as clinical or counseling psychologists but specialize through pre- and postdoctoral work in preventive health and the psychological needs of general medical and surgical patients.

Health psychologists work in a variety of hospital and medical settings. Forensic psychologists are clinical or counseling psychologists who further specialize in forensic issues and typically work in penal, law enforcement, or psychiatric hospital settings. Individuals trained at the master's level in psychology may be identified as psychological assistants or associates and are licensed by many states to provide limited psychological services under the supervision of a licensed doctoral-level psychologist.

As previously discussed, social workers are also major providers of mental health services. Social workers often have unique skills and training qualifying them for roles as case managers (Richardson, 1988). They may also be trained as psychotherapists or counselors. Psychiatric nurses are also important providers of mental health services. Nursing training is heterogeneous, and as a result there are multiple levels of training that may qualify a nurse to provide psychiatric services. The term Psychiatric Clinical Nurse Specialist has been suggested as designating an R.N. with a master's degree in psychiatric services. Such qualified nursing personnel may play an increasing role in the delivery and coordination of mental health services, especially in hospital settings (Richardson, 1988).

Finally, counselors and family therapists are important mental health professionals. The titles counselor, therapist, and family therapist are generic terms and have only recently begun to be defined and licensed by states. Typically a counselor or family therapist has a master's degree in counseling or family therapy from an accredited college or university and has received a minimum of 6 months to a year of supervised clinical experience on at least a half-time basis. There are two major organizations that credential and monitor the training of these professionals, the American Association of Counseling and Development and the American Association of Marriage and Family Therapy.

Counselors are usually affiliated with the American Association of Counseling and Development. Counselors may specialize through graduate study and work experience in a variety of areas such as mental health counseling, counseling of children, marriage and family counseling, school counseling, or rehabilitation counseling. Counselors who work with persons experiencing mental health problems should be further certified by the National Academy of Certified Clinical Mental Health Counselors. Certified Clinical Mental Health Counselors are licensed for independent practice in 28 states (Weikel & Palmo, 1989).

Family therapists are usually affiliated with and should be certified by the American Association of Marriage and Family Therapy (Nichols, 1984). Often counselors and family therapists belong to both organizations but may prefer to refer to their work as either counseling or family therapy. A limited number of practicing counselors and family therapists hold doctoral degrees. Counselors and family therapists are employed in a variety of settings including mental health centers, guidance and counseling agencies, schools, and increasingly in private practice.

THE HEALTH CARE TEAM

Case 11-7. Mrs. G.M. was a 78-year-old widowed woman who lived alone. Because of frequent falls and increasing forgetfulness, she had become essentially homebound by choice. She came to the attention of Dr. R., a general internist, on referral from a social worker from Adult Protective Services (APS) who requested a medical evaluation for her falls, forgetfulness, and the recent onset of a bloody discharge from one of her breasts. The APS became involved because of the neighbors' concerns that Mrs. M. was in need of assistance.

Dr. S., after a careful evaluation, concluded that there was a possibility of significant heart disease as well as a breast nodule, bilateral cataracts, and mild dementia. He referred her to a general surgeon for breast biopsy, an ophthalmologist for evaluation of the cataracts, and arranged for her to have some cardiac studies (echocardiogram and 24-h Holter monitoring).

The breast nodule was biopsied and proved to be malignant. The consulting surgeon suggested a modified radical mastectomy. The ophthalmologist confirmed the presence of cataracts but was not convinced that removing them would prevent further falls. The cardiac studies were normal.

Mrs. M. was admitted to the hospital for breast surgery. Dr. S. visited her in the hospital and met with the nurses to develop a plan of care that would prevent falls and minimize the confusion that he anticipated might result from the unfamiliar hospital environment. He asked that the surgeon request a physical therapy consult to help with the evaluation of the falls and to assure that Mrs. M. remained as active as possible during the hospitalization. The surgery was a success, no complications occurred, and Mrs. M. was discharged to her home. Dr. S. then scheduled a house call and invited the social worker from Adult Protective Services to be present for a discussion of further health care needs.

Patients like Mrs. M. require the services of a variety of health professionals simultaneously. How should these services be coordinated? In the above case, Dr. S. took it upon himself to coordinate Mrs. M.'s care. However, even though his efforts appeared to have been successful, at no time were more than two professionals able to engage in a discussion of Mrs. M.'s situation at the same time, and there were professionals who were excluded from even those discussions (the hospital pharmacist, the hospital social worker, the cardiologist who read the cardiac studies, and the anesthesiologist). Who will coordinate Mrs. M.'s health care once her biomedical problems have been fully evaluated and treated?

Interdisciplinary teamwork in health care as a concept has been described and advocated for at least 20 years. Enthusiasm was particularly high in the 1960s, when several large demonstration projects were funded. Unfortunately, because of the difficulties involved in implementation and a relative shortage of convincing data proving increased efficacy, the movement lost momentum. However, as health professionals find that they are caring for increasing numbers of chronically ill and disabled patients, there has been a resurgence of interest in interdisciplinary approaches to health care. Interdisciplinary teams are now the rule in rehabilitation (Rothberg, 1981), home health care, and geriatrics (Rubenstein, 1983), where there is now some reasonably good evidence that team care is superior to nonteam care (Williams & Williams, 1986).

Of course, any setting in which professionals from more than one discipline work side by side could be considered interdisciplinary teamwork, and that is probably true to a degree. Outpatient clinics, operating rooms, and hospital wards all require interdisciplinary collaboration. However, teamwork in these settings generally means that physicians give orders to the other professionals on the team, who dutifully carry them out. There is very little collaborative decision making.

What are the barriers to true interdisciplinary teamwork? Several have already been mentioned. Professionals from the different disciplines are trained separately in their own specialized fields with little chance to learn about or even interact with professionals from other disciplines until after they graduate. By that time, "turf" boundaries are well established. Specialization tends to emphasize differences more than similarities between professionals (French, 1979). Issues of power, prestige, financial compensation, sexism, and racism also contribute to defensive and distancing behaviors. Attitudes that develop within a group become firmly entrenched through social support and affiliation (French, 1979).

Physicians in particular are trained to be action-oriented, self-contained, autonomous decision makers. Thus, they are systematically educated to be poor team players (Goldstein, 1989). If being a member of an interdisciplinary team means being responsible to other team members, then physicians, whether by selection or training, are often unwilling and ill prepared to do so (Charns, 1976). In addition, teamwork results in significant loss of power and control, items valued highly by many physicians, particularly in today's liability conscious society.

Perhaps the most important obstacle to a team approach is the traditional departmental organizational structure that exists in nearly all health care institutions. Hospitals, for instance, usually have separate departments of nursing, social work, occupational therapy, physical therapy, radiology, laboratory, and pathology. Garner states that "the departmental model places the clients in the middle, where they become pawns in territorial battles for power, control, status, and financial resources. Staff members who serve the same clients are not obliged to know each other, to communicate, to plan together, or to support one another" (Garner, 1988). He describes teams and departments as being like oil and water.

The basic requirements for interdisciplinary teamwork are mutual respect and an understanding of the potential contributions of team members from other disciplines, communication through use of a commonly understood language, and an interdisciplinary decision-making process that facilitates the formation of mutually agreed-on goals and strategies. Teamwork also requires training and practice; it does not occur automatically. For interdisciplinary health care to become a universal reality, a great deal more interaction must occur between disciplines at every stage of training, and administrators must recognize the need to reorganize health care systems into interdisciplinary teams rather than discipline-specific departments. The time required for team meetings must be reimbursed by third-party payers. Liability issues must be explored and addressed. If physicians are to function as leaders of interdisciplinary health care teams, strategies will need to be developed at both the selection and training stages that will foster appropriate attitudes and skills.

CONCLUSIONS

As modern health care has become more complex because of broader definitions of health, increased medical knowledge, technological advances, and changes in the spectrum of illnesses, so too has the health care system become increasingly complex. One aspect of this complexity is the dramatic increase over the last half century in the number of different health care disciplines and in the degree of specialization within the more traditional disciplines, particularly medicine, nursing, and dentistry. In order for such a complicated system to function effectively and efficiently to the benefit of individual patients, teamwork is required.

Effective interdisciplinary teamwork requires that professionals from the various health care disciplines understand and respect each other, that there be a common language and method of communication between them, and that the goals of treatment and the roles played by each team member can be agreed on by all. To become an effective team member, a health care professional must learn his own discipline well and feel comfortable within its boundaries. In addition, he must learn enough about each of the other disciplines to allow colleague-to-colleague communication, consultation, and referral. The consultative process must be mastered. In situations requiring particularly close and frequent interdisciplinary collaboration, such as geriatrics and rehabilitation, group process skills must also be learned.

This chapter has provided a brief introduction to the concept of teamwork within the health care system and to some of the requirements for it to function optimally. In addition, basic information was provided about each of a number of health care disciplines and about the consultative process. Barriers to effective teamwork and consultation have been mentioned not so much to discourage but to stimulate creative solutions to these problems.

CASES FOR DISCUSSION

Case 1

K.S., a 42-year-old man who had no regular physician, saw a plastic surgeon to have a large lipoma removed from his back. Because of the size of the lesion, which would have required a fairly large dose of local anesthetic, the surgeon ordered an ECG to reassure himself that no heart disease was present. The ECG report was equivocal, showing some minor ST–T wave changes possibly caused by ischemia. He recommended and made arrangements for a consultation with a cardiologist.

The cardiologist took a more complete cardiac history and learned that the patient had had a long history of occasional episodes of palpitations, never severe enough to require treatment. In fact, he had never before mentioned them to a physician. The cardiologist ordered some blood tests and recommended an exercise tolerance test and a 24-h Holter monitor study. The blood work was normal except for a fasting serum cholesterol of 250 mg/dl. The exercise test was equivocal with 1.5-mm ST depressions at maximal exercise. He recommended that K.S. begin a low-cholesterol and low-saturated-fat diet.

Before the Holter tracing could be done, K.S. had to be seen in the emergency room with the worst episode of palpitations that he had ever had. A rhythm strip showed paroxysmal supraventricular tachycardia. He was converted using digoxin and carotid massage and was sent home only to return several days later with another episode, which was converted similarly. He was then told to continue to take digoxin indefinitely. The Holter moniter was canceled.

The cardiologist then requested an echocardiogram to look for valvular disease and chamber enlargement and an exercise nuclear ventriculogram to further evaluate the possibility of ischemia. These studies demonstrated no chamber enlargement, normal valves, but a borderline low left ventricular ejection fraction of 50% (normal 60% or greater) and no real evidence for ischemia. However, because of the low ejection fraction and atrial arrhythmia as well as the elevated serum cholesterol, the cardiologist suggested going ahead with a cardiac catheterization, which demonstrated clean coronary arteries and again a borderline low ejection fraction.

One year later, K.S. now follows a low-cholesterol, low-saturated-fat diet to which his wife compulsively forces him to adhere, niacin three times daily to further lower his cholesterol, which remained elevated despite the diet, once-daily digoxin, and once-daily baby aspirin. He has had two more episodes of palpitations requiring emergency room conversions, and he anxiously awaits the results of his follow-up nuclear ventriculogram to see if his "idiopathic cardiomyopathy" has worsened. His lipoma remains intact.

1. What happened? In what ways is K.D. better off for having had the cardiac evaluation? In what ways is he worse off? What do you suspect the impact has been on his family?
2. At what points in this clinical cascade could it have been stopped? Who could have stopped it most effectively?
3. Can too much information ever be harmful? If so, how can we decide how much is enough?
4. What do you suspect would happen if K.S. now developed postprandial epigastric pain?

Case 2

Dr. F.L. was fit to be tied when he learned while examining his long-time patient T.Y. that the consultation he had requested 9 months earlier from an endocrinologist (T.Y.'s blood pressure had been difficult to control, and his serum calcium level was borderline high) had led to a cardiology consultation for a heart murmur, which Dr. L. knew to be benign and of long standing, and an orthopedic consultation for evaluation of low back pain, which Dr. L. had previously evaluated and found to be associated with marital and job-related stress. Neither of the secondary consultants had known to send the results of their evaluations to Dr. L., since they were unaware that he was the primary physician. Furthermore, the endocrinologist who had handled the blood pressure and calcium questions with the patient had not communicated with Dr. L.

1. Why did the endocrinologist probably act in this way? What kind of trouble did it cause?
2. What do you think Dr. L. should do about it?
3. Why didn't T.Y. keep it from happening?

Case 3

When Dr. D.W. decided to admit R.P. to the coronary care unit of the county hospital to rule out an acute myocardial infarction, he was told that he would have to speak with the charge nurse in the CCU. When he was informed by the charge nurse that although there was one open bed, there were not enough nurses available to properly care for any additional patients, and she therefore could not authorize the admission, he was livid. How dare a nurse tell him whether or not he could admit a patient to the CCU? He called the cardiologist in charge of the CCU but to his surprise was informed that the nurse's decision was correct and would be upheld.

1. Should nurses be making this kind of decision? Was the nurse's decision in this case an appropriate one?
2. Why was Dr. W. so angry?

Case 4

A 46-year-old woman suffered a left hemispheric stroke. After a brief hospitalization, she was referred to an inpatient rehabilitation facility. There she was found to have a right hemiparesis, a moderately severe aphasia, some difficulty swallowing, urinary incontinence, and elevated blood pressure and blood glucose.

1. Which health care professionals should be involved in this patient's care? What would each be expected to contribute to her management?
2. Who should be the coordinator of the rehabilitation team? Suggest a method of care that would allow interdisciplinary teamwork.

Case 5

S.R., a pharmacist, called Dr. W.G. to clarify a prescription that Dr. G. had written for D.D. for a potassium-sparing diuretic. He wanted to make Dr. G. aware of the fact that Mr. D. was also taking a potassium supplement and an ACE inhibitor and had just bought a box of Lite Salt, all of which, in combination with the diuretic, might be expected to increase D.D.'s risk of hyperkalemia. He was not terribly surprised when Dr. G. seemed somewhat annoyed and told him in essence to quit practicing medicine. Dr. G. added that he had told Mr. D. not to take any more of the potassium supplement. However, when S.R. had asked D.D. earlier, he had not remembered that advice.

1. What should the pharmacist's role be on the health care team? What, if anything, should the pharmacist have done differently in this case?
2. What obstacles, if any, exist that prevent pharmacists from taking a more active role in patient care?

RECOMMENDED READINGS

Lecca, P. J., & McNiel, J. S. (Eds.). (1985). *Interdisciplinary team practice: Issues and trends*. New York: Praeger.

This text is a state-of-the-art review of interdisciplinary team practice, including rationale for development of such an approach, models, and projections for the future. Specific chapters describe various types of team care, including rehabilitation, mental health, and hospice care.

Mechanic, D. (Ed.). (1983). *Handbook of health, health care, and the health professions*. New York: The Free Press.

This text is a broad-based book on the determinants of health and illness and the organization and provision of health care in this country. Two sections on health care delivery and management and health occupations are especially pertinent to this chapter.

Williams, S. J., & Torrens, R. R. (Eds.). (1988). *Introduction to health services*, 3rd ed. New York: John Wiley & Sons.

This text describes the major features of the American health care system from a macro level and thus serves as a nice complement to this chapter's microview. It also addressed several economic issues, such as health manpower and the evaluation and regulation of health care programs, and concludes with a discussion on health policy.

Wynne, L. C., McDaniel, S. H., & Weber, T. T. (Eds.). (1986). *Systems consultation: A new perspective for family therapy.* New York: Guilford Press.

This text views organizations, using health care organizations in the majority of their chapters, from a systemic viewpoint. It describes a method for consultation when such systems are dysfunctional that derives from family therapy. Case examples show that this approach can be remarkably fruitful when other approaches have failed.

PART IV

Values in Clinical Practice

As technology has expanded the boundaries of life, what patients hold dear and how they view the world have come to assume more importance, expecially as society is learning that resources devoted to medical care are not inexhaustable. Although patients clearly want top-quality health care, as evidenced by the increasing incidence of malpractice claims, the extension of life at all costs is clearly not a top priority for all patients. Learning to recognize where the values of the physician and patient conflict and then negotiating an effective solution that respects the values of both parties is becoming an important skill that physicians must master.

CHAPTER 12

Medical Ethics

James W. Mold and Richard A. Wright

Case 12-1. An elderly couple has come to your clinic at the suggestion of a case worker from Adult Protective Services for complete evaluations and recommendation regarding placement. The wife is basically healthy but has severe dementia of the Alzheimer's type. Her husband, on the other hand, is quite frail, with multiple chronic medical problems. He has had an increasingly difficult time handling his wife, who clings to him constantly and has knocked him to the floor on several occasions, resulting in contusions and lacerations that required emergency room treatment. He is unable to bathe her or get her to take her medications. The case worker would like to obtain temporary guardianship and place her in a nursing home. The husband says that he would rather die from injuries than put her in a nursing home.

INTRODUCTION

Ethically difficult cases such as the one above have always occurred in medicine, but for a number of reasons they are becoming more common and are certainly receiving more intense interest. Some of these reasons include advancements in medical treatment, increasing moral pluralism, increased involvement of the law in medicine, the rising cost of medical care, better informed and more involved patients, and changing and often unclear concepts of the role of health professionals in society.

The purposes of this chapter are (1) to introduce the language of medical ethics, (2) to introduce and discuss several ethical principles important in medical practice, (3) to present several different conceptual models used for making and for judging the quality of ethical decisions, and (4) to describe a process for making ethically sound decisions in everyday medical practice.

MEDICAL ETHICS

Medical ethics is a field of study within ethics, which is in turn a branch of philosophy. It is the study of medical decision making in situations involving principles of good and evil and of moral rights and duties, particularly when a conflict exists between two or more competing principles or between two or more decision-making models. Such situations are called ethical dilemmas. For purposes of this chapter, "ethical" and "moral" principles, values, and beliefs are considered to be the same, although some would argue that the word "moral" more specifically relates to religious doctrine.

The expansion of scientific knowledge is occurring so rapidly that individuals and societies are having a difficult time adjusting to the new ethical questions arising as a direct result of this new knowledge (McCormick, 1974). It has become possible to intervene in even the most basic events of life, including conception (*in vitro* fertilization, artificial insemination, genetic engineering), birth (prenatal medical and surgical treatment, abortion, salvaging of very premature infants), and death (cardiopulmonary resuscitation, respirators, organ transplantation, artificial organs, artificial nutrition and hydration). In 1988 the director of the National Institutes of Health appointed an *ad hoc* advisory panel to address ethical questions related to research involving fetal tissue obtained as a result of abortions (Human Fetal Tissue Transplantation Research Panel, 1988). These questions had become of particular importance because of early reports of successful treatment or at least the potential utility of fetal tissue transplants in the treatment of such problems as Parkinson's disease, Alzheimer's disease, Huntington's disease, and diabetes mellitus (Walters, 1988). Of course, this expansion of knowledge is not unique to medicine. Similar ethical struggles are occurring in other arenas as well, such as nuclear weapons development, use of biological and chemical weapons, and the development and use of genetically designed animals and plants.

There is a basic human tendency to want to be in control of ourselves and our environment. As more and more people become concerned that concepts and values are changing too rapidly, there will be efforts to slow things down or to "return to basic values." This societal trend will inevitably result in the formation of factions within society with very different sets of beliefs to which they hold firmly. Organizations such as the "right to life" groups and the "moral majority" may be examples of this phenomenon. Equally adamant in their beliefs are those who welcome change, often because they stand to benefit in some way, and object to attempts to slow it down. Organizations such as The Hemlock Society (an organization advocating more individual control over the circumstances of one's death), women's rights groups, and certain scientific organizations are examples. Advances in the fields of transportation and communication have served to further increase the "moral pluralism" within societies. Medical decisions take on greater complexity when the values of different participants vary considerably.

One mechanism by which societies are able to keep some control over societal change is by the enactment, interpretation, and enforcement of laws. The increasing involvement of the law in medical practice has increased the awareness of physicians and the public about ethical issues. However, ethical decision making is complex, situation dependent, and often must be done quickly. The legal system, however, tends to act very slowly and by its adversarial nature may undermine the physician–patient relationship. Therefore, legislation, legal precedent, and court action are usually unsatisfactory for dealing with current clinical problems, although they may tend to reflect the general feelings of a society regarding its ethical values. Worse, the knowledge and views of physicians may not always be adequately represented in this legal process.

It is becoming clear that the cost of unrestricted modern medical care will soon outstrip the ability of anyone, including the federal government, to pay for it. This realization can be expected to have profound effects on the practice of medicine. Issues of cost containment have already led to sweeping changes in the Medicare reimbursement system. Medical students and residents are being encouraged to be cost effective in their use of tests and procedures. Leading ethicists have begun to suggest that certain high-priced procedures should not be performed on patients beyond a certain age (Relman, 1980, 1987).

Additionally, people are becoming more involved in their own medical care. They are better informed and less willing to relinquish complete control of health-related decisions to their physicians. This has forced a change in the traditional physician–patient relationship from paternalism toward equality and negotiation. It has resulted in a heightened awareness of issues such as informed consent and autonomy. It has also highlighted the fact that patients' values often differ from those of their physicians (Brett & McCullough, 1986; Siegler, 1981).

Finally, and perhaps most importantly, there appears to be considerable confusion regarding the roles and duties of a physician today (Cassell, 1982). Clearly, most physicians are unwilling to devote their lives totally to the care of the sick, preferring to balance work with family life and other social activities (Berrien, 1987; Kralewski, Dowd, Feldman, & Shapiro, 1987). Is medicine then a business like any other, with a product to sell and willing buyers who are free to shop around for the best value (Egdahl & Taft, 1986)? Are physicians obliged to care for patients who can't afford to pay or have a dangerous communicable disease or have a history of suing another physician or are old and likely to take more time (Pellegrino, 1987)?

Alternatively, are physicians more like applied scientists whose primary responsibility is to discover the biomedical abnormalities that are causing the patient's symptoms and then provide treatment to correct the identified problem? If so, are physicians obliged to care for dying patients once all treatment options have failed, to attempt to uncover psychosocial problems that may be at the root of a patient's distress, or to take into account the patient's values and goals when deciding on treatment suggestions? What are the boundaries of the physician's responsibilities (Childress & Siegler, 1984; Pellegrino, 1983b)?

Do physicians owe a debt to society? After all, the cost of medical training is borne to a great extent by state governments from tax revenues. Further, physicians have been granted special rights and privileges not afforded to others in the society, including the right to ask questions about very intimate matters, the right to examine and touch all parts of another's person, and the right to invade another person's body surgically. Physicians are held in high esteem generally and are paid well for what they do. Does society then have the right to expect that physicians will be willing to make some sacrifices if necessary to repay this debt, such as treatment of AIDS patients, assisting at the scene of a car accident, and treatment of indigent patients (Council on Ethical and Judicial Affairs, 1988)?

ETHICAL PRINCIPLES

Case 12-2. A 34-year-old married man with gonorrhea, which he contracted from a prostitute during a sales convention in another city, asks that you not tell his wife the truth about his infection. Since she has now been exposed and could therefore contract the disease, he asks that you treat her for a "vaginal infection" if he can convince her to come to your office for a visit. He says that he has learned his lesson and that the marriage might not survive if his wife knew about his indiscretion.

Before describing the process of ethical reasoning and decision making, it is necessary to define and discuss some fundamental values that are particularly important in medical ethics: autonomy, beneficence, nonmaleficence, truth telling, confidentiality, and justice.

Autonomy is a value that is particularly strongly held in our society. It is the belief that each person has a right to decide what he or she wants to do or have done for or to him or her. It is the principle of freedom, of being one's own person, able to accept or refuse medical treatment, for example, even if refusal may result in personal injury or death. According to this principle, physicians also have the right to choose what kinds of care they are willing to provide and to whom. In Case 12-1, the principle of autonomy dictates that the husband has the right to keep his wife with him as long as he chooses even though it may result in further injury to himself. The clearest limit to autonomy is the point at which an individual's choice causes harm to or limits the freedom of others (Siegler, 1977). An important issue in Case 12-2 is the potential harm that would be done to the wife by the husband's unwillingness to warn her about her exposure to his sexually transmitted disease.

A second important ethical principle is **beneficence,** or doing good. Physicians are expected to do things that will benefit their patients. In fact, they have a *duty* to do so according to every code of medical ethics since Hippocrates. Thus, the failure of a physician to do good when in a position to do so violates professional codes (Kass, 1980). Before recommending a particular form of treatment, a physician must be convinced, and convince his or her patient, that the potential benefits of the treatment outweigh the possible risks. In Case 12-1, the principle of beneficence argues for placement of the wife in a nursing home to provide better care for her and to prevent further injury to her husband, although one could argue that the separation might be injurious to the husband's psychological health.

Closely related to but subtly different from beneficence is the principle of **nonmaleficence,** or not doing harm, another fundamental ethical principle of medical practice (*primum non nocere*—first do no harm) (Jonson, 1978). In fact, the duty not to do harm is stronger than the responsibility to do good. For instance, it would be considered worse to cause harm by prescribing a toxic drug inappropriately than to fail through ignorance or oversight to give a potentially beneficial one. In Case 12-2, it is certainly tempting to go along with the patient's proposed deceit in order to prevent possible adverse consequences to the marriage. Unfortunately, given the highly invasive and technical nature of medical practice today, it is not always possible to avoid doing harm. About the most that can be hoped for in some cases is that physicians choose actions that will on balance result in more good than harm being done to patients.

Truth telling is another important ethical principle in medicine. Physicians should tell their patients the truth about their conditions and the prospects for treatment (Brody, 1982; Sheldon, 1982). If patients cannot count on their physicians to be honest, the physician–patient relationship is seriously compromised. However, truth is sometimes a slippery concept. Should physicians always tell *everything* that they know about the situation? Does the physician have an obligation to communicate more than the literal truth; that is, is he or she obliged to communicate effectively his or her own level of concern and uncertainty about the information (Childress & Siegler, 1984; Cross & Churchill, 1982)?

As with beneficence and maleficence, the reverse principle, not telling a lie, is clearly a stronger obligation. What would the patient in Case 12-2 learn about the physician if he were to go along with his plan? How might this affect their relationship in the future? Would telling the patient's wife that she has a "vaginal infection" when, in fact, she may have gonorrhea be fair to her? How might this affect the physician's future relationship with her?

Privacy or **confidentiality** is also obviously important to the doctor–patient relationship. Patients must be able to share sensitive information freely with their physicians without fear that it will be disclosed to others. The patient in Case 12-2 might not have come to his personal physician at all if he had not trusted his physician to keep their conversations confidential. However, privacy seems to be more and more difficult to protect as more and more people and agencies feel that they have a right to the information contained in the physician's medical record, such as insurance carriers, peer review and utilization review committees, administrators of health maintenance organizations (HMOs) and preferred provider organizations (PPOs), and employers (Siegler, 1982). Also, just as with the principle of autonomy, it is not always appropriate to keep information confidential when doing so may cause significant harm to others. For instance, physicians are required by law to report suspected child abuse to the appropriate authorities.

Case 12-3. There is one unoccupied cardiac-monitored bed available in your hospital. Two patients are in the Emergency Department with acute myocardial infarctions. The next nearest hospital is 1 hour away.

One final ethical principle that requires explanation and discussion is the principle of **justice.** In medical practice, the principle of justice is important primarily when decisions must be made regarding the distribution of limited resources. A variety of methods could be and have been used to allocate scarce medical resources, including first come–first served, random lottery, distribution based on ability to pay, distribution based on social status (value to society), and distribution based on medical need (severity of illness) as well as formulas taking into account these and other factors weighted in various ways. Case 12-3 is an example of such a situation. Adequate treatment for myocardial infarction today requires the use of cardiac monitoring equipment. However, this equipment and the staff to operate it are expensive.

The high cost of certain types of medical care creates the need for just methods for rationing these types of care (e.g., intensive care for patients with a life expectancy less than 2 years). Instituting such allocation schemes, which leave some patients without potentially life-saving procedures, are clearly both politically difficult and agonizing for physicians, who are faced with the difficult prospect of saying "No" to very ill patients. For these reasons, formal resolution of such issues has been and will probably continue to be delayed as long as possible. Of course, rationing occurs regularly on an informal basis, but it is usually not officially recognized as such. Hospitals and physicians make decisions about which patients will be cared for and which diagnostic or therapeutic procedures will be used based on the ability of patients to pay for the services.

Examples of formal rationing projects are beginning to appear, and indications suggest that more will follow. The state of Oregon made a decision in 1987 to deny Medicaid funds for soft organ transplantation in order to be able to reimburse for more prenatal care. The state legislature undertook an extensive review of its Medicaid spending and then ranked health care services in order of perceived importance, with expenditures to be based on this ranking (Merrill, 1989). Alameda County, California has since followed a similar strategy to develop a rationing plan that will apply to its uninsured and underinsured population (Cotton, 1989).

ISSUES REGARDING LIFE AND DEATH

Case 12-4. Lenora is an 85-year-old woman who was living in a senior citizen's apartment until she suffered a stroke and was taken by ambulance to the hospital. It is now 8 days since the stroke. Lenora remains semicomatose and unable to take food or fluids by mouth. She has developed pneumonia and will almost certainly die if not treated with intravenous antibiotics and nasogastric or intravenous feedings as soon as possible. Her daughter says that her mother had many times expressed her strong wish that if faced with a serious illness, she wished not be kept alive if, after recovery, she would be unable to return to her independent life style. In fact, she completed a living will document specifically expressing the same request. On the basis of this information and the opinion of the neurologist involved in the case, who estimates Lenora's chance of recovery to independent functioning following the stroke, which was quite extensive, to be less than 5%, the daughter has requested that the pneumonia not be treated and that Lenora be allowed to die.

As a result of advances in medical knowledge and technology, it has become possible to influence the timing, setting, and circumstances surrounding both the beginning and the end of life. This capability has resulted in a multitude of ethical questions involving such issues as abortion, surrogate parenting, *in vitro* fertilization, genetic engineering, and experimentation involving aborted fetuses as well as advance directives, living wills, limited care plans, do not resuscitate orders, withdrawal of food and fluid orders, and euthanasia (Kolder, Gallagher, & Parsons, 1987; Lo & Johnson, 1980).

Most experts are in agreement that the rights of a competent, informed person to accept or reject medical treatment should be respected. Parents of minors are generally allowed to make informed decisions regarding the treatment of their children, although controversies still arise occasionally when the choices made seem to be very unwise and likely to cause serious injury to the child (Holder, 1987; Kopelman, Irons, & Kopelman, 1988). The greatest difficulties occur in cases involving incompetent adults (comatose, delirious, demented, retarded, etc.) and those that involve "premature" termination of life such as abortion, euthanasia, and withdrawal of life support including food and nutrition. As the technology of genetic engineering progresses, issues related to genetic manipulation will also become increasingly important.

If an informed, competent adult can decide to accept or refuse medical treatment, then it makes rational sense that such an adult should be able to make decisions in advance about future treatments. Such decisions are called *advance directives*. *Living wills* are examples of advance directives regarding the use of heroic measures and withdrawal of life supports in the event of a terminal illness if the individual is no longer competent to make or communicate such decisions at that time. Decisions made in advance of a situation, however, are often not the same ones that an individual would make when faced with the actual situation. Also, individual life circumstances are constantly changing; therefore, people may change their minds more often than they change their living wills.

An alternative form of advance directive is a legal device called a *durable power of attorney*. A power of attorney is a person appointed by a competent adult to manage his or her affairs, usually financial. It is only applicable to competent adults and becomes null and void if the individual becomes incompetent. A durable power of attorney, on the other hand, is durable and continues in force even after the individual becomes incompetent. Some state legislatures have allowed the use of durable powers of attorney as a way for individuals to designate proxy decision makers in the event that they become incompetent.

A question critically important to ethical discussions of these issues has to do with the definition of human life: when does it begin, and when does it end? Is a fertilized ovum human, and if so, does first-trimester abortion represent murder? Can ova fertilized *in vitro* and not used for some reason then be discarded, or must they be frozen for later "adoption." Is the use of intrauterine devices, which prevent implantation of fertilized ova in the uterus, ethically acceptable (Elias & Annas, 1986)?

Likewise, when is a person dead? Must all organs cease to function, or is cessation of brain activity sufficient? Is a person whose cardiovascular and respiratory systems are being artificially maintained by machinery still alive? If so, does removal of these devices constitute murder? One might also ask, is murder always unacceptable (Black, 1983)?

An alternative definition of life that has gained considerable support and has significantly affected ethical decision making is that human life depends on the ability of a person to interact in a meaningful way with other persons and their environment. By this definition, those people who are in a permanent vegetative state would not be felt to have a meaningful life.

If an individual has the right to refuse medical treatment even if doing so may result in his or her death, does that individual also have the right to choose to end his or her own life by taking an overdose of pills? If so, then can an individual who does not have access to a means to end his or her life, for example a quadriplegic or bedfast person, ask for assistance from a family member or a physician? Should an individual be able to give advance directives regarding circumstances under which he or she would find life unacceptable and would want measures taken to end it? Should a terminally ill and incompetent patient who is refusing to eat be forced to receive food and fluids through a nasogastric tube until the terminal illness actually causes death (Micetich, Steinecker, & Thomasma, 1983; Steinbrook & Lo, 1988)? Such questions are obviously difficult and disturbing. Where is the line to be drawn, and if we cross over a particular line are we headed down a slippery slope toward moral chaos?

ETHICAL DILEMMAS

Case 12-5. Diane has recently become pregnant. Although she is married with two children, the pregnancy was unplanned and unwanted. She is now 40 years old, and her youngest child is 16. Diane's husband's (Bill) father has had Parkinson's disease for 10 years. The disease has progressed to the point that Bill's father is no longer controlled by medications. He is confined to a wheelchair, unable to take care of his basic needs. As a result, he has become quite depressed. A neurosurgical procedure has become available that significantly benefits 50% of Parkinson's disease victims such as Bill's father. The procedure involves implantation of fetal adrenal gland tissue into the brain of an afflicted individual. Diane and Bill were seriously considering an abortion but were having difficulty making up their minds. When they learned about the neurosurgical procedure, they decided that the aborted fetus could give new life to Bill's father. This thought caused them to decide in favor of abortion. They want to specify that the fetus be used to supply Bill's father with an adrenal tissue implant.

An "ethical dilemma" is a situation in which no alternative for action seems wholly satisfactory because, no matter what is done, there appears to be a contradiction of some ethical principle, value, or framework. As a result, the alternatives for action seem to be irreconcilable. For example, in Case 12-2, the principles of confidentiality and nonmaleficence seem to dictate that the physician try to help the patient keep his secret. However, the principle of honesty requires that the physician not become a party to deception, and the principle of beneficence toward the patient's wife, who is also a patient, suggests that the physician tell her of her exposure to a potentially serious venereal disease. If the physician tells the wife, he upholds the principles of honesty and beneficence but violates confidentiality and nonmaleficence; if he does not tell the wife, he upholds confidentiality and nonmaleficence but violates the principles of honesty and beneficence.

Case 12-4 presents a conflict between the principles of autonomy and beneficence as well as questions about the role of individual values in quality-of-life decision making. For if Lenora's wishes would have been honored before she was incompetent, why not after she is incompetent? More importantly, the physician's professional values seem to require the preservation of life, whereas the patient's values, as expressed by the daughter, require that value to be set aside.

Case 12-5 is a dilemma involving the ethical frameworks of consequences and rights (discussed later in this chapter) as well as the principles of autonomy and beneficence. For involved here are questions about the rights of the fetus to life as well as the right of the woman to terminate her pregnancy for the end of potentially producing good consequences for the father with Parkinson's. Also involved are questions about using one person as a means to effect a good end for another person.

The resolution of such dilemmas is always difficult because each of us usually feels particularly strongly about one or two of the ethical principles just described. For example, some might say that "honesty is *always* the best policy" or that the principle of autonomy takes precedence over all others. Firm rules such as these make ethical decision making much simpler. However, the quality of such decisions usually suffers, since there will be situations in which other considerations should take precedence. If, for example, you think that the decision makers in Case 12-1 should honor the husband's right to keep his wife at home, would your opinion change if you knew that his decision is based on a promise he made to her never to place her in a nursing home, but that he nonetheless hopes that someone will take the matter out of his hands so that he will not be the one who puts her in the nursing home? Decisions involving ethical dilemmas are never simple and should not be treated as if they were (Miles, 1988).

In Case 12-4, is a physician compelled to treat the pneumonia and provide nutrition even if the patient would only recover sufficiently to live the sort of dependent life style that she specifically said she did not want to live. The acute infection may be the last chance for her to die a natural death for some time. What if the odds for the patient's recovery to independence were one in four, one in a thousand, or one in a million rather than one in twenty? It would be helpful if Lenora were able to state what odds she felt would justify treatment. Her best efforts to give advance directives were simply not sufficient to solve the current dilemma. Did Lenora really know what it would be like to live in a somewhat dependent situation? If she were able to communicate now, would she still choose death over life in a dependent state? How should Lenora's physician attempt to determine the answers to these questions?

Case 12-5 raises a number of difficult ethical issues including the time of onset of life and the acceptability of abortion for other than medical reasons relating to the health of the mother. It also introduces the question of the importance of motives. Is abortion more acceptable in this situation, where there are apparent altruistic motives, than in a situation in which the reasons are more a matter of convenience? Does the possibility of benefit to another, Bill's father in this case, make the decision more acceptable?

THE FRAMEWORK OF ETHICAL DECISIONS

Most people assume, because individuals have different sets of beliefs and values, that nothing definitive can be said about ethics in general. As a result, it is assumed that ethical decisions are solely a matter of individual preferences. The systematic study of medical ethics over the past 20 years has shown that these assumptions are incorrect. Rather, ethics has as its correct focus the commonalities that form a basis for the perceived differences between individual viewpoints. Thus, for example, no matter what particular set of beliefs an individual holds, almost *all* ethical decisions focus in one of three ways, called "frameworks" for ethical decisions (Wright, 1987). The frameworks differ according to whether the focus of decision making is on the consequences of an act, the duties of the persons involved, or the rights of the persons involved.

The person who focuses on consequences determines what is "right" by choosing from among all possible actions the one that will most likely produce the greatest amount of good and least amount of harm. The consequences framework thus requires *weighing risks and benefits*, goods and harms, according to an identified set of values that define "good," "harm," "benefit," etc. These are then balanced against other things, such as institutional rules or professional duties, according to some scheme of relative values or "weights" for individual considerations.

A physician utilizing the consequences framework for decisions would make a decision about treating Lenora (Case 12-4) by weighing and balancing the risks and benefits of that treatment. Should the causative organism be highly resistant and virulent, the powerful antibiotics necessary might be judged too dangerous to her fragile balance. Or, it might be decided that Lenora's 5% probability of full recovery is too small to outweigh the much greater probability of life in a dependent, seriously debilitated state should she survive her acute infection. In either case, the physician might decide not to treat Lenora, as her daughter has requested.

The second focus, duties, is based on the concept that physicians have obligations to themselves, their patients, and society. The duties framework assumes that a physician must act in accordance with moral duty, as determined by sets of rules, moral beliefs, and professional norms. Determining what is "right" depends on identifying which duties may not be neglected, regardless of the consequences. If there are conflicting duties, then they must be balanced against each other so that the most important duty may be upheld.

If Lenora's case were to be reviewed on the basis of physician duties, a decision might be made to treat regardless of the risk/benefit analysis. This decision could be based on the belief that a physician always has a duty to treat because no one can ever be certain how things will turn out; thus, patients deserve every chance to live. Or, it could be decided based on the belief that a physician has the duty always to use ordinary means of care, and antibiotics are surely ordinary in their usage.

The third focus, on rights, derives from our common understanding that individuals have rights that must be honored and respected. Within this framework, the physician is required to uphold those rights, with the consequences of doing so being a secondary concern. Whenever rights conflict, a decision must be made about which are the most important and thus are to be upheld despite the others.

An examination of Lenora's case from the rights framework could also result in a decision to withhold treatment, based on an understanding of the right to autonomy. For if Lenora's daughter is expressing Lenora's wishes as her proxy, then Lenora's right to consent to or refuse treatment would be violated if she were treated.

It should be clear by now that dilemmas may easily arise in applying any of the three frameworks for decision making. This does not mean that none of them is any good; rather, it means that the framework within which decisions are made affects the decision outcome. Each of the three ethical frameworks has its advantages and disadvantages, but they are far from equal. For although a consequences approach seems most "scientific," it also does the greatest disservice to our basic conceptions of individual rights and duties. It is also somewhat misleading, since real knowledge of consequences can only occur after the fact. The rights and duties frameworks, however, require more sophistication in determining which rights and duties in fact exist and which are most important when there is a conflict.

Because ethical decisions are quite complex, care and consideration are always necessary. The thinking physician must decide within which framework he or she is operating and be prepared to assess the validity of decisions in comparison to the other frameworks. Only then can a decision be truly well thought out.

THE PROCESS OF ETHICAL DECISION MAKING IN CLINICAL CARE

Regardless of the conceptual model that one uses in a particular case, the most important aspect of ethical decision making is the *process* that one goes through to reach a decision. In fact, the general process of ethical decision making is the same regardless of the specific case or the conceptual model used. It includes information gathering, an assessment of the values involved, clarification of the ethical principles that pertain, determination of all relevant options, and, finally, deciding.

One of the most frequently made errors in decision making is failure to spend enough time and energy collecting information. There is no question that this step can be time consuming, but it is also essential and almost always well worth the effort. One method for gathering more information about a particular case is to formulate a list of questions about the case and then search for the answers to those questions. It is important to avoid making too many assumptions. For example, in Case 12-4, the following categories of questions might have relevance:

1. Clarify the medical information.
   - How serious is Lenora's condition at the moment?
   - Regarding her long-term prognosis, how certain is the neurologist

about his estimate that Lenora has a 5% probability for recovery to an independent functional state? What is her prognosis for survival if the acute infection is treated with antibiotics?
   - What is Lenora's overall life expectancy assuming survival from the acute infection and the acute stroke?
2. Identify action constraints.
   - How much time can be taken to make a decision?
   - How recently did Lenora express her views regarding life in a dependent state? Has anything occurred since then that might have changed her mind?
   - If Lenora did survive and was dependent, where would she live? The daughter's home? A nursing home?
3. Identify the decision components.
   - How much did she know about dependency? Did she ever know or care for a stroke victim?
   - How might she feel about these options?
   - Who is involved in the decision?
   - How will they be affected by the decision?
   - Who should be making the decision?

The second step in the decision-making process is an assessment of the values involved for the people who would be affected by the decision. What are their values? What are their motives? In Case 12-4, the relevant parties include the patient, her daughter, other family members, and the physicians, nurses, and other health professionals involved in her care. To the extent that the decision represents a precedent for other similar situations, society as a whole also has a stake in the outcome (but not the decision). The insurance carrier has a conflict of interest and should therefore have no involvement in the decision-making process. The hospital administration may also have a financial conflict of interest and most likely a concern that adverse legal consequences be avoided. Once the relevant parties have been identified, their values must be determined in order to understand their effect on the decision.

The third step involves clarification of the ethical principles and framework involved. In Case 12-4, the principles of autonomy, beneficence, and nonmaleficence are most certainly involved. The strength of the arguments for autonomy may rest on the daughter's knowledge of her mother's wishes as well as Lenora's probable understanding of the matters about which she gave advance directives. Arguments for beneficence must take into account the impact of alternative decisions on Lenora primarily but also on the other parties involved. For instance, what effect might a decision not to give antibiotics and nasogastric feedings have on Lenora's comfort acutely and on her daughter's mental state? In addition, questions must be raised about the meaning of life and the obligation of physicians to preserve it, thus what duties the physician has and what rights the patient has.

The next step, second in importance only to information gathering and just as frequently neglected, is determination of all possible options. There are almost always more options available than are immediately apparent. It is usually essential to ask for opinions from all relevant sources regarding possible options. Often a dilemma that seemed impossible to resolve becomes amazingly straightforward when the right option has been discovered. Even when this is not the case, consideration of every relevant option helps to insure that the best possible decision is made and that people do not have avoidable regrets later. In Case 12-4, the major options are:

1. Continue basic supportive care. Do not start antibiotics or nasogastric feedings.
2. Start nasogastric feedings but not antibiotics.
3. Start antibiotics but not nasogastric feedings.
4. Start both nasogastric feedings and antibiotics.
5. Start antibiotics and parenteral (intravenous) feedings.
6. Begin treatment immediately to allow time for thoughtful decision making to occur.
7. Treat aggressively, hoping that Lenora regains enough cognitive ability to have input into the decision regarding a full course of treatment.
8. Agree to treat the acute infection to allow more time to determine an accurate prognosis before making final decisions regarding limiting interventions.

The final step is making the decision. Decisions involving ethical issues are usually very hard emotionally on everyone involved. To some degree, sharing responsibility among those involved is useful. However, when it comes down to actually making the decision, it is often most helpful for the physician to bear a larger portion of the emotional burden by making a suggestion to the patient and family. This is particularly true in a case such as Case 12-4 in which the patient cannot actively participate and the family will feel the greatest anguish over the decision. The physician might, for example, say to Lenora's daughter, "It appears to me that in view of all of the information that we have discussed, and considering your mother's strong feelings about independence and autonomy, we should not treat her pneumonia and allow her to die. How do you feel about that?" The daughter then has the opportunity to agree or disagree without appearing to be the one who is actually "pulling the plug" on her mother if she agrees to nontreatment.

Several methods can be used in specific situations to gather the relevant information, assess values and motives, clarify the ethical issues, and identify potential options. Often the physician can meet individually or in a group setting with all concerned parties. Sometimes another health professional can take on this responsibility. Consultations may be requested of colleagues (Pellegrino, 1977). A very useful method, which is becoming increasingly available in hospitals and to a lesser extent in nursing homes, is presentation of the case to an ethics committee (Lo, 1987).

Ethics committees are made up of people from various disciplines within the health care facility who might be expected to have different perspectives on ethical issues in medicine. There is generally a chairman who convenes the group and organizes the discussion. Patients, family members, and other involved parties are often asked to join the group for discussion of a specific case. The committee usually tries to reach a decision, although it may serve only to clarify important issues. Any decision reached by the committee is only a recommendation and is in no way binding on the involved parties.

The process of decision making should be fully and carefully documented in the patient's medical record. An important interface between ethics and law is liability for decisions that have been made. The best insurance against successful litigation is a proper decision-making process that is well documented. Proper documentation also facilitates communication among health care personnel involved in the case and can prevent misunderstandings regarding motives and decision-making methods, which are often the cause of litigation.

CONCLUSIONS

Medical ethics is a field of study with direct importance to medical care. Knowledge of the language, principles, and process of ethical reasoning can improve the quality of the decisions physicians make in their everyday practice of medicine. Recognition of personal ethical values and their influence on decision making as well as respect for those with different ethical values are prerequisites for quality patient care. Ethical decision making is often quite challenging and usually requires the effort and cooperation of not only patient and physician but family members, significant others, and other health care providers as well.

A systematic stepwise process can help to assure that decisions are made properly. All relevant information should be collected. Time is frequently a factor, but temporizing measures should be taken when possible to allow sufficient time to gather information from the patient, family, other health professionals, and other appropriate sources. Decisions that at first appear to be difficult often become much simpler when additional information is obtained. All persons who have a stake in the decision should be acknowledged, and their opinions, biases, and motives should be considered. A decision should be made regarding who should be involved in the decision-making process. The ethical principles involved in the decision should be clarified. All options should be elucidated and considered. There are almost always more options than were apparent initially. Finally, a decision must be made.

Appropriate documentation of the decision and the decision-making process is essential to insure adequate communication among health care providers and for protection for future liability. Physicians have a central role in making ethically difficult decisions and should be well trained and experienced to direct and coordinate the process. Patients, families, and other health care professionals look to physicians to weigh the available information, consider the options, and make wise recommendations. Physicians should not underestimate the importance of this responsibility in patient care or avoid it out of fear of liability or accusation of paternalism.

Case 1

A 30-year-old man comes to your office, referred from the local emergency room for evaluation of a generalized seizure following the use of free-base cocaine. The seizure had been witnessed by the patient's girlfriend. Both claim that this is the only time that he has ever experimented with illicit drugs. He had one previous seizure at age 14 and took medications for 3 years following that seizure. There have been no seizures off of medications from then until the present time. He is otherwise in good health.

The medical evaluation is unremarkable; there are no signs of chronic drug abuse. A CAT scan of the head and an EEG are normal.

1. He is employed as a commercial truck driver. Should you report this to his employer?
2. Should he be allowed to drive?
3. What other options do you have?
4. Since there is no law requiring you to report the seizure to anyone, why should you get involved at all beyond the medical evaluation?

Case 2

You are a family practitioner in a three-man group practice. One of your partners, Dr. M., does not take care of hospitalized patients. You have been asked by a general surgeon to see a patient of Dr. M. who has been admitted to the hospital on his surgery service. It seems that this patient was admitted with an acute surgical abdomen that resulted from the perforation of a sigmoid diverticulum. The surgeon asks you to consult because the patient has an abnormal electrocardiogram (ECG), and the surgeon is concerned that he may have had an acute myocardial infarction.

In gathering data about the patient's medical history, you learn that the patient had seen Dr. M. several days prior to the present admission, complaining of shortness of breath and dizziness. An ECG was done at that time. When you review the ECG, it is apparent that the patient had an acute myocardial infarction at that time, a finding obviously missed by Dr. M. The ECG in the office did not have a formal reading on it but had been placed in the chart along with the progress note, which indicated that it showed only atrial fibrillation, which in fact was an incorrect interpretation.

The patient was treated instead for what Dr. M. thought was bronchitis with a codeine-containing cough suppressant. On further reflection, you postulate that the codeine could have caused constipation, which resulted in the patient's use of some powerful enemas and laxatives that may have resulted in the perforated diverticulum.

Dr. M. is an older physician who received mostly pediatric training, but as he practiced in a small town he eventually began to take care of patients of all ages. He has been in this town for 26 years. A number of his patients have grown older with him.

1. In view of the above information, what should you share with the patient?
2. What should you do about the error that your partner has made in terms of preventing future similar errors?

Case 3

A healthy couple in their early 30s has come to your *in vitro* fertilization clinic to ask that you help them have a test-tube baby. They have been through several complete infertility workups and multiple trials of medications and other procedures and have been unsuccessful in conceiving. Their gynecologist has indicated to them that they would be ideal candidates for your *in vitro* fertilization program. After reviewing their records, you agree to accept them as patient in your program.

On their second visit to the clinic, they indicate to you that, having read the information that you have given them regarding the procedure involved, they have decided that they would prefer that you not insert more than two fertilized eggs into the uterus because they do not want to take the chance of having more than twins. Ordinarily, all of the suitable fertilized eggs are injected because the average "take rate" is only 25%. However, there certainly have been cases where twins, triplets, and even quadruplets have resulted from the procedure.

Another problem with injecting less than the full number of fertilized eggs is the issue of what to do with the rest of them. They could be frozen in liquid nitrogen and used in a subsequent procedure in the same woman, but what if this couple decides for some reason not to have another procedure?

1. What would become of the unused frozen embryos, and would this in some way represent wasting or murdering unborn human life?
2. The couple has an unusually good insurance policy that will cover the cost of the procedure up to the point of one successful delivery. Of course, they would like to see success on the first try. What is your obligation to the insurance carrier?
3. There are a limited number of procedures that can be performed each year because of limited trained professionals. Should that influence your decision in this case?
4. What would you do if you were the physician in this case?

Case 4

John K., a 32-year-old lawyer, worried for several years about developing Huntington's chorea, a neurological disorder that appears when a person is in his or her 30s to 40s, bringing rapid uncontrollable twitching and contractions, progressive, irreversible dementia, leading to death in approximately 10 years. John K.'s mother died from this disease, which is autosomal dominant and afflicts 50% of an affected parents' offspring. Often parents have children before they are aware that they have the disease. John K. and his wife have a child because of a contraceptive failure and an unwillingness to have an abortion because of his wife's religious convictions.

John K. has indicated to many people that he would prefer to die rather than to live and die as his mother had lived and subsequently died. He has been chronically anxious, drinks heavily, and has had intermittent depression for which he sees a psychiatrist. Nevertheless, he is a productive lawyer.

John K. first noted facial twitching 3 months ago. Two neurologists independently confirmed the diagnosis of Huntington's chorea. John explained this situation to his psychiatrist and requested help in committing suicide. When the psychiatrist refused, John reassured him that he did not plan to attempt suicide any time soon.

But when John went home, he ingested all of his antidepressant medication after pinning a note to his shirt explaining his actions and refusing any medical assistance that might be offered. His wife, whom he had not told about the diagnosis, found him unconscious and rushed him to the emergency room without removing the note.

1. Should he be resuscitated?
2. How much should his wife's opinion count in the decision-making process?
3. What could have been done to prevent this situation from occurring?

Case 5

Two businessmen have made application for admission to your local hospital's hemodialysis program at approximately the same time. In order to survive, each must use the dialysis machines 12 to 14 h twice a week. Unfortunately, when they apply the available dialysis machines are all in use. Time is available for only one of them. The nearest hospital with a similar machine is more than 200 miles away.

1. Which of the following should be taken into consideration when deciding which of the men should be admitted into the program, and how should the factors be ranked in order of importance?
   a. Severity of illness.
   b. Severity of symptoms, nausea, itching, lethargy, etc.
   c. Access to transportation (ability to make the 200 mile trip to the other hospital).
   d. Ability to pay, insurance coverage, income, etc.
   e. Social standing in the community.
   f. Past contributions to the hospital.
   g. Long-term prognosis for survival.
   h. Which application was submitted first.
   i. Age.
2. Would your decision-making process differ if you used a less utilitarian model? How?

RECOMMENDED READINGS

Beauchamp, T., & McCullough, L. B. (1984). *Medical ethics: The moral responsibilities of physicians*. Englewood Cliffs, NJ: Prentice Hall.

This nicely written book is a good basic introduction to the ethical dimensions of medical practice. It is a valuable book both because its presentation is so clear and also because it puts the current understanding of medical practice into its appropriate historical perspective. By focusing on the physician–patient relationship as the basis for medical ethics, this book nicely ties together the discussion of the PPR in Chapter 2 and the discussion of foundational ethics in this chapter.

Veatch, R. (1977). *Case studies in medical ethics.* Boston: Harvard University Press.

Consisting entirely of case studies and their analyses, this book helps enlighten the physician's understanding of the role of ethics in medical practices. In addition, the discussions are focused on assisting the development of a physician's understanding of issues that may have been previously hidden in commonly occurring cases. The book also serves as a good reference for looking up analysis of cases that may be similar to a current problem. This aids an enlightened decision process in handling the current case and improves one's understanding of the ethical dimensions of practices.

Wright, R. A. (1987). *Human values in health care: The practice of ethics.* New York; McGraw-Hill.

This book serves as a primer on both the ethical components of medical practice and the process of ethical decision making. By focusing on the decision-making process, this book avoids getting bogged down in disagreements over particular issues. Instead, the process of decision making is presented in a way that permits its application to any circumstances within the physician's practice. In addition, the book contains a number of readings that emphasize the importance and role of ethics in medical decision making.

CHAPTER 13

Medical Malpractice

Steven A. Crawford

Case 13-1. A 28-year-old woman, pregnant for the third time, consented to voluntary permanent sterilization following the birth of her child. Her physician, a close personal friend, had explained the risks, benefits, and alternatives, which she understood. Subsequently, she delivered a healthy infant and underwent a bilateral tubal ligation 24 h later. Four months afterward she returned to her physician because she had missed her period two months in a row and felt as though she might be pregnant. A urine pregnancy test was positive, and the exam confirmed the existence of an intrauterine pregnancy. Her physician, feeling bad that her close friend had become pregnant, offered to provide obstetrical care for free. The woman accepted and subsequently delivered a fourth healthy infant. Two months later, the physician was sued by her friend for malpractice because of the failure of the permanent sterilization.

INTRODUCTION

As can be seen from the above true case, even being a "good friend" does not prevent a physician from being sued for medical malpractice. Malpractice, according to Webster's dictionary, is a "dereliction from professional duty or failure to exercise an accepted degree of professional skill or learning by rendering professional services which result in injury, loss, or damage."

This chapter discusses medical malpractice. An overview of the current malpractice climate is presented first, followed by a brief review of the legal system and how it affects the practice of medicine. Then a review of some of the basic concepts of medical malpractice is presented, including informed consent, negligence, and liability for the acts of others. A discussion of medical malpractice insurance is presented next. Some ways to avoid a malpractice suit conclude the chapter.

Interpreting malpractice claims data is no small task, since there is no standard reporting system. The American Medical Association uses data obtained from surveys of physicians to determine the extent of malpractice cases. These surveys reveal that the chance of having a malpractice claim filed against a physician in 1985 was 10.1%, which compares with a chance of 3.2% before 1981. A physician in 1985 could therefore expect to have one claim filed against him every 10 years compared to one every 31 years before 1981. The rate ranges by specialty in 1985 from 2.4% for psychiatrists to 26.6% for obstetrician/gyneologists. Family physicians, internists, pediatricians, and anesthesiologists had rates between 5.5% and 7.6%. Older physicians, who are supposedly not keeping up with current medical knowledge, were not the most likely age group to be sued. Physicians aged 40 to 45 had the highest rates and the largest losses.

Because of the ever-increasing frequency of malpractice suits and settlements, the costs of medical liability insurance have risen steadily. At the same time there has been a corresponding decrease in its availability. As of 1984, 41 physician-sponsored insurance companies have emerged to provide relief. They too must maintain healthy premiums to insure themselves against the possibility of going out of business (Robertson, 1985). Significant differences exist in premiums among different states, as can be seen in Table 13-1, and among different specialities (Table 13-2).

The rise in frequency of malpractice claims against physicians has led many doctors to adopt a "defensive" style of practice. Such physicians order many more lab tests and x rays than are medically sound to "just make sure" they don't miss a diagnosis, no matter how unlikely. When tests and x rays are done to look for unusual or rare conditions on patients who have a low prevalence of a particular disease or condition, the likelihood of false positive results increases. If action is taken on these results, the risk of unnecessary adverse effects and increased costs to the patient occurs. This tactic, therefore, has the potential to increase the physician's risk of a malpractice claim rather than decrease it.

Table 13-1
Cost of Annual Malpractice Premium for Obstetrician/Gynecologist Performing Surgery Covered for $1 Million Liability Based on 1985 Data

Location	Amount
Oklahoma (PLICO)	$10,357
Michigan	$38,268
Detroit	$57,979
Minnesota	$10,149
Wisconsin	$29,773
Utah	$23,983
Missouri	$26,187
Colorado	$24,312

Table 13-2
Medical Professional Liability Premium Rates for Different Specialists, 1987[a]

Class	Examples	Liability limits single event/ annual aggregate limits		
		100,000/ 300,000	1,000,000/ 1,000,000	5,000,000/ 5,000,000
I	Physicians performing no surgery	953	2,154	2,802
IA	Urgent care physicians	1,451	2,668	4,268
II	Physicians performing only minor surgeries and doing no obstetrics	1,586	2,915	4,664
III	Family physicians assisting with major surgery and doing nonoperative obstetrics	2,026	3,724	5,958
IV	Otorhinolaryngologists performing major but no plastic surgery	3,694	7,684	13,522
V	Anesthesiologists or general surgeons	4,183	8,702	15,315
VI	Plastic surgeons	4,455	9,268	16,311
VII	Thoracic surgeons	4,674	9,721	17,108
VIII	Neurosurgeons, orthopedic sureons, and obstetrician/gynecologists performing major surgery	5,477	11,393	21,305

[a]Rates obtained from the Physician Liability Insurance Company of Oklahoma.

The rise in the number of physicians subspecializing may be partially attributable to the malpractice problem. Physicians can limit their exposure to risk by limiting their practice to a certain very limited specialty area, the theory being that such physicians have less chance of missing something "important" within their subspecialty area. For example, family physicians and even "general" obstetrician/gynecologists are giving up obstetrics in increasing numbers to maternal–fetal medicine specialists (Smucker, 1988; Weiss, 1986). Although this trend may decrease individual malpractice risks, it has the potential of fragmenting care further, weakening the doctor–patient relationship, and thus also has the potential of actually increasing the risk of malpractice claims for the profession overall.

MEDICAL MALPRACTICE

Medical malpractice suits are civil proceedings that generally involve either tort or contract law. Tort proceedings involve individuals, groups, or other parties acting in a nonpublic capacity seeking compensation for injuries suffered through the wrongful acts of another. Contract law suits involve consensual agreements between two or more parties whereby one party seeks damages because another party has failed to undertake defined obligations to the other. Criminal suits differ from both types in that they are brought by a governmental entity to enforce laws that exist for the protection of society at large. A defendant who loses a civil suit is said to be liable for damages but is not considered guilty as in a criminal one. In addition, the standard of proof in criminal prosecutions is higher than the standard required in civil litigation. The prosecution in a criminal case must prove its case beyond a reasonable doubt rather than by a preponderance of evidence as in a civil suit (Rosoff, 1987).

Torts involve either deliberate or negligent liability. For a negligent tort to be successful, the injured patient must show that the physician had established a *duty* or obligation to the patient; the physician must be shown to have been *derelict* in this duty, performing significantly below the legally required standard of care; the patient must prove that he or she was harmed or that *damage* occurred and that the physician's negligence was a *direct causation* of the patient's injuries. In deliberate torts, it is not necessary to show that the physician meant to injure the patient but only that the physician deliberately performed the wrongful act. Battery is a type of deliberate tort that involves touching an individual without his or her permission or consent. Other types of deliberate torts include fraud and deceit and breach of confidentiality (Rosoff, 1987).

Contracts are legally binding if two elements are present. *Consideration* consists of performing an act that one party is not otherwise bound to perform or refraining from an act that the party otherwise is entitled to do. This consideration must be mutual for the contract to be binding. An *offer* by one party and an *acceptance* by the other, a bargained-for exchange or "*quid pro quo*," must also occur. Contracts can be either expressed or implied. Most contracts for health care are implied by presenting to a health care provider for care who agrees to enter into a contract by providing that care. An important application of contract law to the health care setting is illustrated by suits brought by patients against health care providers for failure to obtain the positive results that the providers allegedly contracted to deliver, a *breach of warranty of cure* (Rosoff, 1987).

Most malpractice cases are tried before a judge alone, unless one of the parties named in the suit makes a request for a jury trial. In a jury trial, the jury's purpose is to decide disputed issues of fact. A judge can make a summary judgment without resorting to a jury when there are not factual issues to be decided. A judge's function is to control the trial's procedural aspects, to supply the applicable law, and to decide disputed issues of law. The jury may announce the verdict, but it is bound to apply the law as instructed by the trial judge (Rosoff, 1987).

A statute of limitations is present in most jurisdictions that establishes a maximum period of time during which a legal suit may be initiated. This period may vary for suits concerning different legal matters. Usually, the statute of limitations for personal injury actions is 1 to 3 years. For contract suits, the statute of limitations is usually longer, 4 to 6 years. The beginning of the statutory period for medical malpractice actions is defined variously as the date the alleged malpractice took place, the physician–patient relationship was terminated, the patient discovered the alleged malpractice, or the patient discovered, by exercise of due care, or should have discovered the alleged malpractice

(Rosoff, 1987). An example of the latter would be the discovery of a subtle mental impairment in a teenager as a result of a preventable birth injury.

If a physician is held liable in a malpractice suit, the amount of damage is determined by a number of different measures. Compensatory damages compensate the injured patient financially for the tangible harm caused by the defendant. Tangible economic losses, such as expenses for remedial care, loss of wages, and future loss of earnings because of physical impairment, are the principal elements of compensatory damages. Pain and suffering, mental anguish, and loss of consortium damages attempt to provide financial compensation for losses that are real and discernible but that cannot be readily measured in financial terms. Punitive damages may be awarded against a physician who acted in a grossly negligent manner or with deliberate wrongful intent. Their purpose is to punish wrongdoers and to deter them, and others, from acting similarly in the future. The amount is usually computed by assessing the degree of culpability of the physician's actions and the defendant's ability to pay. Nominal damages are awarded when the injured patient has been able to establish the physician's negligence and, thus, his liability but has not been able to prove that he suffered any compensable damages. In addition, each party bears its own legal expenses, regardless of who won the litigation (Rosoff, 1987).

If a physician loses a breach of contract suit, the measure or purpose of the damages is to place the patient as nearly as possible in the position he or she would have enjoyed had the contract been performed as agreed. In general, only economic losses are considered in awarding damages for a contract breach. Emotional distress and other intangible harms are not compensable. In addition, punitive damages are generally not awarded for a breach of contract (Rosoff, 1987).

IMPORTANT MALPRACTICE ISSUES

Case 13-2: Consent. A 27-year-old woman delivered her first-born son in the hospital without any unusual occurrences. He weighed 8 lb 2 oz. His hospital course was also uneventful save for the occurrence of an unrequested circumcision. Retrospectively, it was determined that his mother had been approached by a hospital staff member with the familiar questions of whether the mother would feed by breast or bottle and whether she desired the baby to be circumcised. Although the mother's negative answer was documented in the chart, somehow a slip-up occurred, and the child was circumcised on the morning of discharge without any additional discussion with the mother. The mother and father alleged both a lack of consent and a disregard for their wishes.

Most cases of medical malpractice occur because of improper diagnostic evaluation leading to misdiagnosis or late diagnosis, improperly performed diagnostic or treatment procedures, medication injuries, and nonmedical injuries such as breach of confidentiality. To avoid these possibilities, a physician must keep abreast of new information in his specialty field. The physician's education only starts with medical school and should continue throughout his entire professional career. In addition, if a diagnosis is not forthcoming in a patient who clinically worsens, consultation should be obtained.

If a physician does not have the training, experience, or skill to perform a particular procedure, then an appropriately trained physician should be consulted. It is foolhardy for a physician to try to perform a procedure for which he has had no training. It is also risky to promise unwarranted results.

When prescribing pharmaceutical agents, physicians should be aware of the indications for which they are approved by the Federal Food and Drug Administration and be cautious in their use in "nonapproved" situations. They should also be aware of any contraindications to their use and be sure that the patient is informed about the potential of adverse effects and drug interactions that may occur. Many physicians use the same informed consent principles in the prescribing of drugs as they would with a surgical procedure. Drug information sheets are most helpful in these instances.

Confidentiality is a hallmark of a physician's responsibilities. A physician has the societal privilege to delve into a person's most intimate thoughts and feelings and be allowed to view and touch a person's body. With this privilege comes society's mandate that this information be held strictly confidential, except when specifically released by the patient himself or herself or under very unusual circumstances, such as potential grave harm by a patient against another person.

As can be seen in Case 13-2, a physician must obtain consent before touching a patient, even if no harm was meant or occurred. Our society places high value on the physical integrity and inviolablity of the individual, treating such contact as a breach of a person's legal rights to privacy. The practice of medicine requires physicians to touch patients in many ways, including diagnostic examination, withdrawal of body fluids, and treatment by manipulation, punctures, incisions, and excisions. Imaging procedures such as x rays and ultrasound also constitute contact and therefore require consent. Even the collection and analysis of a urine sample requires the consent of the patient. There are four ways in which a consent can be given:

1. It may be expressed consent, as when a patient gives consent orally or when a patient signs a consent form for his child.
2. Consent may be implied by actions, as when a patient rolls up his sleeve to receive an injection or when a patient brings his child to the doctor's office.
3. Consent is also implied in emergency. When a patient needs immediate treatment but is physically or mentally unable to give consent, the physician is considered to be justified in assuming that he has the patient's consent to give the treatment. Consequently, this type of consent could well be considered a form of "consent implied in law."
4. Except in emergency, consent of a parent or guardian is required for a minor, and consent of a guardian is required for the mentally incompetent. The law assumes that the consent of a parent or guardian is equivalent to the patient's own consent. This is another type of what is known as "consent implied in law" (Oklahoma State Medical Association, 1986).

Case 13-3: Informed Consent. A 34-year-old massively obese male underwent an intestinal bypass procedure to lose weight. The surgical event itself was complicated only by a mild suture line infection, which responded quickly to treatment. The postoperative year, however, was a disaster in the patient's eyes in that he had debilitating diarrhea and was totally unable to work. He filed a malpractice suit alleging not only faulty surgical technique but also failure to inform him of the possible negative consequences. Unfortunately, no record documenting an informed consent discussion was found; a prompt out-of-court settlement followed (Robertson, 1985).

Case 13-3 illustrates how important the concept of *informed consent* is in the eyes of patients and their attorneys. Informed consent in most states requires the physician to disclose and explain to the patient what is wrong with him or her, what type of treatment or operation is being suggested, the chances for success of this treatment, any other methods of treatment, including no treatment, and their attendant risks. The risks to be included in the discussion with the patient are usually taken to be those risks that a reasonable person would need to know to make a decision. For example, most courts would acknowledge that no discussion of the risks of anesthesia would need to take place, as a "reasonable" person would know of these risks.

To emphasize these points, Leslie J. Miller (1986), a member of the AMA Division of Corporate Law, recommended that when a physician obtains informed consent:

1. The doctor should personally talk with the patient.
2. The information conveyed should be in intelligible form.
3. Promises of "no risk" should be avoided.
4. If an emergency exists so that the patient is unable to consent, a spouse or relative should be informed; this act will help establish the doctor's concern about the patient's welfare.
5. All discussions and procedures should be documented.

Before performing a consequential procedure, the physician should have the patient sign a consent form that gives evidence that informed consent has been given; an example from the Oklahoma State Medical Association is contained in Fig. 13-1. "Consequential" has a relative meaning, but for most cases it would imply any procedure or treatment that may result in injury, impairment, or death. After the patient signs the consent, the physician should retain a copy of that consent form in the office file. The physician should then make a notation in the office record that the discussion was held, when and where, and that the physician feels that the patient or patient's representative really did understand the information. Lastly, if the procedure is to take place in a different setting than the office, a copy of the consent should be placed in that facility's record for that patient. It is important to note, though, that the signing of a piece of paper in and of itself does not prove informed consent. The signed consent form is simply evidence that the discussion took place and that the patient or legal representative indicated agreement.

Case 13-4: Discreet Disclosure. A 10-year-old asthmatic with chronic tonsillitis was referred by his pediatrician to an ear, nose, and throat (ENT) specialist. This physician decided to admit him to the hospital for a tonsillectomy and adenoidectomy. The pediatrician and ENT specialist, being con-

REQUEST AND CONSENT FOR SURGICAL, MEDICAL OR DIAGNOSTIC PROCEDURES AND ACKNOWLEDGEMENT OF RECEIPT OF INFORMATION

PATIENT: ____________________

PATIENT NO: ____________ DATE: ____________ TIME: ____________

The hospital and your physician are required by law to obtain your consent to perform the surgical, medical or diagnostic procedure(s) listed below. Signing this form will acknowledge that you request and consent to your physician performing the recommended procedure(s). Your signature also confirms that your physician has explained to you the procedure(s), the risks of the procedure(s), the alternatives, if any, and risks of the alternatives and the risks or consequences of foregoing all treatment. Please READ THIS ENTIRE FORM CAREFULLY and then before signing it, ask your physician any additional questions you may have. Your request and consent is valid until you withdraw it.

1. I hereby request and authorize ____________ with hospital personnel and/or other trained persons of his/her choice to perform upon (patient) ____________ the following surgical, medical or diagnostic procedure(s) ____________

   ____

   to include any necessary or advisable anesthesia and disposal of tissue removed during surgery. I further request and authorize my physician and his assistant(s) to perform any other procedure that in his or their judgment is advisable for my wellbeing. This additional request and authority is extended as I recognize that during the above listed procedure(s), unforeseen conditions may require different or additional procedures.

2. I hereby request and consent to the administration of such anesthetics as are necessary. I further request that the choice of anesthetic to be used shall be made by professional anesthesia personnel.

3. I acknowledge that some of the risks known to be associated with surgery and anesthesia and which may be applicable to the proposed procedure(s) are:

INFECTION	LOSS OF ARM OR LEG
SEVERE BLOOD LOSS	LOSS OF BLADDER FUNCTION
IMPOTENCE	LOSS OF BOWEL FUNCTION
DISFIGURING SCARS	PARALYSIS BELOW THE WAIST
LOSS OF FUNCTION OF AN ORGAN	PARALYSIS BELOW THE NECK
LOSS OF FUNCTION OF AN ARM OR LEG	BRAIN DAMAGE
LOSS OF AN ORGAN	DEATH

4. I am aware that the practice of medicine and surgery is not an exact science and acknowledge that no guarantees or warranties have been made to me concerning the results of the procedure(s). I acknowledge that even though my physician has advised me of all known risks, up to and including the rare but possible severe risks as revealed in item 3 of this form, that additional unforeseeable and unpreventable situations could arise in the course of my care which might result in injury.

5. I HEREBY STATE THAT I HAVE READ AND UNDERSTAND THIS REQUEST AND CONSENT AND THAT ALL MY QUESTIONS ABOUT THE PROCEDURE(S), ALTERNATIVE PROCEDURE(S), AND RISKS OF EACH HAVE BEEN ANSWERED IN LANGUAGE THAT I UNDERSTOOD AND THAT ALL BLANKS WERE FILLED IN PRIOR TO MY SIGNATURE.

Signed: ____________

Patient or person authorized
to request procedures for patient: ____________

Relationship or Capacity: ____________

Witness to signature: ____________

I have explained the procedure(s), alternative(s) and risks to the person or persons whose signature or signatures are affixed above.

____
Signature of Physician

PL 0487-1

Figure 13-1. An informed consent document developed by the Oklahoma State Medical Association. Reprinted with permission.

cerned that the patient was quite excitable and that his apprehension might provoke an asthmatic attack, consulted with the anesthesiologist. They also noted that the mother was prone to hysteria and was equally excitable. They expressed to the anesthesiologist their feeling that if the mother became distraught, it would probably affect her son and cause the undesired asthmatic attack. The anesthesiologist devised the following solution to the problem: He would go the room the evening before and start an intravenous line with the idea in mind that the patient would not be so apprehensive in the comfort of his room, with his family present. On the morning of the surgery, he would go to the room and inject through the intravenous line a drug that would put the patient in a trance-like state so that he could be transported to the operating room where anesthesia would then be induced.

The anesthesiologist went to the room the night before surgery and explained to the mother that he intended to insert the intravenous line, and she agreed. The intravenous line was inserted uneventfully. The next morning he went to the room and, while engaging the patient in conversation, injected the drug in the intravenous line. The patient's eyes rolled back in his head, and he fell back on the pillow in the expected trance-like state. The mother, present in the room, was not prepared for this event and became hysterical and fainted. She struck her head on the windowsill and opened a small gash on her forehead. At the sight of the blood, the patient's grandmother, also in the room, developed palpitations of the heart and had to be seen in the emergency room. The surgery was subsequently performed uneventfully. The family of the patient claimed damages against all three doctors. The suit was eventually won by the defendant physicians based on the doctrine of discreet disclosure.

Even though a patient's consent to treatment should be informed, it is sometimes medically wise for a physician to exercise discretion as to what is disclosed to the patient. The law recognizes the validity of "discreet disclosure" if it is consistent with accepted medical practice in the physician's locality. In other words, the physician need not reveal to the patient everything that is known or suspected about his illness if in the physician's opinion it would not be in the patient's best medical interest. However, the physician may not be so discreet in his disclosure that the patient is thereby misled into giving consent that he would not otherwise have given. In the climate of the 1980s, a physician would be unwise to invoke the discreet disclosure defense in not seeking an informed consent, i.e., claiming that a complete and candid disclosure was not possible because of the possible effects on the physical or emotional well-being of the patient, unless a carefully documented second, third, or even fourth opinion have been obtained (Robertson, 1985).

Case 13-5: Negligence. A 35-year-old man presented to the emergency room of his local hospital because of the sudden onset of left substernal chest pain that radiated down his left arm. It had begun to ease as he was being checked in and evaluated by the ER nurse. The doctor's history revealed that the patient had never had a similar problem until now and that the pain had started only 30 min prior to ER admission. The patient smoked three packs of cigarettes a day and had a father who died suddenly at age 50 of an undetermined cause. The doctor's exam revealed no significant problems except for some left chest wall tenderness. An electrocardiogram had significant ST-segment elevation in several of the leads (an indication of acute myocardial injury), but the doctor thought it was within normal limits. The doctor ordered some pain medication for the patient, discharged the patient from the ER, and told him to return to see his doctor in 1 week for follow-up. While walking out to his car, the patient collapsed and was found about a half an hour after he was dismissed from the ER without pulse or spontaneous respirations. All attempts at resuscitation were unsuccessful. An autopsy showed that the patient had suffered an acute myocardial infarction (MI) of recent onset. The deceased patient's family sued the ER physician for negligence in not detecting the MI, and the physician's insurance company settled out of court for a substantial damage award.

This obvious case of negligence or "malpractice" is the type of suit most frequently brought against physicians. The misdiagnoses of myocardial infarction, ectopic or tubal pregnancy, appendicitis, fetal distress, childhood meningitis, and cancer are several of the most common forms of negligence suits brought against physicians. Medicine is not an exact science, and no physician can or should guarantee successful results after treatment. However, if a patient has been harmed because a physician failed to exercise the care and skill that under the circumstances could reasonably be expected of a physician with his experience and learning, then he may be liable for negligence.

The quality of a physician's care is measured based on a principle called "standard of care." This principle implies that physicians employ recognized and accepted treatments. However, a given treatment need not be accepted by all medical practitioners; it need only have the approval of a significant minority of licensed medical practitioners. Ordinarily, only a physician could be expected to state what treatments meet approved standards of care under a given set of circumstances. Therefore, in the trial of most malpractice cases, the evidence of a physician's negligence must be established by the testimony of other physicians, referred to as "expert witnesses."

Several different rules have been applied by courts to determine what standard of care should apply in a certain case. In the late 1800s, a *strict locality rule* was used that required that the expert testimony in a case be drawn from the geographic community in which the alleged malpractice occurred. More recently, a *same or similar community standard* has been used, allowing the expert witness to be drawn from a closely comparable medical community. This change obviously made it easier for the injured patient to obtain expert testimony. In addition, *national standards* have been adopted by some jurisdictions, especially in cases where specialty care is rendered by board-certified physicians (Rosoff, 1987).

When a physician claims the ability to provide the type of care that normally is rendered by a limited-care specialist, the standard of care applied is that of the appropriately trained limited-care specialist. Under emergency circumstances in which specialty care is not available, a primary-care specialist standard is applied to measure the adequacy of care rendered. Failure to refer a patient to a limited-care specialist when more in-depth care is indicated subjects the physician to liability, a case sometimes referred to as *negligent nonreferral* (Rosoff, 1987).

Also involved in the issue of standard care is the principle of duty. If a physician agrees to care for a person and subsequently terminates that relationship without giving the patient "reasonable" notice to acquire additional medical care, and injury results, then a breach of duty occurred. In addition, a physician may acquire a duty toward people who are not his patients, such as a potentially violent patient who injures others. The physician may be held liable for not warning responsible parties about the patient's potential for violence.

Case 13-6: "*Res Ipsa Loquitur.*" A 68-year-old man had been an insulin-dependent diabetic for many years. He had developed severe peripheral vascular disease with extensive skin ulcers on both lower extremities and chronic osteomyelitis (bone infection) on the left. Unresponsive to continued medical management, he was scheduled for amputation after full discussion of the alternatives with him and his relatives. Carefully prepared, he was brought into the operating room and positioned for surgery. Despite the following of traditional routine steps, the surgeon proceeded to amputate the wrong lower extremity. A financial settlement followed (Robertson, 1985).

Sometimes the care rendered by a physician may have been so negligent that a judge or lay jury may infer negligence even in the absence of expert testimony under the doctrine of "*res ipsa loquitur,*" Latin for "the thing speaks for itself." In these cases, the courts have held that the very occurrence of certain types of injury during the course of medical treatment creates a presumption of negligence on the part of the physician, and a judge or jury may decide the question of liability on the basis of injury alone. This principle is usually presented by the injured patient's attorney, and the judge rules whether the doctrine applies. Given two cases with identical circumstances, this doctrine may be applied by a judge in one case and rejected by a judge in another. When the rule is applied in a negligence case, the physician must actively defend himself by proving that the accident or injury was not caused by his failure to exercise proper skill or care.

Case 13-7: Liability for the Acts of Others. A 26-year-old woman was admitted to a small rural hospital for an elective hysterectomy. While the surgeon was scrubbing up, the certified registered nurse anesthetist (CRNA) began putting the patient under anesthesia. After a few minutes, the CRNA noted that the patient's blood pressure had dropped. The CRNA attempted to correct the problem but was unsuccessful, and the patient's heart stopped beating. She called the surgeon, who attempted to resuscitate the patient but to no avail. The patient's family brought a successful suit against the surgeon, noting that the CRNA was under the supervision and control of the attending surgeon.

As can be seen from the above case, a physician may incur liability because of the acts of other people even though the doctor does not commit the acts himself. This type of liability is known as "vicarous liability" or by its Latin term, *respondeat superior* ("let the higher up answer for it"), because it involves responsibility for wrong committed by another. As applied to the practice of medicine, this principle means that the doctor may be held liable for the acts of those whom he has duty to train or supervise in the care and treatment of his patients. However, he is subject to this liability only if the wrong is committed by the employee acting "within the scope of his employment." Even though this "scope" is often difficult to determine, one frequently used criterion is whether or not the employee's acts are intended to serve the employer's interest or business.

In addition, a doctor may be held liable for the acts of someone else's employees, including other physicians or hospital personnel. This principle, commonly known as the "captain of the ship doctrine," holds that ". . . in the course of an operation . . . he is in the same complete charge of those who are present and assisting him as is the captain of a ship over all on board" (OSMA, 1986). In many states this doctrine is not followed, and in some, the courts have applied it inconsistently.

Case 13-8: Treatment of Minors. In a local hospital emergency room, S.C., a single 16-year-old male, presented for the treatment of a dog bite. His parents were not with him. The doctor quickly assessed that he was not in any acute distress and told him that he could not be treated unless one of his parents consented to his being treated. S.C. told the physician that he did not want him to call his parents because the dog bite occurred while he should have been in school. If his parents found out that he had skipped school, they would get very angry. S.C. refused to give the doctor his home phone number or his last name. The doctor informed him that if the wound was not treated properly, it might get infected, or, worse, he might get rabies. The doctor informed S.C. that his parents must personally consent or he must bring a note from them to be treated in the emergency room. S.C. left the ER and did not tell his parents about the dog bite for several days, until he subsequently developed a serious wound infection that required hospitalization. His parents brought a suit against the ER physician and the hospital for refusing to care for their son. Their suit was unsuccessful.

The above case illustrates how physicians may be placed in difficult legal situations. Physicians may be prevented legally from treating a minor for a nonemergent problem, realizing that harm may come to the minor without such treatment. The legal age of majority varies from state to state but is usually 18 or 19 years of age. Individuals who have not attained this age cannot give legally effective consent except in the following situations (these may vary from state to state):

1. Any minor on active duty in the armed services in the United States.
2. Any married minor.
3. Any minor who has a dependent child.
4. Any emancipated (legally separated) minor.
5. Any minor who is separated from his or her parents or legal guardian for whatever reason and is not supported by the parents or guardian.
6. Any minor parent as to his or her own child.
7. Any spouse of a minor when the minor is unable to give consent by reason of physical or mental incapacity.
8. Any minor requiring emergency care to treat a life-threatening condition.

In all of the above situations, the physician is free to accept the minor's consent for the service just as if he or she were an adult. The state laws usually provide that if a minor falsely represents his or her situation regarding the ability to give consent, and a health professional provides health services in good faith based on that misrepresentation, the minor shall receive full services without the consent of the minor's parent or legal guardian, and the health professional shall incur no liability except, of course, for negligence or intentional harm.

In many states, limited consent by a minor may also be allowed in the following situations:

1. Any minor who is or has been pregnant.
2. A minor afflicted with any reportable communicable disease.
3. A minor abusing drugs or alcohol.

This consent is commonly applicable only to the prevention, diagnosis, and treatment of those specific conditions. If a health professional accepts the responsibility of providing such health services, he also assumes the obligation to provide counseling for the minor by a health professional. If a minor is found not to be pregnant or suffering from a communicable disease nor drug or substance abuse nor abusive use of alcohol, the health professional usually cannot reveal any information whatsoever to the spouse, parent, or legal guardian without the consent of the minor. Whenever a physician treats a minor under any of the self-consent statutes, the laws commonly provide that the minor is liable for payment and not the spouse, parents, or legal guardian.

MEDICAL MALPRACTICE INSURANCE

Professional liability insurance for physicians is considered by most medical management consultants to be a necessary expense of practice. Because of the high probability of being sued despite practicing high quality medicine, and the risk of financial ruin if found liable for damages, almost all physicians carry some form of protection against liability.

Medical malpractice insurance, in general, covers claims made against a physician for medical negligence, improper or lack of obtaining consent, breaches of confidentiality, and improper treatment of minors. It does not protect against personal claims of liability such as causing an injury to a person in a motor vehicle accident. It also does not cover suits claiming defamation, libel, or punitive damages, those claimed to punish a person for "gross, malicious, or wanton misconduct." In addition, it does not cover against criminal acts.

Many state medical associations have developed their own insurance companies to provide an economical alternative to the commercial insurance industry. They can offer lower rates because the income from surpluses goes back into the company to help defray claim expenses and operating costs. Other important features that some of these policies have include never settling a claim that does not have merit, use of defense attorneys who do not pursue suits against insured physicians, and an underwriting committee made up entirely of physicians. This last feature helps to eliminate the often arbitrary decisions that are made by commercial insurers regarding premium surcharges or coverage suspension and termination. Such decisions are made only after thorough investigation into all open, settled, or litigated claims by this physician-peer group, with action taken only when there has been actual negligence. Decisions are not based solely on the number of lawsuits or the dollar amount involved.

Medical liability insurance is generally available in two forms: the more available "claims-made" coverage and the more desirable "occurrence" coverage. Occurrence coverage provides the physician with protection against any suits brought at any time for cases occurring during the year the premium was paid. This contrasts with the less desirable claims-made coverage in which the insurance must be in force at the time when the claim is actually made. Therefore, if a physician decides to leave practice for any reason, i.e., retirement or moving to another state, the physician would have to buy a rider, or what is called a "tail," to protect against claims brought after the end of the premium-paid year of coverage for occurrences during the "covered" time period. A tail policy commonly costs two to three times the last year's premium.

SOME WAYS TO AVOID MALPRACTICE

After all of the above discussion, it would not be surprising if the medical student reading this chapter should want to leave medical school and become a lawyer. However, there are many simple ways that a physician can prevent claims from being brought or can at least make a claim easier to defend. The following list may help in this regard:

1. *Communicate with your patient.* This issue is important not only at the time of seeing a patient but also when obtaining informed consent, when you will be unavailable to your practice, and when talking on the telephone. You and your staff should be alert to the dissatisfied patient and attempt to resolve the dispute with tact and professionalism.
2. *Keep detailed records.* These records should contain summaries of all patient communications including office visits and telephone calls, procedures, failure to keep an appointment or to maintain prescribed therapy, and results of tests and consultations or referrals.
3. *Keep only appropriate records.* Care should be used in how summaries are phrased. Remember that an attorney may some day read the record, and written arguments regarding a case, statements of fault, or superfluous details may draw an attorney's attention.
4. *Keep up medically.* As the standard of care imposed on physicians extends to national levels, it becomes especially important for a physician to keep abreast of developments in medical knowledge, attend continuing medical education programs on a regular basis, and keep a record of attendance for future reference.
5. *When in doubt, consult.* The use of a consultant affords great protection against a claim or suit. If you are uncertain about a patient's complaint, a diagnostic test, a particular treatment, or if the patient has not responded appropriately to a prescribed treatment, then consultation should be obtained. In addition, if a patient or his or her family insists

on a consultation, it is foolhardy to refuse unless the request is obviously unreasonable.

6. *Never admit fault.* An admission of fault or guilt may be damaging to the physician even though it has been made to a third party rather than to the patient, and even though it was made in private or before there was any indication of a malpractice suit.
7. *Do not make warranties.* Physicians should never guarantee a result of treatment. This admonition does not imply that a physician must be totally pessimistic about the treatment being prescribed.
8. *Avoid accusing others of malpractice.* A physician seeing a patient who has been seen by another physician or hearing of a case "second-hand" rarely has all the information about a case. Accusations of malpractice based on such information may lead to unwarranted suits.
9. *Be definite about instructions.* A physician should always tell a patient or guardian all the details of medical treatments including what side effects may occur. Instruction sheets can be very helpful in this regard. Document their use in the medical record.
10. *Do not abandon patients.* A physician should take appropriate measures to insure that patients are notified about his or her unavailability and who will be caring for them until he or she is available again.
11. *Select appropriate staff.* A physician's staff can be one of the best protections against malpractice if appropriately chosen. These individuals should be able to communicate well and manifest the proper attitude and caring behavior toward patients.
12. *Avoid undue familiarity.* A physician should always have a staff member of the opposite sex present in an exam room when examining a patient of the opposite sex.
13. *Involve patients and other physicians in decision making.* Physicians should allow patients to be involved in decisions regarding their treatments as much as possible. Informed patients are usually not surprised regarding the possible outcomes of treatments.
14. *Never mention malpractice insurance.* Physicians only raise the idea of bringing suit by mentioning they carry liability insurance to a patient, the patient's family or friends, or the patient's attorney.
15. *Advise patients about services and fees.* Physicians should be sure that patients are aware of the scope of their practices including what facilities they use to avoid unmet expectations. This advisement also includes a tactful discussion of what fees will be charged and the practice's payment policies.
16. *Inform the insurance company immediately if sued.* If a physician is notified of a possible suit, or if he feels one may occur because of an untoward event, he should notify the company immediately. It is extremely helpful to write out a detailed narrative of the exact sequence of events involving the possible suit as soon as a physician is notified or feels a suit may occur because important details may be difficult to remember by the time a suit is brought or actually comes to trial. This narrative would be in addition to the appropriately detailed medical record that should be kept. The existence of this narrative should only be mentioned to the physician's insurer and designated defense attorney.

CONCLUSIONS

The incidence of medical malpractice claims and settlements has increased over the last several years. These claims have led to an increase in the cost for medical liability insurance and a corresponding decrease in its availability. Though the incidence of malpractice suits is high, many physicians are learning how to lessen their risks of being sued by taking to heart information similar to that presented in this chapter. Many liability insurance companies now require all physicians to attend risk reduction seminars to obtain coverage.

Medical malpractice suits are civil proceedings that generally involve either tort or contract law. Torts involve either deliberate or negligent liability. For a negligent tort to be successful, such as missing an easily diagnosed cancer, the patient must show that the physician established a *duty* to him and was *derelict* in this duty by performing below a legally required standard of care, prove that *damage* occurred, and prove that the damage was a *direct consequence* of the physician's negligence. A deliberate tort, such as battery, requires only that the physician deliberately performed the wrongful act. A legally binding contract requires that mutual *consideration* occurred and that an *offer* by one party and an *acceptance* by the other also occurred.

Several important legal concepts were presented in this chapter. *Consent*, which may be expressed or implied, is required before a physician may touch a patient. *Informed consent* requires that before performing any consequential procedure on a patient, the physician must explain the nature of the ailment, the nature of the proposed treatment or operation and the probability of success, any alternative methods of treatment and their risks, including the risk of doing nothing, and any material risk of unfortunate results and unforeseen conditions within the body. *Discreet disclosure* allows the physician in very special situations to exercise discretion as to what is disclosed to the patient. *Negligence* suits are the most frequent type of suit brought against physicians. The doctrine of *res ipsa loquitur* involves certain types of injury during the course of medical treatment, such as amputating the wrong leg, that create a presumption of physician negligence so that the judge or jury may decide the question of liability on the basis of the injury alone. The concept of *respondeat superior* means that the physician can be held liable for the acts of others if the doctor has a duty to train or supervise the care given by another. The treatment of *minors* without parental consent is restricted to certain very limited circumstances in most states.

There are several simple ways to prevent medical malpractice claims from being brought or to make them easier to defend. These include clearly communicating with patients, keeping appropriate and detailed records, keeping up medically, consulting when in doubt, and never admitting fault.

Because the cost of physician liability insurance is high and continues to increase, many groups are advocating "tort reform" legislation to lessen the financial burden that is ultimately passed onto the patient. Unfortunately, the two groups that benefit the most from the "malpractice crisis," trial lawyers and insurance companies, blame each other for the problem, and therefore the reform process is slow and tedious. However, progress is being made in this arena in many states with the active participation of physicians, their patients, and many other groups.

Case 1: Laceration of Forearm in a Minor

Scott is a 16-year-old high school student who lacerated his forearm on the way home from school and came to Dr. Jones's office asking that Dr. Jones suture the laceration. The office personnel attempted to contact Scott's parents, but apparently they would be unavailable until about 5:30 that evening. Dr. Jones had seen Scott before for minor problems but had not seen his parents as patients. He went ahead and sutured Scott's laceration and saw him back in follow-up. The wound seemed to be healing satisfactorily, and the sutures were removed. One year later Scott's parents sued Dr. Jones, saying that the scar that resulted from the laceration was unsightly, that they had not given their consent for Dr. Jones to repair the laceration, and that they would have taken him to a plastic surgeon had they been notified of the injury.

1. Does this represent malpractice?
2. Which legal doctrine(s) applies?
3. At what age does a minor become an adult?

Case 2: Goiter Removal/Nerve Damage

Hazel had thyroid surgery recently in Los Angeles. She had had previous thyroid surgery because of pressure caused by her enlarged thyroid gland on the esophagus and the trachea. The surgeon who performed surgery on Hazel previously did not mention finding, or even looking for, the recurrent laryngeal nerves.

A second operation was felt to be indicated because of a recurrence of some difficulty with swallowing and pressure in her neck and some gradually increasing recurrence of enlargement of the gland. Dr. Ross, a surgical resident, performed that second operation with Dr. Hartline as his teacher.

With any thyroid operation there is a potential for damage to the recurrent laryngeal nerve, which may cause permanent hoarseness. The risk of this complication in this case was somewhat greater since there had been a previous surgery performed in the area. Hazel did, in fact, develop this complication and was left with permanent hoarseness. She sued Dr. Hartline, Dr. Ross, and the hospital, stating that she had not been informed of this particular complication prior to the surgery and that she would not have had the operation had she known about this possibility.

The consent form she signed prior to surgery indicated that hoarseness was listed as one of the possible complications, but without any specific mention of damage to a nerve or the permanency of the hoarseness. Hazel contended that she was simply asked to sign the form and that the specifics of the form were not discussed with her.

1. Was this malpractice?
2. What legal doctrine(s) applies?
3. Does the fact that Hazel signed an informed consent document in which hoarse-

ness was mentioned as a possible complication vindicate the physicians and the hospital?

Case 3: Baby–Mother Blood Incompatibility

Melanie has Rh-negative blood. Her first child was Rh-positive. Her attending physician was Dr. Lee, but the delivering physician, who was on weekend call for Dr. Lee, was Dr. Murray.

When a baby has Rh-positive blood and the mother Rh-negative blood, some of the baby's blood often gets into the mother's circulation during the delivery. Three days after delivery, the mother's body begins to build antibodies against the Rh-positive blood. Subsequent Rh-positive children are liable to suffer damage from those maternal antibodies.

Rhogam, a specific antibody to the Rh antigen, can be given to a mother to effectively destroy the Rh-positive red blood cells in her circulatory system before antibodies can be formed. It does not persist in the mother's system. The Rhogam must be given within 72 h of the birth to be effective. Melanie had a second child. The second child, Delbert, is experiencing medical problems because his mother was not given the Rhogam injection at the time that her first child was born. She developed antibodies against Rh-positive blood, his blood type, the same as that of her first child. She brought suit against all of the involved physicians and the hospital.

Dr. Lee blamed the laboratory, which was under the direct control of Dr. Kasper, for giving faulty information about the blood type of the child. Dr. Kasper, however, claimed that he gave the correct information to Dr. Lee but that Dr. Lee neglected to review the results of the laboratory work on both the mother and child. Dr. Murray contended that he was not responsible because he was relieved of duty as soon as Dr. Lee returned on the scene, 14 h after the delivery.

1. Does this represent malpractice?
2. Which legal doctrine(s) applies?
3. Who was primarily at fault (responsible)?

Case 4: Discovery of Lung Cancer

Angelo was 52 years old when he injured his back. He was admitted to a Detroit hospital, placed on bed rest, and had special x rays taken of his back. The x rays revealed a ruptured disk, and subsequently he underwent an operation to repair the disk. After surgery, Angelo's temperature was slightly elevated. A portable chest x ray showed no signs of pneumonia. There had been no chest x ray taken on admission.

Ten days after his discharge from the hospital, Angelo developed right-sided chest pains and was taken to an emergency room, where a chest x ray showed a tumor in his right lung. The x ray showed a 1-inch rounded area that was highly suspicious, and Angelo was readmitted to the hospital. A thorough examination and evaluation, including studies inside the lung with a bronchoscope, multiple special x rays, and other studies did not reveal any cancer. Angelo also had a lump at the junction between the collarbone and breastbone areas, and it was quite tender. However, it was not biopsied. Angelo had a past history of tuberculosis, and it was felt that the abnormality on the chest x ray could have been from an old, healed tuberculosis scar. Angelo was discharged from the hospital but 4 days later was readmitted to another hospital because he was dehydrated and severely ill. The calcium in his blood was elevated significantly because of a widespread and virulent lung cancer, which was spreading throughout his body. During the 3 weeks Angelo was hospitalized, he had x rays taken that showed cancer involving many bones and the bone marrow. Angelo finally succumbed to his illness.

Angelo's family sued his physicians at the first hospital for negligence in not making the diagnosis of lung cancer and specifically for not biopsying the tender area at the sternoclavicular junction.

1. Do they have a case?
2. What legal doctrine(s) applies?

Case 5: A Physician/Insurance Company Disagreement

Dr. Lambert was served notice by authorities that he was being sued by a former patient for medical malpractice. After reviewing his records, Dr. Lambert felt that he had done nothing wrong. His malpractice insurance carrier recommended that they settle out of court for $40,000 since they said that the cost of pursuing the case through the courts would be greater than that and since there would be a small chance that he might lose the case in court even though they agreed that he was not guilty.

Dr. Lambert was quite upset about the situation and decided to pursue the case in court to vindicate his reputation and to serve notice that patients should not expect to win lawsuits unless the physician was at fault.

1. What is Dr. Lambert's malpractice insurance carrier's responsibility in this situation? Can they refuse to represent him in court?
2. How often do physicians lose cases in which they and their insurance carrier feel ahead of time that they are not guilty? Is there any type of review board that looks at malpractice claims and decides whether they have any merit?

RECOMMENDED READINGS

Belli, M., Sr. (1989). *Belli for your malpractice defense,* 2nd ed. Oradell, NJ: Medical Economics.

A very entertaining book describing all aspects of a malpractice defense written by the "King of Torts" himself. Excellent case examples and the many chapters on prevention will be helpful to the practitioner not involved in a malpractice case.

Monagle, J. F. (1985). *Risk management: A guide for health care professionals.* Rockville, MD: Aspen Systems.

This book describes all aspects of developing, implementing, and evaluating hospital-based risk management programs. Although it is clearly for the more advanced reader, certain sections are appropriate for the novice.

Robertson, W. O. (1985). *Medical malpractice: A preventive approach*. Seattle: University of Washington Press.

An excellent, concise description of the malpractice problem with many illustrative cases throughout the text. An appendix contains 30 risk management review units that describe specific actions practitioners can take to reduce their malpractice risk.

CHAPTER 14

Medical Economics

Garth L. Splinter

Case 14-1: Managed Care Involvement. Dr. O. L. Fashioned has been in practice for 15 years in a suburban area of a large metropolitan city. He has a stable core of patients but has recently noted that his number of new patients has been declining. He believes that this is mainly caused by managed care plans (HMOs, PPOs), which are now operating in his community and tend to absorb employees transferred into the community.

Although Dr. Fashioned has resisted joining a managed care program in the past, he is now concerned about the future of his practice. He has recently received an offer to participate in a PPO program that would pay him on a fee schedule equivalent to approximately 80% of his usual and customary fees. In addition to the lower prices, he would also have to meet certain quality-of-care review processes on both his use of specialists and hospitalizations.

Dr. Fashioned is concerned about his decreasing volume of patients but is also concerned about receiving lower fees and having someone "look over his shoulder" if he joined a PPO.

INTRODUCTION

The economics of the practice of medicine are changing along many dimensions, with most of these changes not currently under the control of physicians. Cost containment is the largest force driving these changes and has spawned a multitude of new medical institutions. These institutions include alternative delivery systems (e.g., HMOs, PPOs) and the creation of peer review organizations that monitor utilization and quality of care. Additionally, various payer groups are demanding a decrease in "cost shifting," so that their expenses reflect more truly the cost of care to the patients that they serve rather than including the cost of care for the poor through inflated charges to those who can pay. Outcomes of these changes include an increasing concern over the quality of health care being rendered within the United States health care system, the possibility of rationing of health care (including provision of care to indigent patients), and decreased physician self-determination.

All of the above economic changes are causing changes in physician behavior. The broadest of these changes concern methods of practice (including a greater number of physicians now being salaried employees), greater concerns about the business aspects of medicine, and greater competitive stresses between the various specialty groups within medicine. The hypothesized glut of physicians that may occur in the near future only heightens these competitive stresses.

This chapter is concerned with detailing some of these recent changes and discussing current economic trends. Basic financial terminology with which physicians should be familiar is also described. The medical environment 5 to 10 years from now will probably be substantially different from the current one. Thus, today's medical students should be prepared to practice in an environment different from what they anticipated when they entered medical school.

HEALTH CARE ECONOMICS

Much of the motivation behind cost containment in medicine can be understood by looking at total expenditures for health care in the United States. These have grown from $12.7 billion in 1950 to $500.3 billion in 1987 (National Center for Health Statistics, 1989). This growth has been much more than a secondary

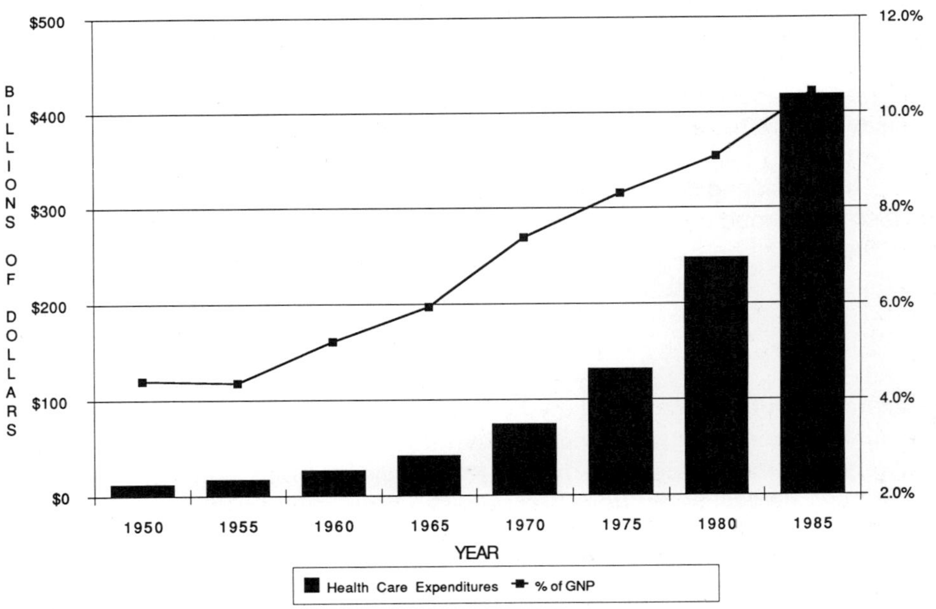

Figure 14-1. United States health care expenditures in billions of dollars (left axis) and as a percentage of GNP (right axis). Source: National Center for Health Statistics, 1989.

effect of inflation, since the total percentage of gross national product that is spent on health care has grown from 4.4% in 1950 to 11.1% in 1987. Future health care expenditures are projected to continue along the same growth curve (see Fig. 14-1).

The source of payment for health expenditures is shown in Fig. 14-2. Governments (federal, state, and local) account for approximately 40% of expenditures, and private health insurance and direct payment are each approximately 30%. Figure 14-3 shows that approximately 40% of health care expenditures are for hospital care, approximately 20% is for physician services, and the rest is divided among various other sources of care, none of which exceed 10%.

Medicare

In 1965, the program of national health insurance for the aged, now known as "Medicare," was passed as an amendment to the Social Security Act. There are two main parts to Medicare; the first, Part A, covers hospital benefits, and the second, Part B, covers physician services and other supplemental benefits. Part A has provisions for cost sharing by the beneficiaries (deductibles and coinsurance) and is financed by the Social Security earnings tax. Part B is a voluntary program financed by premiums from the beneficiaries with matching payments from government general revenues.

Part A of Medicare for hospital care is now paid under the DRG system, as explained below. Historically, payments under Part B (for physician services) have been by a method based on "usual, customary, and reasonable" fees

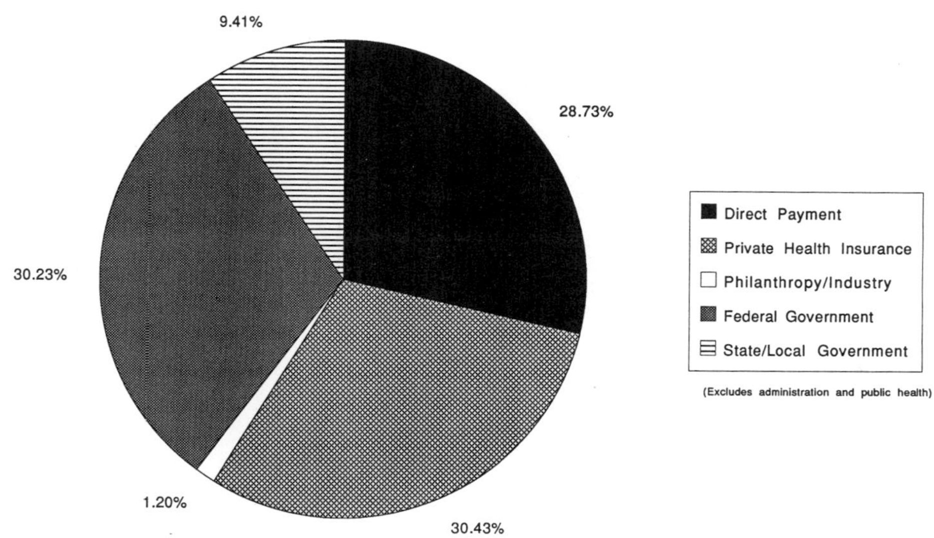

Figure 14-2. Sources of health expenditures in the United States in 1989. Source: National Center for Health Statistics, 1989.

(UCR). However, beginning in 1991, payment will be based on the resource-based relative value scale.

Medicaid

Case 14-2: Medicaid Participation. Dr. Mercy is a family physician recently in practice who is trying to decide whether to participate in the Medicaid program. He is aware that because of the low reimbursement from the state for these patients, many other physicians in the community refuse to accept them. He is torn between his compassion as a physician and his belief that he should see all patients regardless of their ability to pay and the economic realities of his practice (including his desire to make a reasonable income).

The 1965 amendments to the Social Security Act also included provisions for the expansion of the Kerr–Mills Medical Assistance Program to groups other than the elderly, a program now known as "Medicaid." This became Title 19 of the Social Security Act. This program is a federal–state matching grant program covering some medically indigent, usually single-parent families with dependents whose income is below the poverty line. It is administered by state agencies.

Health Maintenance Organizations

Health maintenance organizations (HMOs) combine insurance and health care delivery in one organization. An HMO will provide all medical care needed

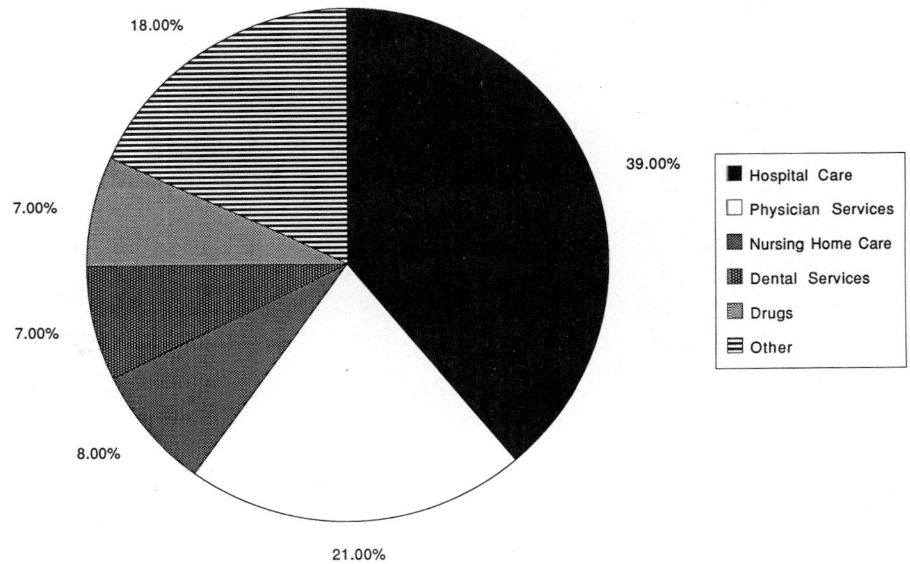

Figure 14-3. Distribution of health expenditures in the United States in 1989. Source: National Center for Health Statistics, 1989.

for the covered services for a fixed payment over a fixed period of time. Although, as the name implies, prevention would ideally be a major focus of these plans, in practice they often only provide traditional medical services, but with savings resulting from decreased hospitalization. Supporters claim they offer quality health care more efficiently. Critics claim they lead to substandard care. HMO plans have grown in both number and enrollment and have largely been concentrated in the western United States. As a percentage of the total private spending on health care, it is estimated that HMOs have grown from approximately 2% in 1965 to over 6% in 1983 (Jonas, 1986). More recent data indicate that the growth has continued, with there being an estimated 650 HMOs with enrollment at 29.3 million at the end of 1987 (Kenkel, 1988).

There is a great deal of disagreement about the ultimate future of HMOs. Some experts predict that they will be the dominant form of health care delivery in the future, but others believe that they have reached their maximum growth. In 1987, only about half of the HMOs in operation were profitable (Kenkel, 1988). Whether this represents a signal that HMOs have reached the limit of their ability to cut costs (which is the major reason for their existence) or represents the expected consolidation or shake-out phase of a new industry remains to be seen.

Physician participants in HMOs work under several different formats. In staff-model HMOs, physicians are salaried employees of the HMO and work at one location. In panel-type HMOs, physicians contract to see HMO patients but also see other (non-HMO) patients in their private offices. The legal organization of panel-type HMOs is usually as an independent practice association (IPA), which is a contractual arrangement and a type of joint venture.

Preferred Provider Organizations

Preferred provider organizations (PPOs) are insurance plans that are distinguished by being fee-for-service but with contracts between the insurance company and health care providers that limit fees and may address quality issues. Patients under PPOs are given financial incentives to use the "preferred" providers but may choose other providers if they wish. Hospitals are compensated under this system either on a fee-for-service basis, usually with a percentage reduction, or by a DRG payment system. The incentive for health care providers and hospitals to join a PPO is to capture the patient volume the plan brings.

The PPOs are rapidly growing in number. It is estimated that in 1986 there were 535 PPOs. The number of PPOs grew to 608, covering more than 35 million people, by the end of 1987 (Kenkel, 1988). PPOs are most commonly seen in workplace situations, where they are offered by employers. A recent trend is for employers to offer a triple-option plan in which an employee can choose among a PPO, an HMO, or traditional indemnity insurance, all managed by one insurance company.

Capitation

Capitation refers to payment for medical services based on a predetermined per-patient amount for a specified period of time. This is most common in capitated HMO plans wherein private physicians receive payments for their patients based on the number enrolled and not on services provided. One outcome of this type of system is that physicians assume a greater portion of the financial risks associated with the care of the patients, in some ways functioning as a small insurance company. These plans are often criticized as changing physician financial incentives in a manner that may result in decreased quality of care. Also, since primary care physicians are usually used as the "gatekeepers" in these plans, specialists generally dislike capitated plans. Supporters argue that having a single physician responsible for a patient's care can result in improved care with less use of medical resources.

Capitation of Medicare patients has been proposed as a possible future payer method by the Health Care Financing Administration (HCFA), and several pilot programs have tested the idea. However, it now appears very unlikely that it will be implemented on a large scale. Even some HMO plans have removed referral coverage from the capitation payment, thus decreasing the gatekeeper role of the involved primary care physicians.

Diagnosis-Related Groups

Case 14-3: Diagnosis-Related Groups. Dr. Good is a general internist who has hospitalized a patient with diverticulitis. He has been notified by the hospital that the allowable length of stay used to calculate the DRG payment for this Medicare patient is 4 days. The patient has reached the fourth day and has been afebrile for 24 h off of his intravenous antibiotics. However, he is still having some abdominal pain, and Dr. Good is worried that he might be discharging him too early if he lets him go home now.

Dr. Good knows that under the DRG payment there is a flat payment for the hospitalization based on diagnosis and that each additional day stay in the hospital will hurt the financial condition of the hospital. Also, if the case in question is reviewed for admission and stay criteria, his patient would not meet the requirements for a fifth day of hospitalization. This could result in additional financial penalties for the hospital. However, he is professionally concerned about his patient's condition and wonders what he should do.

In 1983, the Medicare program began paying hospitals for care based on a prospective payment system (PPS). Under this plan, fixed rates were established for each of approximately 470 diagnosis-related groups (DRGs). It was thought that having a fixed payment based on diagnosis would decrease the cost of health care by removing the financial incentives for long hospital stays and excessive testing. Institution of DRGs represented the end of cost-plus reimbursement, the traditional method of Medicare reimbursement in which all costs of hospitalization plus a reasonable profit were paid to hospitals.

The DRG system has resulted in more cost-effective patient care but has done so by a mechanism of price fixing rather than by changing incentives (McCarthy, 1988). The system will probably change over time, partly because of the criticisms of underpayment, lack of payment predictability (McCarthy, 1988), and decreased quality of care as a result of early discharges (Cotton, 1988). The

American Medical Association (AMA) House of Delegates has recently proposed replacing the present Medicare program with a system of vouchers to older persons that could be used to purchase private insurance (Board of Trustees Report, 1986). Also, DRGs for physicians have been proposed, especially concentrating on the areas of radiology, anesthesiology, and pathology (RAPs).

Utilization Review, Quality Assurance, and Peer Review

Case 14-4: Peer Review Organization Denial. Mr. Smith is a 62-year-old white male with longstanding diabetes mellitus and a previous below-the-knee amputation of his right leg. He recently developed a left foot ulcer and was hospitalized for 10 days for antibiotics and whirlpool treatment. He was then discharged on oral antibiotics. Two weeks later, Mr. Smith was readmitted for a worsening of his diabetic foot ulcer. The orthopedic surgery service decided that the foot could not be saved, and an amputation was performed.

At the time of review by the Medicare peer review organization, the initial hospitalization was denied payment based on the argument that the amputation should have been done at that time. The physicians involved appealed the case but lost.

The rise of nontraditional payment systems and the resulting criticisms about the potential for decreased quality of care have resulted in a new system of checks and balances. Utilization review (UR) retrospectively looks at the use of medical resources by medical providers. Its main purpose is to assure payers (or a medical group with an HMO plan) that medical resources are not being overutilized. Examples of situations that could be reviewed under this system are the use of specialists by primary care physicians or the use of medical technologies such as MRI or CT scanning. Concurrent review is the term used to describe this process when it is done during a hospitalization as opposed to retrospectively.

Quality assurance (QA) looks more from the viewpoint of the patient to assure that adequate medical treatment and use of resources are being employed by medical providers. Examples of this type of system include sampling charts to assure that blood pressures are being taken on every office visit or that a referral to a specialist is made at the appropriate time during the management of a particular disease process.

Peer review refers to groups of physicians reviewing the care rendered by other physicians (both UR and QA); currently, this is usually in conjunction with Medicare admissions. Criteria for appropriate admissions, appropriate discharges, length of stay, and care during hospitalization are used. An important current legal question is whether records of peer review are confidential or may be made available during malpractice lawsuits.

Quality versus Cost Containment

As can be seen from the above discussions, a major issue resulting from the implementation of these new payer systems concerns the quality of care received by patients and whether quality is adversely affected by efforts to contain costs. To date, there are no definitive studies relating outcomes, costs, and patient satisfaction.

Closely related to this issue is the question of rationing of health care. Although to some extent rationing has always existed in the United States health system (e.g., a decision on the part of a hospital to expand a dialysis unit versus adding beds to a pediatric intensive care unit), the current discussion is whether this would be implemented as a matter of national policy.

Effect on Hospitals

The change in payer systems (especially DRGs and managed care systems) has resulted in a shift to ambulatory care, away from hospitalized care. As of 1985 there had been little change in the number of hospitals (a decrease of 2.4%) or the number of hospital beds (an increase of 6.2%). However, Figs. 14-4 and 14-5 show that hospital discharges per 1000 population have decreased from 168 to 118 from 1975 to 1988 (a decrease of 29.8%), and the average length of hospital stay has decreased from 7.1 days to 6.4 days for the same period (a decrease of 9.9%). The result of this has been decreased occupancy of hospitals, with the 75.0% occupancy rate in 1975 decreasing to 69.0% in 1984 and then to 64.8% in 1985 (American Hospital Association, 1986). The result of this has been increased financial strain on hospitals, especially rural hospitals.

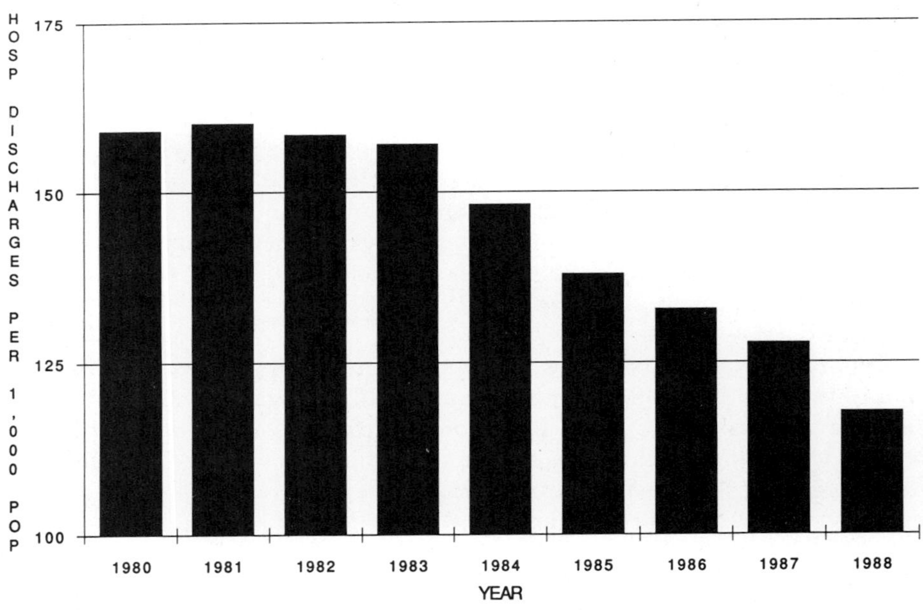

Figure 14-4. U.S. hospital discharges/1000 population. Source: National Center for Health Statistics, 1989.

Relative Value Scale

In addition to payer concerns about the total cost for health care, there have also been concerns about differences in payments between different physician specialties. To address this problem, the U.S. Congress mandated a study to determine the relative values of various physician services. This study was conducted by Harvard University with the AMA as a subcontractor. To determine the relative values of different physician activities, the study looked at intensity of efforts and procedures, the time involved before, after, and during the service, the investment of time, lower earnings during specialty training, and practice overhead costs. In general, the study found that procedures were overvalued compared to cognitive services with the result that primary-care physicians' incomes would rise while some specialists' incomes would decline if payments were made based on relative values (Hsiao, Braun, Dunn, Becker, DeNicola, & Ketchum, 1988a; Hsiao, Braun, Yntema, & Becker, 1988b; Kirchner, 1988).

Current plans are to phase in the relative value scale (RVS) system over several years beginning in 1991, replacing the usual, customary, and reasonable (UCR) method of determining Medicare fee schedules. It is likely that private health insurers will adopt similar programs. Some physicians are concerned that this system will be used as a price-fixing mechanism rather than being used to realign payments between medical specialties. This could occur through a large reduction in payments for technical procedures with a small increase in payments for cognitive services, thus decreasing total expenditures.

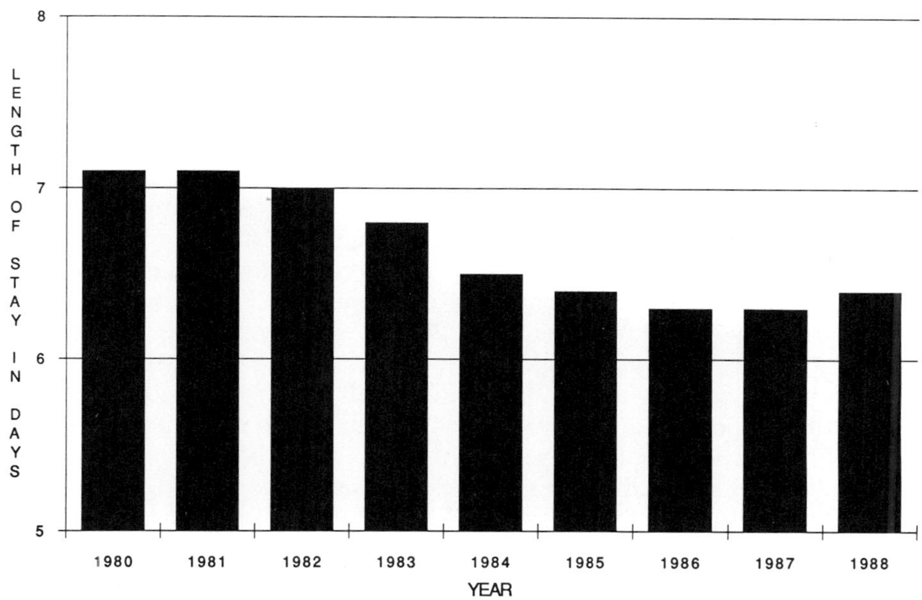

Figure 14-5. Average length of U.S. hospital stay in days. Source: National Center for Health Statistics, 1987.

Care of the Uninsured/Working Poor

The payment methods listed above have the common feature of attempting to decrease the cost of health care to the purchaser by decreasing the amount paid for medical services. In the process of trying to receive the least expensive health care possible, payers (often large corporations) have also been demanding that their costs be truly reflective of the services received by covered patients. Indigent care has traditionally been paid for by shifting costs to paying patients. However, this is becoming more difficult under current economic conditions. It is estimated that 35 to 40 million U.S. citizens are without any form of health insurance and that approximately 75 to 80 million persons are not covered by major medical policies. In addition, most major medical policies do not provide coverage for extended nursing home and home care services (Ginzberg, 1988). Private hospitals, both profit and nonprofit, have an increasing financial incentive to discourage admission of medically indigent patients. This obviously increases the financial strain on public hospital systems. The situation is certain to become more critical as the United States population ages and as the number of AIDS patients increases.

These changes are creating a multitiered health care system with categories of adequate insurance coverage, inadequate insurance coverage (e.g., Medicare, Medicaid, many small companies), and no insurance coverage. This situation has raised moral questions about the right to health care and the use of rationing. Proposed solutions to this problem vary, but most involve either a much increased role for the federal government in financing indigent care or mandating worker coverage by companies.

PHYSICIAN MANPOWER ISSUES

Health manpower forecasting has been a common practice for the last 50 years. The most recent concern began with the 1980 report from the Graduate Medical Education National Advisory Committee (GMENAC), which had been commissioned by the U.S. Congress in 1976 to determine the future supply and needs for physicians in the United States. In the report they estimated that by 1990 there would be an overall surplus of approximately 70,000 physicians and that the surplus would be approximately 145,000 by the year 2000 (Department of Health and Human Services, 1981). The methodology of the GMENAC report came under close scrutiny and criticism; Reinhardt (1981) analyzed the process and stated that it left "one with serious doubts about the reliability of the ultimate GMENAC projections." More recently, the AMA began an ongoing research effort to determine the future of physician manpower. Their most realistic option analyzed (scenario D) assumed a continued modest decline in U.S. medical school class size. This analysis showed that even if the number of new physicians were restricted, the total active physician population would continue to grow through the year 2000 (Kletke, Marder, & Silberger, 1987).

Figure 14-6 shows the AMA scenario D projection for the number of active physicians per 100,000 U.S. population. The 1985 ratio of 214.2 physicians per 100,000 U.S. population is projected to increase to 250.4 physicians per 100,000

U.S. population by the year 2000. For comparison, the GMENAC report recommended an ideal ratio of physicians to population of 191 per 100,000.

In a recent forecast, Schwartz, Sloan, and Mendelson (1988) concluded that "a substantial surplus is likely to occur only if cost containment efforts lead to considerable rationing of beneficial services." They estimated that in the year 2000, physician demand would exceed supply by 7000 physicians, based on the number of nonclinical physicians, the number and workload of residents, and the percentage of female physicians (who tend to work 8% to 10% fewer hours than male physicians); by varying the assumptions, they showed that physician supply fluctuated between a shortage of as much as 60,000 and a surplus of 40,000 physicians in the year 2000. The basic difference in their model from previous ones was their belief that the demand for physician services would grow substantially in the next 12 years.

A possible physician shortage by the year 2000 is thought likely by Schloss (1988), who states that with "general population growth, the aging of the baby boom generation, declining enrollments in medical schools, the shrinking labor pool, lower physician productivity, and the increasing unattractiveness of medicine as compared with other professions," there may be a physician shortage of approximately 42,000 starting in 2010. He anticipates that this may increase to a shortage of approximately 82,000 physicians by 2030.

There are also approximately 22,000 active osteopathic physicians (D.Os) in the United States. Available data indicate that the osteopathic physician population grew 21.1% between 1980 and 1984, compared to 14.2% in the number of active M.D.s. It is anticipated that this differential will continue in the future, with approximately 44,000 active D.O.s by the year 2000.

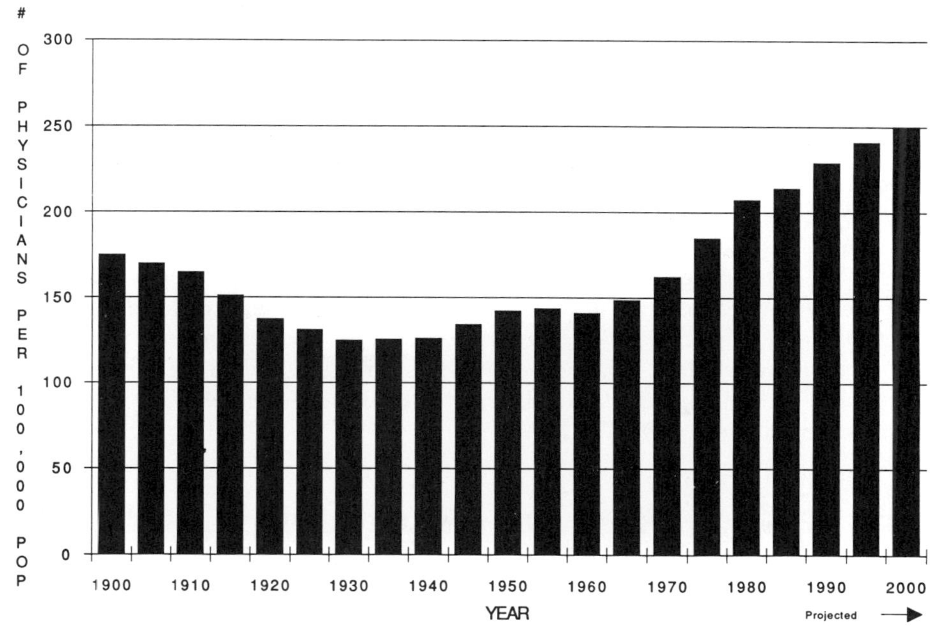

Figure 14-6. Number of active U.S. physicians/100,000 population. Source: Kleike *et al.*, 1987.

The issue of physician manpower projections is important because it is intricately involved in public policy decision making and also may lead to both decreased residency slots in certain specialties and increased competition in practice. As the above review indicates, the true situation is far from being fully understood.

Physician Incomes

The AMA (Gonzalez & Emmons, 1986) reports that the average net income of physicians in 1985 was $113,200 compared to $56,400 in 1975. After adjustment for inflation, the 1985 figure was essentially equal at $56,600. However, relative to the average salary and wages of all full-time-equivalent workers in the United States, physician average net income rose by 4% from 1975 to 1985. There is also substantial variation by specialty, with general/family practice and pediatrics having 1985 average net incomes of $77,900 and $77,100, respectively, as compared to surgery and radiology having 1985 average net incomes of $155,400 and $150,800, respectively. As mentioned above, these comparisons may change significantly if an RVS payment system is fully implemented.

Physician Employment Status

Recent surveys show that a greater number of physicians are opting for employee status as opposed to traditional fee-for-service self-employment. A recent AMA survey (Gonzalez, 1986) showed that the percentage of employee physicians among nonfederal patient care physicians, excluding residents, grew from 23.4% in 1983 to 25.7% in 1985. The most significant changes occurred in young physicians and female physicians. Among physicians under 36 years of age, 47.0% were employees in 1985 compared to only 19.4% of physicians over age 55. Also, in 1985, 45.4% of females were employees compared to 23.5% of males. Self-employed physicians earned nearly $38,000 more per year than employed physicians; however, they worked an average of 1.5 weeks more per year and spent 4 h more per week in practice care activities. Currently it is not possible to determine to what extent this income difference reflects purely a difference in employment status and to what extent it reflects differences in age, experience, and specialty between self-employed and employed physicians. Also, as explained below, self-employed physicians usually have their own capital invested in their practice, and thus some of the difference could represent a return on their investment.

PRACTICE MANAGEMENT

Many of the issues discussed above directly affect the doctor–patient relationship. Additionally, there are effects on the management of the physician's practice. These include increased use of computers for information management, better understanding of contracts and negotiating, increased paperwork, and improved skills in staff management. However, the most critical management skills required of new physicians will be the ability to understand financial issues and make appropriate financial decisions.

Financial Statements

Physicians in private practice have always had to be concerned with the financial viability of their practice. Therefore, the use of accounting and financial control is not new to medical practice, but, in the new cost containment environment, it has taken on a greater importance.

There are three types of financial statements (see Tables 14-1 through 14-3): income statement, cash flow statement, and balance sheet. When a business venture is being anticipated, and these statements are created based on assumptions, they are known as *pro forma* financial statements. For a physician wishing to obtain a loan to start up a practice or to expand an existing practice, the use of *pro forma* financial statements and accompanying assumptions in discussions with bankers will greatly improve the chances of success.

For an ongoing practice, the use of regular financial statements allows physicians to know the financial viability and financial trends of their practice. Accounting systems that track cost data by various services (cost accounting) also allow physicians to determine whether subcomponents of their practices are profitable. For instance, a physician who is in a capitated HMO program and is therefore responsible for referral costs may want to know what the net income is for that one portion of her practice. The information used to create income statements can also be used to determine the productivity of various providers, either M.D.s or ancillary personnel. As can be anticipated, this is very common in organizations that employ physicians or in physicians' offices that employ a large number of ancillary care providers.

Not all of the items in an income statement are true cash items. For instance, accounts receivable shows what money is owed to the physician, but until it is collected, it is not available to be spent. Therefore, an increase in accounts receivable (as in a growing practice) results in the income statement understating the cash available. Likewise, depreciation (an expense item) or an increase in accounts payable creates available cash that will not be reflected in net income. The result of all of this is that a separate statement called the cash flow statement must be created to determine exactly what cash is available from the practice. This becomes extremely important in a start-up situation, where total income is small and items such as accounts receivables are growing. Also, for existing practices, decisions to purchase new, expensive equipment must consider the methods that will be used to pay for it. Payment may be out of available cash but can also be from new loans, which will require debt service and therefore increase cash flow needs.

The final common financial statement is the balance sheet. This statement shows assets and liabilities and the difference between these two, which is the equity in the practice. It is important to remember that the value shown on the balance sheet probably does not represent the true value of an ongoing practice. This is because the true amount at which assets can be sold may at times be much below or much above the book value (i.e., the amount shown on the balance sheet). Also, the method of valuing a practice according to what the pieces could be sold for, known as liquidation value, is usually not the true value of a company. More commonly used for valuation is the current value of the future earnings of the practice, which is called the discounted net present value of future earnings. This concept is explained in somewhat more detail later in this chapter.

The issue of productivity is taking on greater importance in organizations

Table 14-1
Income Statement (Idealized Solo Practice)

Revenue	
Office visits	$119,000
OB	16,000
Emergency room visits	1,200
Hospital admissions/visits	30,000
Nursing home visits	1,700
Office lab services	24,300
Office x ray	11,200
Office procedures	12,300
Total	$215,700
Collections (%)	93.0%
Total collections	$200,601
HMO capitation payments[a]	22,500
Total income	$223,101
Expenses	
Personnel	$64,660
Lab	7,000
Radiology	3,500
Medical and surgical supplies	4,300
Building and equipment depreciation[b]	11,600
Interest on loan	5,200
Furniture and equipment[c]	3,300
Office supplies and services	3,000
Telephone	2,000
Insurance	10,000
Outside professional services	2,400
PR and marketing	1,000
Miscellaneous	5,500
Subtotal	$123,460
HMO consultant expenses[d]	7,600
Total expenses	$131,060
Net income	$92,041

[a] Payments to M.D. from insurance company to provide all medical care for covered patients.
[b] Depreciation is a noncash expense allowed by the tax code to reflect decreasing value of capitalized items (capital items are those that retain most value and are shown on the balance sheet as a shift in categories, e.g., from cash to buildings).
[c] Replacement, repair, or small items that do not qualify as a capital item.
[d] M.D. expenses under a capital HMO plan for referral costs for covered patients.

that use employed physicians or in practices involved with managed care systems. The most common types of control for productivity involve such measures as number of clinic visits per session, average dollars billed per clinic visit, and measurements of total referrals for other services. There are, of course, many others that can be used depending on the specific aspects of behavior that are to be monitored.

The above discussion of finance and financial controls is very superficial. Since the use of financial controls is gaining greater importance in medical practice, it is probable that in the future many physicians will elect to learn a great deal more about formal accounting systems. This can be accomplished either through self-learning from accounting and finance textbooks or through enrollment in medical economics courses, some offered through medical societies.

Financial Concepts

The following concepts are included so that the terms will be familiar when used by the physician's CPA or investment advisor. To gain a good working knowledge of the concepts would probably require taking a course in finance.

Time Value of Money

Because of interest that can be earned on money over time, money in the future is worth less than current money. The amount by which they differ varies

Table 14-2
Cash Flow Statement (Idealized Solo Practice)

Net income	$92,041
Plus depreciation[a]	11,600
Plus new loans	20,000
Plus increase in accounts payable[b]	2,200
Less increase in accounts receivable[c]	(6,100)
Less loan repayments	(3,000)
Less new equipment purchases[d]	(29,500)
Total cash flow	$87,241

[a] Depreciation is a noncash expense allowed by the tax code to reflect decreasing value of capitalized items (capital items are those that retain most value and are shown on the balance sheet as a shift in categories, e.g., from cash to buildings). Because it is a noncash expense, it is added back to net income.

[b] Accounts payable is the amount of money owed by the practice. Because it is subtracted as an expense before being paid, it is added back to net income. When accounts payable decreases, the amount of the decrease is subtracted from net income (since the cash would have been paid out without an expense shown in net income).

[c] Accounts receivable is the amount of money owed to the practice. Because it is added as a revenue before being received, it is subtracted from net income. When accounts receivable decreases, the amount of the decrease is added to net income (since the cash would be received without a revenue being shown in net income).

[d] Capital items are not shown on the income statement as an expense but require cash to purchase. Therefore, the amount required is shown as a cash outflow. If a loan is used in the purchase, the loan is shown as a cash inflow (as in the above case).

by the interest rate. For instance, at 10% interest, $1.00 at time zero (the present) is worth $1.10 1 year from now. Likewise, in two years, $1.00 now would be worth $1.21 (or the receipt of $1.21 in 2 years is equivalent to $1.00 now). The important implication of this is that for investment or business opportunities that have various cash flows over time to be compared on an equal basis, all cash flows must be related to the same particular point in time.

Net Present Value

Given the concept of time value of money and a given interest rate (which would be set by the other possible returns available to the investor in question), the net present value of an investment is the time-zero value of all discounted cash inflows and outflows.

Table 14-3
Balance Sheet (Idealized Solo Practice)

Assets	
Short term	
Cash	$14,200
Accounts receivable[a]	29,367
Total short-term assets	$43,567
Long term	
Land	$6,200
Buildings	80,800
Equipment	15,000
Less accumulated depreciation[b]	(35,600)
Total long-term assets	$137,600
Total assets	$181,167
Liabilities and equity	
Current liabilities	
Accounts payable[c]	$10,772
Payroll due	2,487
Total current liabilities	$13,259
Long-term liabilities	
Loan: building, land	$52,100
Loan: equipment	17,000
Total long-term liabilities	$69,100
Equity	
Capital account[d]	$15,000
Retained Earnings[e]	83,808
Total equity	$98,808
Total liability and equity	$181,167

[a] Accounts receivable is the amount of money owed to the practice.
[b] Accumulated depreciation is the total of current and past depreciation for all items on the balance sheet.
[c] Accounts payable is the amount of money owed by the practice.
[d] A capital account shows the value of the initial contributions put into a practice by the owner (may be cash, land, equipment, etc.).
[e] Retained earnings are the past earnings (net income) that have been left in the practice and used to finance growth (e.g., increase in accounts receivable, equipment).

Example 1. You invest $1,000 in an antique desk now (time 0) and sell it for $1,300 in 2 years. At a 10% interest rate, the net present value (NPV) is $74.38
[NPV = $1,300/(1.10 × 1.10) − $1,000].
Example 2. You lend $1,000 to your college roommate and hope to receive $620 at the end of year 1 and $620 at the end of year 2 (a total of $1,240). At a 10% interest rate the net present value is $76.03
[NPV = $620/1.100 + $620/(1.10 × 1.10) − $1,000].
If in fact your roommate pays you back the $1,240 at the end of year 3, the net present value is *negative* $68.37
[NPV = $1,240/(1.10 × 1.10 × 1.10) − $1,000].

Expected Value

When a physician prescribes a particular treatment for a patient, he knows that he is dealing with a range of possible outcomes, with each outcome having a given probability and the sum of all probabilities being equal to 1. In a like manner, when certain financial decisions are made, there is a range of possible outcomes, each one having a probability of occurrence, and the sum of all of these probabilities is equal to 1. By determining the final financial result of each possible outcome and the probability of each outcome occurring, multiplying them by each other, and then adding them, it is possible to come up with the weighted or expected value of the overall decision.

Example. In the above example of the loan to a roommate, the two possible outcomes are NPV = $76.04 or NPV = $(68.37). If the probability of the first occurring is 60% and the probability of the second is 40%, then the expected value is $18.27 [EV = 0.60 × $76.04 − 0.40 × $68.37].

Sunk Costs

Once an investment is made, the amount invested, for most practical purposes, becomes unimportant to future economic decisions. This is because the value of an asset at a particular time is what the marketplace determines as a value for that asset rather than what was initially invested (i.e., the initial cost is a sunk cost). For example, a physician who is moving and wishes to sell a house is constrained by the marketplace as to what price he can charge for his house, even if this price is below what he originally paid.

Liquidity

Liquidity refers to the amount of cash that can be raised quickly by a particular person or organization. It is important to differentiate this from total assets, since many times financial circumstances demand that transactions be handled in cash. For example, a large clinic may buy a variety of very expensive equipment, thereby generating a large debt service. If they experience a downturn in their clinical production, they may have a cash shortage and be unable to meet financial obligations, even though they have a positive equity on their balance sheet.

Financial Incentives

This is included as a financial concept to highlight the fact that along with issues of service to others, self-fulfillment, personal recognition, and other positive motivations, physicians are also motivated (in varying degree) by financial return. This fact is used in many medical organizations to help motivate physicians and is also used as a strong motivator for medical office staff. The usual practice is to tie financial incentives to objective measurements of desired behavior, thereby modifying that behavior in a way positive for the organization. The physician should be aware of the financial motivators in his environment and how they effect his practice of medicine.

Fixed versus Variable Costs

It is important to recognize that the expenses (overhead) of an organization are usually broken into two broad categories: fixed costs and variable costs. Fixed costs are those expenses that do not vary with the amount of production done in the clinic, for example, rent, utilities, insurance, and staff salaries. Variable expenses would be items such as PT or OT personnel (used on an as-needed basis), referrals under a capitated HMO plan, and consumables such as sutures. As could be seen from the above examples, most of the expenses in a physician's practice are fixed. An important implication of this is that a set number of patients must be seen to cover the fixed expenses and that each additional patient after this fixed number is usually very profitable for the practice.

Incremental Economics

The economics of providing services are different for an ongoing business than they are for a start-up business. For instance, an entrepreneur who decided to start a service that would provide nutritional counseling would need to look at the costs of providing a set of rooms, furniture, utilities, brochures, and staff (including receptionist and a dietitian). This would then be compared with the expected return from patient fees. However, a physician who currently has an ongoing practice would be able to look at providing the same service for only the costs of brochures and additional staff. This assumes that the physician's office has adequate space in which to conduct the service and that there would be no additional cost for utilities. The revenue side may also be increased for the physician since she already has a patient base to whom the service would be offered.

Return on Investment

It is important to remember that a self-employed physician or a physician in a partnership will have a certain amount of personal assets invested in the practice. Return on investment (ROI) refers to the amount of income that is derived from the use of these assets or, alternatively, could be derived from the use of them if they were invested in another area. For instance, a physician who has assets of $100,000 invested in his practice and the option of investing in bonds at a 9% annual return, should consider $9,000 of his income as return on investment. It is thus important to separate out the total income from a practice into the amount that can be considered equivalent to "salary" and the amount that is returned on investment. This may be one of the factors that cause employed physicians to earn less in salary than the earnings of their self-employed counterparts in private practice.

IMPLICATIONS FOR PHYSICIAN BEHAVIOR

Self-Determination

The traditional role of a physician as a solo practitioner or member of a small group having one-on-one relationships with his patients, with payment coming either from a third party or from the patient, is rapidly changing to a system in which physicians have less autonomy. This is because of both professional affiliations within larger groups or being a salaried physician and the intrusion of managed care systems (through mechanisms such as quality assurance, utilization review, and peer review). It is still unclear what the limit of this trend will be.

M.D. versus M.D.

Much of the past political power of physicians has been diminished because of divisions between physicians resulting in less unification. A few of the major divisions are primary care versus specialists, salaried physicians versus fee-for-services physicians, cognitive services versus procedures, community-based practitioners versus academic-based practitioners, and rural physicians versus urban physicians. Current changes in the health care system such as gatekeeper plans and the proposed relative value scale will tend to exacerbate these conflicts.

Negotiating/Strategic Planning

The increase in the business aspects of medical practice has made it more important for physicians to be comfortable with certain business principles. What many residents realize as they prepare to go into practice is that they must now negotiate with a group, a hospital, or another potential employer concerning terms of employment, guarantee of salary, and other aspects of practice. Many books or professional advisors are available to help in this activity. A basic tenet is to know your own position in terms of what you want and the economic impact of your practice. Knowing the motivations and economics of the other side is also important.

Physician Managers

One side effect of the business changes in the medical environment is the rise of "physician executives." The American College of Physician Executives (previously named the American Academy of Medical Directors) is an organization of physicians who are involved in the management of the business side of medicine with approximately 5000 members.

M.D. Responses

The above major forces in the national health care system are, of course, eliciting responses from physicians. To the extent that physicians are able to agree on solutions, organizations such as the AMA and state medical associations attempt to influence legislation. In the "medical marketplace," physicians are responding by forming larger economic entities that are able to compete with the other large entities involved in health care (hospital chains, insurance companies, governments). This has usually taken the form of large clinics or more loosely affiliated networks of independent providers.

As the above figures indicate, many physicians are also opting for salaried positions, which relieve them of the problems of risk assumption and business management. These same concerns also are motivating factors to join large groups or to affiliate with hospitals for practice management services.

CONCLUSIONS

This chapter has attempted to show how many of the current changes in the practice of medicine are being driven by the increased costs of medical care. These increased costs have led to efforts by various payers to exert more control and have therefore resulted in changed payer systems. Combined with a perceived surplus of physicians, this has resulted in increased competition in the medical marketplace.

There is much this chapter has not tried to cover or explain, including the economics of increased medical costs, the substantially increased role of corporations in trying to control their medical costs, the role of marketing in medical practices, or the role of non-M.D.s in providing medical services. However, it is hoped that with the areas covered, the student will appreciate that there are significant changes occurring in the environment of the physician and that some knowledge of general business management will be needed to function effectively.

Case 1: Employment Decision

Dr. Sally Smart is nearing the completion of her residency in family medicine. She plans to practice in the town in which she has been doing residency and has developed the following options:

1. Go into solo practice.
2. Form a partnership with a friend of hers who has been in practice for 2 years.
3. Sign a contract with a local hospital to staff an ambulatory care center, where she would receive 45% of practice income with a $70,000 per year practice guarantee from the hospital.
4. Join a large multispecialty group with a first-year guarantee of $65,000 and a potential for profit sharing.
5. Join an HMO as a staff physician at a salary of $55,000 per year.

In considering her situation, she notes the following facts:

1. She desires to have control over her own life.
2. She knows that she enjoys the security of quickly being able to call on specialists for rare or complicated cases.
3. She has large medical school debts to pay.
4. She dislikes frequent calls.
5. She plans to be married in the near future and desires to have children.
6. She enjoys the comradery of her peers.

1. If you were Dr. Smart, how would your list of concerns differ?
2. What would you decide to do?

Case 2: DRGs

Mr. Prudent is hospital administrator of a large suburban hospital with a large inpatient population covered by Medicare. It has recently come to his attention that the average length of stay for these patients is exceeding the averages used to calculate payments under the DRG system. He wants to bring this to the attention of the medical staff in order to enlist their aid in decreasing average lengths of stay.

1. If you were Mr. Prudent, how would you proceed?

Case 3: Peer Review Organization

Dr. B. S. Driver has been in practice for 15 years and is well respected by the physicians in his community. Recently he has been asked to participate as a reviewing physician in a peer review group (to review Medicare hospitalizations). Dr. Driver believes in maintaining high standards for medical care, but he feels uncomfortable being in a position to pass judgment on other physicians. He is also somewhat concerned that the legal status of the confidentiality of the proceedings is unclear.

1. If you were Dr. Driver, would you join the PRO?

Case 4: Financial Control

Dr. Marx is a primary care physician practicing in a large staff model HMO. Recently the financial controller of the organization came to him and said that through their monitoring, they have decided that he is not productive enough. His average number of visits per session has only been 14 per half day over the last 3 months, and they think that this should be raised to 17. Furthermore, the implication is that failure to achieve this goal may result in his termination of employment.

Dr. Marx is very concerned about whether his quality of care and personal preference in practice will suffer as a result of trying to see more patients.

1. What would you do?
2. What issues do you see being involved?

Case 5: Indigent Care

Dr. Rand is chief of staff for a large not-for-profit hospital. He has recently been asked to comment on a proposed policy by the board of directors that the hospital attempt to limit the amount of indigent care. Dr. Rand knows that the hospital is under financial constraints because of decreased payments from the Medicare DRG system and the hospital's participation in several PPO plans (with the hospital pricing based on incremental economics). At the same time, though, he is concerned that this is a partial abandonment of the hospital's mission to serve the sick, and he knows that institution of the policy would result in some patients being diverted from the emergency room and possibly receiving less adequate care at a different location or being placed in life-threatening situations as a result of the increased transport time.

1. If you were Dr. Rand, what would you do?
2. What other information would you wish to have?
3. How would that affect your decision?

RECOMMENDED READINGS

Aluise, J. J. (1986). *The physician as manager.* New York: Springer-Verlag.

This textbook of management is oriented toward the physician in medical practice who must be involved in managing his or her own practice. Covered areas include marketing, choosing a practice site, financial management, personnel management, computerization, and professional relations. It is written at a level and in a style such that concepts can be easily grasped by physicians who do not have formal business training.

Curry, W. (Ed.). (1988). *The physician executive.* Tampa, FL: American Academy of Medical Directors.

This text described the progress in the field of physician management that has been made over the past few years and describes skills required to be a successful manager. Covered areas include (1) the future of medicine, (2) career positioning, (3) marketing, (4) finance, (5) hiring and firing, (6) recruiting, (7) legal issues, and (8) communication.

Farber, L. (Ed.). (1988). *Medical economics: Encyclopedia of practice and financial management*, 2nd ed. Oradell, NJ: Medical Economics Books.

This text is a very detailed and clear reference on practice management. It provides multiple beneficial suggestions on this difficult topic. It also includes a large section on personal financial management for the practicing physician.

Heskett, J. L. (1986). *Managing in the service economy.* Boston: Harvard Business School Press.

In this book, Heskett presents the results of an intensive analysis of many case studies to determine which management strategies have given leading service companies their clear competitive advantages. Heskett develops a four-point blueprint for service managers: (1) targeting on a marketing segment, (2) conceptualizing how the service will be perceived by consumers, (3) focusing on an operating strategy, and (4) designing an efficient service delivery system that transforms vision into action. Many examples are given as well as a structured set of guidelines for developing and maintaining a competitive advantage.

PART V

Conclusions

Even though the science of clinical practice is in its infancy, that science is pointing to the need for a new approach to medical care. This section details the outlines of that new approach in an attempt to integrate the many clinical practice themes developed in this text. This integration will not end with this chapter, however, not only because knowledge is rapidly expanding in this area but because the principles of clinical practice described in this text will need to be integrated with specific medical knowledge and skills as the student progresses through medical school and because the practice of medicine itself will need to be integrated with the practitioner's life. Integration therefore becomes a lifelong task for the student of medicine. Why do you think they call it the *practice* of medicine?

CHAPTER 15

Patient-Centered Care

Mark B. Mengel and Richard A. Wright

> Mastery is central to any scholarly or professional discipline. Mastery of a discipline requires mastery of a method. . . .
>
> Ian McWhinney, M.D., 1989

Case 15-1. Dr. G.H. is a third-year family practice resident. As a part of her residency training, she is assigned to spend 2 months in a small rural community working with a group of primary care physicians. It's a rainy Saturday afternoon, and G.H. is on call.

Suddenly, G.H.'s beeper summons her to the emergency room. On arrival, the nurse informs her that the ambulance has called and is bringing a 6-year-old boy in marked respiratory distress to the hospital. Two minutes later the ambulance arrives. The EMTs unload their patient, who is a young boy with severe inspiratory stridor. His parents have followed the ambulance to the emergency room and are outside the exam room.

As G.H. begins to work on the patient, the boy begins to struggle for breath and becomes cyanotic. He is unable to speak. The nurse tells G.H. that he has a fever of 103°F. G.H. notices that his pulse is slow and orders cardiac monitoring in addition to oxygen. As the nurse applies the cardiac electrodes, the patient suffers a respiratory arrest. G.H. attempts to ventilate the patient with mouth-to-mouth resuscitation. Efforts to do so are unsuccessful. She attempts intubation but finds that the epiglottis is severely inflamed and swollen. She is unable to visualize the airway or intubate the patient. As seconds, which seem like hours, tick by, she realizes that she will have to attempt a cricothyroidotomy.

Using a large-gauge IV catheter, she is successful in performing the cricothyroidotomy. Ventilation of the patient through the IV catheter immediately restores his pulse. As he receives some oxygen, spontaneous respirations return. Although he is quite somnolent, he is responsive verbally. A general surgeon is consulted, and a better tracheostomy is established.

Treatment of the patient's epiglottitis with antibiotics and steroids results in rapid resolution of his illness. G.H. removes the patient's tracheostomy 3 days later, and he is able to go home. He is healthy, well, and has suffered no brain damage as a result of his respiratory arrest (contributed by J. Steinbauer).

INTRODUCTION

If method is key to any professional discipline, as McWhinney points out in the above quote, then one can learn a great deal about medicine by studying its method. Medicine's method of taking care of patients has not remained static but has changed over the centuries, as described in Chapter 1. These changes have, by and large, improved the care that physicians have given to their patients, yet each method has gradually been replaced by a newer method as disadvantages of the older one became more apparent.

The Biomedical Model

The dominant method of medicine today arises from the biomedical model, which began its evolution during the 1700s on the foundation of scientific reductionism (White, 1988). Its aim is simple: to interpret the patient's symptoms and signs in terms of physical pathology. The dominance of the biomedical model is easily understood when its strengths are noted: (1) its procedures often yield beneficial results for the patient; (2) procedures are performed in an order that simplifies a otherwise complex and difficult process; (3) objective data, e.g., results of laboratory tests, biopsies, autopsies, validate the method (McWhinney, 1989); and (4) this method enables clinicians to eradicate or cure many previously fatal diseases, as G.H. did in Case 15-1, and successfully control many illnesses for which a cure has not been found (Rogers & Blendon, 1977).

Despite its great strength and dominance, the biomedical method has been seriously critiqued. Ivan Illich, for example, points out that (1) much of what medicine recommends as treatment is based more on tradition than scientific evidence; (2) many epidemiologic studies have revealed that some medical care provided to patients may actually be inadequate or harmful to health; (3) extensive resources are devoted to offsetting iatrogenic (doctor-induced) damage resulting from overaggressive biomedical interventions; and (4) medical care tends to encourage dependency rather than foster patient autonomy (Illich, 1975).

The method's success is also questionable, for although collective health has improved over the past 30 years, surveys of patients continually reveal decreased satisfaction with personal health (Barsky, 1988). Barsky explains this paradoxical finding by the following facts: (1) the increased prevalence of chronic and degenerative diseases impairs patient functional status despite longer lives; (2) a greater self-scrutiny and overall awareness of symptoms has resulted from patients' consciousness of their health; (3) the widespread commercialization of health has fostered a climate of apprehension, insecurity, and alarm; and (4) the medicalization of problems previously thought to be simple matters of daily living has lead to unrealistic hopes of cure.

Recent research has, in addition, pointed out important shortcomings of the biomedical method. Kroenke and Mangelsdorff (1989) reviewed the records of

1000 patients who presented to an internal medicine clinic over 3 years. Five hundred sixty-seven new complaints were noted in these patients' charts. Diagnostic tests were performed in more than two-thirds of cases. An organic disease was discovered in only 16% of these cases. The cost of discovering an organic etiology was high, particularly for patients with headaches ($7778) and back pain ($7263). Furthermore, treatment was instituted for only 55% of symptoms and was often ineffective. The authors concluded that "diagnostic strategies emphasizing organic causes may be inadequate."

Second, the biomedical method provides no means for the physician to assess the meaning of the patient's illness, as recognized by physicians who themselves have become patients (Rabin, Rabin, & Rabin 1982; Sacks, 1984). As Stetten (1981), a physician afflicted with macular degeneration, a disease of the retina, has written:

> Through all of these years and despite many encounters with skilled and experienced professionals, no ophthalmologist has at any time suggested any devices that might be of assistance to me. No ophthalmologist has mentioned any of the many ways in which I could stem the deterioration in the quality of life . . . [The] purpose of this essay is . . . courteously but firmly, to complain of what appears to be the ophthalmologist's attitude: "We are interested in vision but have little interest in blindness."

Failure to recognize the specific "threats to self" that an illness brings to a particular patient, such as disruption in functional status, loss of control, or decreased confidence, only serves to increase patient vulnerability and alienation, further worsening the illness experience (McWhinney, 1989; Toombs, 1987).

Third, the biomedical method does not allow physicians the opportunity to understand the context in which illness occurs. As reviewed in the chapters on the family system and cultural issues (Chapters 9 and 10), contextual influences such as a person's family, work groups, or community can all have profound effects on a person's health. Rather than taking these systemic influences into account, the biomedical method isolates the individual from his or her context as a diseased organism. Although this focusing clearly allows the physician to concentrate on the biological disease process, ignoring contextual influences that maintain unhealthy and problem-producing behaviors limits the effectiveness of interventions designed to promote health.

Paradoxically, it seems that the widespread success of the biomedical method has spawned great societal and physician dissatisfaction with medical care. As a result, clinicians increasingly believe that medicine is on the brink of a major transformation of its basic model into one that will more adequately respond to societal and patient demands (Bloom, 1963; Engel, 1987; McWhinney, 1989; Perkoff, 1985).

The Framework for a New Method

If flaws in the biomedical method are becoming more apparent, is a new medical method available that might correct these flaws? Can a new method maintain the advantages of the biomedical method while correcting its disadvantages? Unfortunately, sufficient work has not yet been done by medical scholars and practitioners at this time to define clearly a new and improved method of medical care. Even so, the rough outlines exist for a new approach to medical care that should develop into medicine's dominant method. Before we describe this approach, we contrast its philosophical characteristics with those of the biomedical method.

The biomedical method emphasizes beneficence and nonmaleficence as principles of practice, rather than autonomy and justice. A disease-oriented framework, as opposed to a person-oriented one, forms the perspective for the biomedical model. Physicians utilize the priestly or engineering models of care while emphasizing competence and diligence as their main obligations to patients.

The newer approach would contrast with the biomedical model by emphasizing patient autonomy and justice as the primary principles of practice. The framework of practice would be person-oriented with quality of life of the person an additional important factor to consider. Because of the focus on autonomy, the physician would operate more from a collegial or contract model of the physician–patient relationship and emphasize the obligations of honesty and candor.

Many clinicians, particularly primary care physicians, are already experimenting with this new approach to medical care. At the same time, many physicians discourage widespread implementation of the new approach, fearing that the "priestly" physician would simply be traded for the "priestly" patient. Physicians worry that they would have to accede to patient demands rather than exercising good biomedical judgment. Granted, if this new clinical approach made patient autonomy supreme, both the patient's health and the professional authority of the physician would suffer. Thus, to achieve widespread acceptance among both practitioners and patients, the new approach must respect physician autonomy as well as patient autonomy. Whatever therapeutic plan then emerged from the dialogue between physician and patient would be because both autonomous parties worked together to improve the patient's health.

The approach that best fits the philosophical framework described above is the patient-centered approach (Benfield, 1979; Engel, 1980; Kleinman *et al.*, 1978; McWhinney, 1989; Pendleton, Scholfield, Tate, & Haveleck, 1984; Stein & Apprey, 1985, 1990; Stein, 1987e). Although this approach has been well described from a philosophical viewpoint, and although many herald it as an approach that will transform clinical practice, how it would actually work in practice is only beginning to be elucidated. The goal of the rest of this chapter is to examine the patient-centered approach in more depth, including new physician and patient roles and the ethics, efficacy, and safety of this approach.

THE PATIENT-CENTERED APPROACH

Physician Roles

Case 15-2. A 29-year-old white female who had recently moved presented to a physician's office complaining of fatigue. Her new physician rapidly uncovered her history of hypothyroidism and her story that her previous physician had recommended a reduction in the frequency with which she took her thyroid medication, from every day to every other day, because her laboratory values had indicated that she was taking too much medication. She complained that since she had reduced her dose of thyroid medication 3 months ago, she had felt progressively more and more fatigued and wondered if she was now taking too little thyroid medication. Her health goal was to feel more "perky" in a month or two.

Even though the patient had noted no weight gain or changes in her skin and hair consistent with hypothyroidism, the physician agreed that her fatigue could be caused by inadequate intake of thyroid medication. He therefore recommended to the patient that a test of her thyroid status be obtained and then presented her the option of either doing nothing until the test returned or increasing her medication intake slightly by taking her medication the first six days of the week but not on the seventh. Because the patient felt strongly that she was taking too little medication, she elected the latter option, asking the physician to write her a letter with the results of the test and agreeing to come back in 6 weeks for another check of her thyroid status.

The physician was concerned that there might be some other reasons for her fatigue, however, particularly given the fact that she had no findings of hypothyroidism on physical examination. On further questioning the physician learned that the patient and her 3-year-old daughter had recently moved in with her sister because she was in the process of obtaining a divorce from her husband, with whom she became "incompatible." She felt that she was rapidly wearing out her welcome, yet without employment she could not support herself and her daughter. Her ex-husband was not willing to provide child support until the divorce was finalized. The physician also learned that she was not hopeful that her situation would improve and was not exercising regularly, even though that previously gave her pleasure. She was not considering suicide.

Given the patient's history of multiple major life events and her depressed mood, the physician presented the patient with two other options, antidepressant medication or a referral to a counselor to aid her in her adjustment to her new situation. The patient thought she was on enough medication already and so declined the option of antidepressant medication but did agree that counseling would help. On referral, a clinical psychologist instituted cognitive–behavioral treatment of the patient's depression after the patient had ruled out the options of family therapy and psychoanalysis.

The patient's initial laboratory work returned showing that she was minimally hypothyroid. The patient was informed of this by letter and urged to continue her current thyroid regime. Six weeks later the patient returned to follow-up. Examination at the time showed a significant improvement in her mood. Although she had still not been able to find employment, she had been successful in obtaining child support from her ex-husband, even though the divorce had not been finalized. A physical exam revealed no physical findings of hypothyroidism; laboratory tests showed normal thyroid functioning. The patient was very positive about her counseling and wanted to continue it; the physician agreed.

The roles of the physician operating under the biomedical method are fairly straightforward: (1) diagnose illness; (2) treat disease; and (3) apply preventive strategies based on the age, sex, and risk factors of the patient (McWhinney, 1989). Although these roles are important within a patient-centered approach, physician roles significantly expand as clinical care takes into account patient autonomy and values, explores the meaning and significance of the illness for the patient, and attempts to understand how the patient's context affects and is affected by the patient's illness. Additional roles include (1) helping the patient to decide what health means to him or her and how best to optimize it; (2) obtaining psychosocial and contextual information from the patient; (3) facilitating the patient's role in the decision-making process through the formation and prioritizing of goals designed to optimize health; and (4) assisting the patient through an effective decision-making process intended to select the best therapeutic options that will attain the patient's goals while respecting his or her values.

Some of these new roles are illustrated in Case 15-2. There, the physician made a biomedical diagnosis (hypothyroidism) but also assessed contextual issues, which led to the discovery of the patient's depression, which probably contributed more to her symptoms than her hypothyroidism. Using the patient's goal that her symptoms of fatigue be relieved in 1 to 2 months, the physician recommended three options to achieve that goal: (1) increase her dose of thyroid medication; (2) refer to a clinical psychologist for counseling designed to help her cope with the many recent changes in her life; and (3) institute a trial of antidepressants. When the patient selected the first two options, the physician took appropriate steps to implement those options.

These new physician's roles clearly require more essential knowledge as well as different attitudes and skills than those needed using the biomedical method. Biomedical knowledge would still be important, but physicians would have to expand their knowledge base beyond disease-process knowledge to include patient-process knowledge, especially psychosocial factors and contextual issues related to the patient's health. Physician self-awareness will also be important, as the physician will need to understand how personal behaviors, values, feelings, and emotional reactions affect and are affected by patient interactions. Empathy, avoidance of premature judgment, and congruence become even more important in a patient-centered approach. Skills of active listening, ability to ask open-ended questions, probabilistic thinking, negotiation, conducting psychosocial and contextual assessments, and taking all this into account while formulating a treatment plan are also important. Given this summary of the knowledge, attitudes, and skills required of physicians under the patient-centered approach, a more detailed exploration of these new roles is in order.

Exploring Health-Related Values

Case 15-3. In April, a 47-year-old wheat farmer came into his physician's office complaining of pain and swelling in his left groin. He told his physician that this pain and swelling had been going on for 3 weeks, that it was worse when he stood up or coughed, but that it became much less painful if he lay down. The physician was concerned that the farmer might have an inguinal hernia, and indeed, on exam, a large reducible inguinal hernia on the left side was discovered. The physician recommended that he come into the hospital the next week and have his hernia repaired, but the farmer flatly refused, saying that harvest time was approaching and that he couldn't take any time off during that activity. The physician then discussed all the potential dangers and possible complications of an inguinal hernia, but to no avail. The farmer kept reiterating that the harvest had to be completed, as that was the time when the farmer made all the money he needed to support himself and his family for the coming year. The physician eventually relented, recommending that the farmer wear a supportive belt and come back for a repair when the harvest was over.

In July the farmer returned, having sustained no complications from his hernia, and asked the physician to repair it. One week later, the physician repaired the farmer's inguinal hernia without difficulty.

Health is a very elusive concept to define. Under the biomedical model health is the absence of disease. In a patient-centered approach, health is defined in a much broader, functional way as the totality of the patient's physical, emotional, and social well-being (WHO, 1947). To add to the confusion surrounding a definition of health, sometimes physicians and patients define health differently, even though a congruence of definition is crucial to shared decision making.

The dichotomy between the narrower absence-of-disease definition of health and the broader quality-of-life definition of health has been recognized throughout the century by physicians when they talk about curing versus healing. "Curing" implies the elimination of a disease state, whereas "healing" implies the restoration of an individual to his or her particular role in the family and community. Clearly, some patients can be cured without being healed, such as a woman with breast cancer who undergoes a radical mastectomy that leaves her with feelings of multilation, grief, and inadequacy concerning sexual functioning. Some patients can be healed but not cured, such as a diabetic patient who effectively maintains her functional status by controlling her disease and actively coping with its ramifications. Obviously most patients would like to be both cured and healed. The patient-centered approach, unlike the biomedical method, recognizes not only physician *curative* abilities but also the potential *healing* capacity that doctors can bring to the encounter with the patient.

Just as important as how the patient defines health is the value placed on that health. Is health the number-one priority, as most doctors would like, or are other values higher? A related question is: What is the patient willing to invest in order to achieve a certain measure of health? This investment is not just economic but also entails psychological and social costs, such as violations of cultural norms, disruptions of family roles and dynamics, or disruptions in the work environment. Not only do patients value health differently, but there are often limits beyond which they would not go in order to improve their health, as in Case 15-3, where the farmer was unwilling to suffer the economic loss of missing the harvest in order to have his hernia repaired immediately. Finding and respecting such limits is absolutely necessary under the patient-centered approach.

Unfortunately, there are also biological limits in the degree to which health can be improved in some patients. A bicyclist who sustained a cervical fracture resulting in quadriplegia is probably not going to bicycle again. Such limits should be respected, but sometimes they prematurely defeat physicians and patients, who give up hope of ever restoring any measure of patient health, particularly physicians and patients who hold to a narrower absence-of-disease definition of health. In such cases, the patient-centered approach allows physicians to help patients, and themselves, by expanding their definition of health and optimizing the patients' health in other ways. The success of many severely injured and disabled patients in achieving happy, productive lives attests to the benefit of this approach.

Obtaining Psychosocial and Contextual Information

Using the processes of interviewing, examining, and laboratory testing, physicians have become very skilled in identifying patients with physiological and pathological abnormalities that may decrease life expectancy. Doctors operating within the biomedical method, however, often ignore important psychosocial and contextual issues. Although searching for physiological and anatomic abnormalities is clearly important, and so the search for these abnormalities should proceed consistent with principles of clinical decision making, the search should not stop there. Psychosocial and contextual issues that bear on the patient's health are also important to assess.

Exploration of psychosocial issues allows the patient-centered physician to travel down many potential avenues. McWhinney (1989) has recently identified the most important psychosocial areas to explore: (1) the patient's expectations about the illness; (2) feelings about the illness; and (3) fears that accompany the illness. Open-ended questions should be asked to explore the significance and meaning of the illness: What bothers you about your illness? What can you no longer do that you used to do before you become ill? What sort of feelings have you noticed since you have become ill? What do you fear will happen to you now that you have this illness? Answers to these questions will give the physician a sense of the patient's adjustment to his or her illness and what issues are important to address when educating the patient about his or her disease. Such an approach would clearly have been of benefit to the physician with macular degeneration described earlier.

Contextual issues are also important to address. The patient and physician are embedded in a web of social relationships because each is a member of multiple systems: family, work, community, etc. (Fig. 15-1). These relationships both affect and are affected by the patient's health because (1) the context often defines healthy and unhealthy behaviors; (2) the context promotes healthy and unhealthy behaviors through behavioral reinforcement and dynamics; (3) context dynamics can have a significant impact on disease outcome through neuroendocrine and immune mechanisms; and (4) contextual issues can have a significant impact on compliance and rehabilitative behavior (Ramsey, 1989).

By limiting the treatment plan to a disease-oriented framework, physicians risk disruptions of the patient's systems or failure because systemic feedback loops perpetuate unhealthy behaviors or disease exacerbations through psychoneuroendocrine mechanisms. For example, if the family meal preparer is not involved in physician–patient discussions about lowering a heart patient's dietary cholesterol, then dietary instructions provided by the physician are less likely to be implemented despite the best intentions of the physician and patient.

Exploring the patient's entire context could be quite time consuming and lead to more confusion than clarification. The physician must develop the skill to identify and explore relevant context to gain an understanding of the problems within the patient's system that may lead to adverse outcomes. A few simple open-ended questions can be asked in order to explore important contextual issues: What have you or those around you suggested or tried to do to improve your condition? Which of those suggestions have you tried? Why have you tried those suggestions? What's worked and what hasn't? How has your illness affected those around you? In what way? If those effects are problems for those around you, how did they respond? How did you respond to their response? These few questions will enable the patient-centered physician to rapidly determine which contextual issues are important. Further assessment of the patient's systems can be guided by answers to those questions.

Formulating Goals to Optimize Health

With the biomedical method, goals are defined by the diseases or deficits uncovered. Since there is such a close correspondence between diagnoses and goals under the biomedical method, treatment goals, such as cure or palliation,

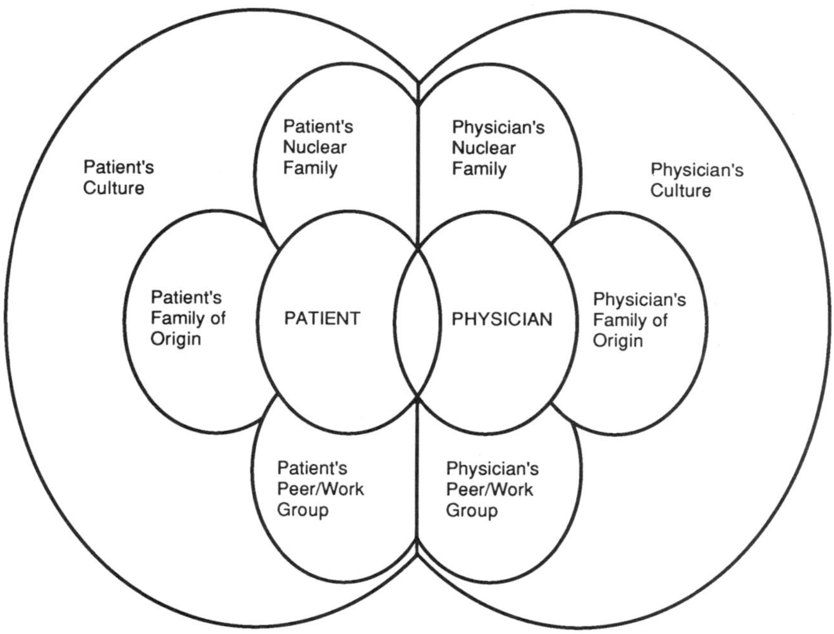

Figure 15-1. The web of social relationships surrounding the doctor–patient relationship.

are not formally mentioned or recorded in the medical record. The patient-centered approach, however, acknowledges the relative nature of health and the "trade-offs" that patients often make in order to optimize their health. Thus, clearly defined, specific, realistic goals that are mutually agreed on by both the patient and doctor (prioritized if multiple or conflicting goals arise) are very important if the patient-centered approach is to work. Often, a physician using the patient-centered approach may recommend fairly traditional biomedical goals, depending on the patient's illness, but the option of negotiating broader life- or health-related goals is also available.

Goal setting also must take into account what each patient is willing to invest in order to achieve a certain degree of health. By setting goals, these "trade-offs" can be brought out into the open and discussed; motivation to achieve goals then increases, and noncompliance decreases, particularly when short-term goals are set, behavioral rewards are included within the plan, and follow-up occurs often to judge if the therapeutic plan is succeeding.

If the patient is unwilling to acknowledge and discuss "trade-offs," or if goals set by the patient are incongruent with the physician's beliefs about how best to optimize the patient's health, then a negotiation process, described in Chapter 6, should ensue. Through this process of negotiation the physician and the patient might find that they can work together on only a few desired goals. If no goals are mutually acceptable to the physician and patient, then the physician or patient should consider terminating the relationship.

Patient-Centered Clinical Decision Making

Case 15-4. Sandra, a 29-year-old female, presented to her physician with pelvic pain of 3 months' duration. Sandra described the pain as an achy sensation on both sides of her pelvis that was constantly present, although it did get worse at times. It particularly got worse during sexual intercourse with her husband. The pain was not associated with any other genitourinary symptoms.

Sandra had been married to her husband for a year and a half. They had a 1-year-old daughter. Sandra said that her father was furious when she became pregnant out of wedlock and demanded that her boyfriend marry her. Her boyfriend, a somewhat passive man, agreed to the union but then became more distant emotionally after their marriage. The patient and her family were also under a financial burden, with her husband working two jobs, one during the week and one on the weekend. Sandra was also taking care of two to three neighbor children during the day while their parents worked.

Given the above information, the physician formed a differential diagnosis that included pregnancy, ectopic pregnancy, chronic pelvic infection, endometriosis, urinary tract infection, gynecologic cancer, depression, alcoholism, and incest. After formulating this differential diagnosis, the physician asked further questions and conducted a physical examination.

Further questioning revealed that Sandra did not think that she was pregnant since she was using vaginal sponges as a contraceptive method, did not have a previous history of a pelvic infection in college, did not feel particularly depressed, did not have any of the somatic symptoms of depression, cried when asked about possible incest and admitted that her father had abused her sexually when she was a young girl, and stated that she had never told anyone this before and had not received any treatment for this condition. Sandra admitted to drinking two to four beers per night, a significant increase for her, as the beer seemed to ease her pain. She stated that her father was also a heavy drinker.

Examination revealed no vaginal discharge or signs of a pelvic infection, although there was significant tenderness on palpation in both adnexa. The uterus was normal size. A urine pregnancy test was negative, and a urinalysis was normal. Samples for a Pap smear and cultures of common pathogens were also taken, all of which were unremarkable.

At the conclusion of his workup, the physician stated that she thought Sandra's pelvic pain was probably linked in some way to her difficult marriage, her past history of incest, and her increasing use of alcohol but admitted that the exact mechanism of such an association had not been elucidated by medical research at this time. The physician also stated that she could not rule out endometriosis as a cause of Sandra's pelvic pain and so recommended an examination by a gynecologist. Sandra and her physician then formulated the goal of getting rid of her pelvic pain and resuming normal sexual relations with her husband. The patient also hoped that her marriage would improve, and she wanted to deal with the issues of incest and potential alcoholism. The physician agreed that those were appropriate goals to accomplish but that Sandra needed to prioritize them since she could probably not accomplish them all at once. The patient then stated that it was most important for her to reduce her pelvic pain and to improve her marriage.

Sandra and her physician then discussed the options of (1) referral to a gynecologist to rule out endometriosis, (2) institution of a trial of antiinflammatory medications to reduce her pelvic pain, (3) institution of a trial of antidepressant therapy to reduce her pelvic pain, (4) referral to a family therapist to improve her marriage, (5) referral to an alcohol treatment facility, and (6) enrollment in a patient support group for survivors of incest. Given the prioritization of her goals, Sandra elected to be referred to a gynecologist since her insurance would cover the referral, try antiinflammatory medications to reduce her pelvic pain, and be referred to a family therapist to improve her marriage.

The gynecologist determined that endometriosis might be present and so scheduled the patient for laparoscopy. Laparoscopy revealed a few adhesions but no signs of endometriosis. The gynecologist lysed the adhesions at the time of the laparoscopy.

After the lysis of adhesions and the trial of antiinflammatory medicine, the patient's pain was significantly reduced but not totally eliminated 6 months later. Also during this time, the patient and her husband received every-other-week marital therapy, which significantly improved their relationship, although Sandra still felt that her husband was too emotionally distant and passive. Their sexual relations had improved substantially, however, as Sandra no longer felt pain on intercourse. Sandra stated that she felt ready to reduce her alcohol intake over the next 6 months but was still not ready to tackle the incest issue.

At a follow-up visit 6 months later, Sandra stated that she had reduced her drinking to only one beer a night and thought she was ready to enroll in the patient support group for survivors of incest. Over the next year the patient attended monthly meetings of the support group. At follow-up 1 year later, Sandra still had occasional episodes of pelvic pain but controlled them through use of antiinflammatory medications. Sandra's marital relationship continued to improve such that now the couple was thinking about having another child. Sandra drank only occasionally now. The physician congratulated Sandra on meeting her goals, and both agreed that family therapy could probably be discontinued but that Sandra should continue to attend the support group since she still had difficulty relating to her father.

Clinical decision making using the biomedical model takes the form of a hypotheticodeductive approach utilizing biomedical data. The patient-centered approach expands clinical decision making to include psychosocial and contextual information as illustrated in Case 15-4. Additionally, the patient plays a larger role in the decision-making process.

The medical decision-making components outlined at the end of Chapter 2 provide an excellent framework on which to build a patient-centered clinical decision-making process. Medical decision making involves multiple components: (1) the data base, (2) values, (3) action constraints, (4) decision theory, and (5) ethical theory. Important people who contribute to this decision-making process are first the physician and patient but also people within the patient's and physician's context. Putting these people together with the essential components of the medical decision-making process yields the patient-centered clinical decision-making matrix shown in Table 15-1. This matrix displays important elements that may affect the decision-making process. Each component of the patient-centered clinical decision-making process is now discussed in more detail.

Data Base

A data base is the information necessary for a medical decision. Obviously no good medical decision can be made in the absence of data; on the other hand, simply gathering data is not the only concern of the patient-centered clinician. How much data to collect is one of the first questions that clinician and patient must answer, since the amount of data that could be collected is vast. The amount of data to be collected can to some extent be determined by the hypotheses that the patient and physician hold with regard to the patient's illness, the amount of psychosocial and contextual information needed to understand the patient's illness and offer the patient an adequate number of treatment options, and the patient's health-related goals.

A medical history, physical examination, and results of appropriate laboratory tests are the essential components of the data base using a biomedical

Table 15-1
Factors Affecting Clinical Decision Making

	Data base	Values	Action constraints	Decision theory	Ethical theory
Patient	History Physical exam Lab tests Feelings Effect of illness on self	Individual values Health Economic Ethical Legal Meaning of illness to self	Time Money Habitual behavior patterns Transference	Hypotheticodeductive approach Clinical management process Health maintenance process	Duties Rights Consequences
Patient's context	Data from/about Family Work group Community Effect of illness on Family Work group Community	Values of Family Work group Community Explanatory models of illness	Family and community resources Systemic feedback loops Erroneous health beliefs	Theory used by Family Work group Community Standardized family, work group, or community protocols	Theory used by Family Work group Community
Physician	Knowledge base Attitudes Skills Feelings Effect on patient	Physician values Health Economic Ethical Legal Effect of patient illness on self	Time Reimbursement for services Lack of knowledge or skill Motivation Countertransference	Hypotheticodeductive approach Clinical management process Health maintenance process	Duties Rights Consequences
Physician's context	Other professionals available to help Technology available Effect of health care system on practice	Values of Family Colleagues Health care system Predominant model of illness, usually biomedical	Poor communication or disagreements among consultants Feedback loops within the health care system Too many helpers	Theory used by Family Colleagues Health care system Standard office or hospital protocols	Theory used by Family Colleagues Health care system

approach but are only several of many important components using the patient-centered approach. Many factors affect the patient's health; thus, an attempt should be made to assess all important factors. Many clinicians suppose that just the biomedical factors are important in all cases and thus relegate other information to the "back burner" to be assessed only if the biomedical method does not work. Such an approach is inefficient, however, since more time is needed to conduct another assessment and, more importantly, the exclusion of contextual data does not reflect clinical reality. For many medical decisions, knowledge of a patient's health-related values and context may be equally or more important. Furthermore, psychosocial and context issues clearly affect patients with "real" biomedical disease.

Also important are data concerning the clinician and the clinician's context. The extent of the physician's medical knowledge and skills is obviously important in formulating a therapeutic plan. For example, the physician in Case 15-4 knew that endometriosis was a diagnostic possibility even though she was not qualified to do the test that would rule it out. Physician contextual issues are also important. A physician's knowledge of available medical and consultative help, consultant's ability to manage patients, and knowledge of the health care system in which the physician operates are all important considerations in the decision-making process. For example, a physician confronted with a patient who has an acute myocardial infarction may make vastly different decisions in a tertiary care center with rapid access to a cardiac catheterization lab than in a small rural community without access to a cardiologist.

The physician's self-knowledge about personal values, attitudes, feelings, expectations, and fears toward specific patients and patients in general is crucial to the physician in understanding his or her own biases and prejudices. For example, a physician strongly opposed to abortion may not be able to adequately counsel an unmarried adolescent with an unexpected pregnancy who wants to be informed about the abortion option. If the physician understood his values, he or she might want to refer the patient to a more unbiased counselor.

Health-related values are probably the most important values to explore with the patient, as discussed earlier in this chapter. Since an individual's values largely come from family and cultural values and traditions, those contexts may be important to explore as a critical component of the decision-making process.

Physician values, particularly health-related values, have great impact on the clinical decision-making process. Even though physicians utilizing the biomedical model believe their decisions are value neutral, their actions and behaviors under the model uphold the eradication of disease as a predominant value. Such values may clash with patients whose health-related values focus more on illness and restoring functional status. Another common clash occurs when physicians place a supreme value on improving health at any cost, whereas patients value other human endeavors and activities more, as in Case 15-3. Finally, the patient-centered approach recognizes the values of involving the patient in decision making through negotiation.

When values come into conflict in a particular situation, it might be beneficial to explore not only the patient's value context but the physician's value context as well. Physician values, like patient values, largely come from the physician's own family and cultural traditions. In addition, physicians utilize values received from the health care system in which they were trained. By conducting an exploration of their value context, physicians may find that their own values have been shaped by systemic processes that may or may not benefit the current clinical situation. For example, a physician who highly values eradicating disease as a way to benefit patient health and who places health as a top priority might demand that a diabetic patient comply with dietary therapy. This demand might actually exacerbate noncompliance because of the physician's authoritarian manner, and an exploration of the physician's values would reveal that they arose from the health-related values of his family and teaching in medical school rather than being formulated individually through his experience as a clinician and his philosophical beliefs. By realizing the origin of his values, the physician might be more willing to explore other options and negotiate rather than demand that patients comply in clinical situations where values are in conflict.

Action Constraints

Action constraints are those factors that impose themselves on us and preclude or demand certain decision-making options. Common action constraints are time and money, but other individual action constraints such as habitual behavior patterns, low motivation, and transference also can block attempts at a solution. Similarly, the individual's context may place action constraints on a particular option or decision, for example, systemic feedback loops that maintain problem behavior, decreased family resources or social support, which preclude complex or difficult decision-making options, and erroneous but powerfully held beliefs that contradict the physician's explanation of the patient's disease state.

Action constraints impose on the physician as well. Time and money are action constraints for physicians, as they must see a certain number of patients per day to earn a living. Likewise, lack of medical knowledge or skills in a certain area will preclude certain decision-making options, as will availability of equipment, such as MRI scanners, and personnel, e.g., cardiologists. Countertransference can actually be a hindrance not only to the doctor–patient relationship but to the decision-making process as well. Physicians may become so frustrated with certain patients because of countertransference arising from family-of-origin issues that they react in ways that preclude rational decision making and only serve to maintain patient problems. For example, the physician son of an alcoholic father may unconsciously be so angry at his father that he cannot establish enough of a therapeutic relationship to encourage his alcoholic patients to quit drinking.

Finally, the physician's own context might impose action constraints on the decision-making process, such as a recurrent poor communication process among health care professionals, consistent disagreements with specific consultants, or systemic feedback loops within the physician's own health care system that may preclude certain options. Too many health care professionals working on a specific case can actually be an action constraint, as responsibility is so diffused that little active decision making is performed.

PATIENT-CENTERED CARE

The ways that patients and physicians make decisions are also a vital part of the clinical decision-making process. Fortunately, since both physicians and patients are human beings, the decision-making processes they use are actually quite similar. It is not clear whether these decision-making processes, such as the hypotheticodeductive approach, are common to all humans because they arise out of the structural makeup of our brains, because they represent learned phenomena common to all humans, or because they are consistent with the logic inherent in a structured system of communication.

Regardless of origin, they hypotheticodeductive approach described in Chapter 5 and the clinical management process described in Chapter 6 are both useful frameworks for guiding medical decision making. Additionally, the process of deciding which patient behaviors should be stopped or decreased in order to improve health seems to be similar between patients and physicians as noted in Chapter 7. Thus, these three processes can also serve as useful decision theory under the patient-centered approach.

As shown in Case 15-4, the process of medical decision making will have to be expanded under the patient-centered approach, but such an expansion can easily take place if all that information, including contextual information, is utilized as cues for hypothesis formation, similar to the way symptoms, signs, and laboratory tests are utilized to form a differential diagnosis. Under the patient-centered approach, however, all factors that might have an impact on the patient's health are assessed at the same time.

Once all patient-centered factors have been assigned, then hypotheses about how those factors affect the patient's health can be formulated. Disease-specific hypotheses may be a part of that information, but only a part. Hypotheses based on nonbiomedical information are also important, even when the patient has a biomedical disease, as in Case 15-4, where the lysis of old pelvic adhesions helped reduce the patient's pelvic pain but did not entirely resolve it. The near-total resolution of the patient's pelvic pain was also based on hypotheses constructed from contextual information.

Once hypotheses have been formed, more information can be gathered or a plan can be formulated, depending on the physician's and patient's level of certainty. Further information gathering, if needed, should not be limited to laboratory tests but should also include other sources of information if the patient consents, such as other family members. Once a comfortable level of certainty has been attained, then a therapeutic plan can be constructed based on the patient's health-related goals.

Construction of a patient-centered therapeutic plan would also not be limited to biomedical options but include other options that might benefit the patient's health. Here again, it is important to consider those options at the same time as more traditional biomedical options. Both types of therapeutic options need to be considered together in order to construct a therapeutic plan that has the highest likelihood of success.

Finally, the process of health maintenance can also be expanded to include patient-centered information in order to change unhealthy patient behavior. In fact, of all the medical decision-making processes, the health maintenance process seems to be one that already incorporates a great deal of patient-centered information within its purview. This inclusion probably occurs because in order to understand human behavior, particularly unhealthy human behavior, knowledge of the patient's values, psychosocial issues, and contextual information is already seen as critical to changing those behaviors.

Case 15-5. A 28-year-old white female is admitted to the labor and delivery ward of a busy tertiary care hospital with premature rupture of membranes (PROM). Her pregnancy is at term, and even though her membranes have ruptured she has no complaints of labor pain. This is her first pregnancy. She has had a benign prenatal course. Examination reveals no signs of infection, a fetus in the vertex position with good fetal heart tones, and a cervix that appears unfavorable for induction. The family physician taking care of this patient obtained a consult from the obstetrician on call, who recommended early induction even though the patient's cervix was not favorable in order to decrease the risk of intraamniotic infections in the mother and sepsis in the infant, a known complication of prolonged rupture of amniotic membranes.

The family physician in this case was uncomfortable with the obstetrician's recommendation because he knew that an induction in the face of an unfavorable cervix would greatly increase the chances of C-section and maternal mortality. Despite his discomfort, the physician, fearing medical–legal complications, did go ahead and induce the woman. Eighteen hours later, the woman failed to progress and underwent a C-section. The C-section was productive of a term, viable, male infant who appeared healthy. Mother and baby were discharged 5 days later having suffered none of the complications of an operative delivery.

Despite the good outcome in this case, the family physician continued to wonder if this case should have been managed in a different way so that the woman would not have had to undergo a C-section. Because of his concerns, he consulted a colleague with expertise in clinical decision making, who agreed that constructing and analyzing a decision tree, an analysis detailing all possible outcomes with their probabilities given certain clinical actions, might be a useful way to analyze the problem.

In order to find the probability of the specific events in women with premature rupture of membranes, the physician's colleague did a literature review in which he found three randomized control trials that examined the management of women with premature rupture of membranes in different settings with different interventions. Two early trials done in 1984 and 1986 concluded that expectant management was the correct course, but one recent trial published in 1989 concluded that early induction was better (Duff, Huff, & Gibbs, 1984; Morales & Lazar, 1986; Wagner, Chin, Peters, Drexler, & Newman, 1989). Because these trials did not solve the controversy, the colleague felt comfortable in constructing a decision tree using probabilities taken from those randomized control trials in order to see which management strategy reduced risk the most.

A decision tree was constructed comparing four options: induction on presentation at the labor deck, induction 6 h after PROM, induction 12 h after PROM, and expectant management (Fig. 15-2). Both maternal and neonatal morbidity and mortality were used as outcome measures. The decision tree produced contradictory results. With regard to maternal morbidity and mortality, the management strategy that best reduced risk and improved outcomes was expectant management, since early induction greatly increased the risk of unnecessary C-sections and maternal mortality.

However, given the hospital's policy of performing a septic workup on all infants born of mothers with premature rupture of membrances for longer than 24 h, the analysis from the perspective of infant morbidity and mortality revealed that early induction was best, since that significantly reduced the risk of iatrogenic complications from the huge number of septic workups that would be performed on infants delivered of women with PROM for greater than 24 h. Even when the model was reanalyzed using a more relaxed policy for requiring septic workups on infants, early induction was still found to be the best way to reduce infant risk.

In trying to formulate a coherent approach to this problem, the physician realized that recommending early induction to all PROM patients would no doubt decrease infant morbidity and mortality, but at the cost of increased maternal morbidity and mortality. Likewise, recommending expectant management would reduce maternal risk, but at the cost of infant morbidity and mortality. The physician also realized that to change the outcome of this

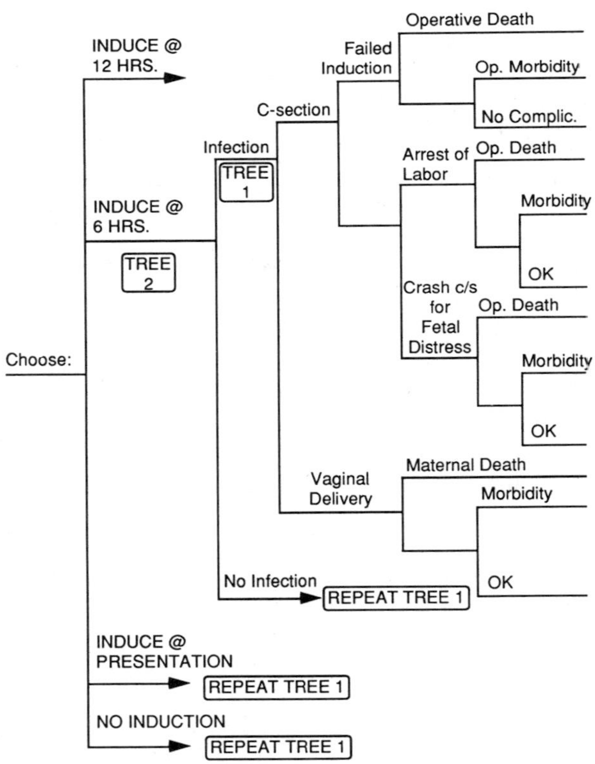

Figure 15-2. Decision tree for patients with premature rupture of membranes.

decision analysis would require a significant relaxation of the septic workup policy, thus going against hospital policy and increasing medical–legal risk, or discussing the conclusions of this analysis with each woman with PROM to formulate an individualized management plan that would balance the trade-offs involved.

In thinking further about this problem, the physician realized that a patient's decision could depend on her own unique situation and values. The physician could envision scenarios in which a woman might elect early induction, for example, a woman who was pregnant for the first time after a long course of fertility drugs, versus a woman who might opt for expectant management, for example, a woman with six children already who fulfilled the vital family role of child caretaker. Despite the fact that it was more time consuming to explain to each patient the details of the decision analysis, the critical importance of the patient's context and values in helping to make the decision convinced the physician that he should take the time to explain the decision analysis to patients with PROM in order to help them make a decision that best fit their situation and respected their values (contribed by D. Marley).

Once important patient values have been identified, they are often easily incorporated into the clinical decision-making process while therapeutic options are being discussed. For example, a patient who is a Jehovah's Witness will quite rapidly rule out any therapeutic option involving a blood transfusion even before the decision-making process begins. In Cases 15-2, 15-3, and 15-4, each patient ruled out certain options because of personal values discovered while negotiating a therapeutic plan with his or her physician. Situations exist, however, as illustrated in Case 15-5, when the integration of patient values into the decision-making process is left until last, usually because the options are few, choosing among them involves a trade-off between values, or because the patient or physician confronts a true ethical dilemma.

Ethical Theory

Physicians and patients also utilize ethical theories to frame their approach to the decisions they make. These ethical theories, introduced at the end of Chapter 2 and extensively discussed in Chapter 12, enable patients and physicians to order their values and judge the rightness or wrongness of their actions. As mentioned in Chapter 2, three different theoretical approaches have been traditionally used by individuals making decisions: (1) consequences based, (2) duty based, and (3) rights based. Also noted in Chapter 2, and very important to the discussion here is the fact that the different models of practice utilize different theoretical bases and are thus influenced differently by the same set of facts. This applies to patients as well. For example, using Case 15-5 as an example, imagine that the pregnant woman was utilizing a duty-based approach to her decision. In that situation, she could believe she had a duty to protect her children, regardless of the risk to herself. She would then opt for early induction because that would enhance her ability to meet her obligation (duty) to her children. On the other hand, if the physician were utilizing a consequences-based approach, she would try to balance the harm to the mother against the harm to the baby and act to minimize the harm. If she believed the potential harm to the mother through induction was greater than the potential harm to the baby, she would then favor not inducing. The resulting conflict between patient and physician would be at the level of ethical theory, however, not medical decision making.

The biomedical model of medicine has traditionally depended on the consequences-based ethical theory. The aim of that model has always been the eradication of a specific disease process (thus producing a good consequence) through practices that emphasize a statistical/scientific concern with outcome (a formal analysis of projected consequences) as their primary focus. Under a patient-centered approach, the rights of the patients (specifically autonomy) become more important, especially with the understanding that patients are not required to accept care that in the best medical knowledge would produce good consequences. Thus, in Case 15-5 as just described, the physician using a patient-centered approach would recognize the patient's right to decide on induction. This also recognizes the patient's values and the patient's basic responsibility for value judgments concerning her own care.

As certain serious issues, such as functional status and quality of life, become crucial in patient-centered decision making, ethical theories play a more helpful role under a patient-centered approach. This is because the patient-centered approach allows the balancing of viewpoints that is so crucial to a good physician–patient relationship. More importantly, the patient-centered approach allows for a more realistic interpretation of physician duties, since the duty is primarily determined by the patient's needs and not by an abstract concept of "disease cure."

The patient-centered approach, with its autonomy orientation, also allows more flexibility in dealing with physician–patient disagreement. Since each participant in the relationship is autonomous, the decision process, not the disease process, becomes the controlling factor in decision making. As a result, if the physician and patient disagree on how to judge the rightness or wrongness of a decision, negotiation with an exploration of contextual issues can easily take place. Under the biomedical model, this negotiation is not possible because the "science" of the "disease cure" does not permit such considerations. Also, under the patient-centered approach, consultation with an ethicist is also an option, since the range of consultation is not (as in the biomedical model) limited to "scientific" specialties.

Patient Role

The patient-centered approach to care will require much more from patients. The biomedical model has been dominant for many years not only because it has spawned a very effective medical method but also because it is very culturally acceptable to if not demanded by patients. Often, patients who are ill view themselves very mechanistically, almost as a car being taken into a shop (the physician's office) where they can be fixed by "looking under the hood" and "tinkering with a few lines or valves." Such a view is very congruent with the biomedical model.

However, the patient-centered approach would discourage patients from holding such a simplist notion of health. Patients would be encouraged to allow the doctor into their world, to explore feelings, meanings, and context. Patients would also be encouraged to assume a greater degree of responsibility for their own health and to exercise that responsibility by formulating goals and negotiating therapeutic plans with their physicians. Finally, patients would be encouraged to develop an awareness of how their own behaviors, feelings, and emotional reactions affect and are affected by their interaction with people around them and work to develop a decision-making process that respects the values of all involved and takes their health and the health of others into account.

For patients able to accept such an approach to health care, the patient-centered approach can be very empowering as patients assume an active role in the medical decision-making process. Such empowerment is also very conducive to the patient's psychological growth and development.

Systemic Change

Physicians who use a patient-centered approach try to change dysfunctional systems in order to improve patient health. Some systems, such as communities or cultural systems, may be so large and powerful that physicians may find themselves frustrated if they attempt to change even a small facet of those systems.

In reality physicians and health care providers are already attempting to change dysfunctional aspects of systems at many levels. Family therapists, as noted in Chapter 9, have become very successful at changing dysfunctional family systems. Physicians in many communities across this country have taken on the responsibility of educating public school students, community groups, and local parent–teacher associations on various health issues including AIDS, the unhealthy effects of certain patient life styles (Doctors Ought to Care), and the medical effects of nuclear war (Physicians for Social Responsibility). Physicians who participate in such activities not only view them as part of their professional role as a health care provider (improving the health of larger groups through systemic involvement) but also view them as a duty or repayment to society for the investment society made in educating them and for the special privileges and respect it has bestowed on them.

Physicians who attempt to work with small and large systems must continually remind themselves that systems are homeostatic and thus resistant to change. "Burnout" and frustration occur at a very high rate not only because of the demands of practice but because of unrealistic expectations in attempting to change patient behavior to improve health. Physicians who lack the skill or motivation to tackle systemic issues should be cognizant of the limitations that are placed on their ability to optimize patient health. Physicians skilled in systemic intervention should work to change systems if they see that such change is a realistic possibility, work on larger systems' issues to improve patient health slowly, particularly if that can be done with a group of like-minded physicians, and accept that some systems are simply beyond the power of an individual physician to change. Acknowledging such limitations to patients, which may be difficult for many physicians, will also go far in helping patients to understand the influences of systems on their own behavior and perhaps will cause them to construct more realistic goals.

Ethics of the Patient-Centered Approach

There are also ethical implications of systemic involvement. Informed consent, confidentiality, and the physician's duty to other members of the patient's system all need to be explored if the patient and the physician agree that a change in a system is warranted. Many physicians are uncomfortable working with larger systems because they perceive their duty to individual patients as supreme. Since systemic interventions are sometimes paradoxical, particularly in the short term, some physicians may find themselves faced with recommending that patients continue or even increase unhealthy behavior for a short time. For example, a physician caring for an obese female who is in a complementary conflicted relationship to her mother might actually counsel against a diet initially, anticipating that a straightforward approach would result in noncompliance and failure.

Although difficult, these problems are not insurmountable if approached in an open fashion. If a family system needs to be changed, the physician can obtain consent from the patient to call all family members together, explain the problem, set goals to solve it, and then explain why the involvement of other family members is necessary. The physician can then describe what needs to be done in order to change the system. All members of the family can then give consent and participate depending on their desires. The envelope of confidentiality would need to be expanded past the individual physician and patient, but that too is not unreasonable as long as the patient agrees.

The physician's duty to an individual patient must still take top priority, but concern, compassion, and professional skills can be directed at other members of the patient's system. Paradoxical systemic interventions can even be used as long as the physician is highly skilled in their use, indications are appropriate, and appropriate follow-up is planned in case the intervention fails. If the physician or patient cannot negotiate these ethical hurdles, then a consultation with an ethicist may be necessary.

Efficacy of the Patient-Centered Approach

One of the first questions physicians ask about a new test or treatment option is, "Does it work?" McWhinney (1989) has recently reviewed studies supporting the efficacy of the patient-centered approach. Although few studies have been done, and almost all have been done in the primary care setting, early indications are that a patient-centered approach results in improvements in health for a variety of conditions, including acute conditions, undifferentiated symptoms in which a traditional biomedical diagnosis cannot be made, and chronic illnesses (Table 15-2).

Furthermore, these studies have found few side effects of the patient-centered approach; in other words, the patient-centered approach is not only effective but safe. However, a review of the potential side effects or disadvantages of the patient-centered approach is in order given the early stage of this research.

Safety of the Patient-Centered Approach

Viewed from the perspective of the biomedical method, many physicians feel that the patient-centered approach may possess some undesirable side effects. The breadth of the patient-centered approach may dilute physician focus on the biomedical aspects of the cases (Seldin, 1981). Physicians would lose some power within the doctor–patient relationship, although physician autono-

Table 15-2
Efficacy of the Patient-Centered Approach[a]

Author	Process variables	Health status measure	Outcome
Comley (1973)	Family conference for patient with emotional problems	Health care utilization over the next year	49% decrease in utilization compared to a matched control group
Stewart *et al.* (1979)	Doctor's knowledge of patient's problem (by questionnaire)	Structured interview at 3 months	Perceived recovery
Headache Study Group (1986)	Patient able to discuss problem fully	Telephone interview at 12 months	Resolution of headache
Bass *et al.* (1986)	Patient's agreement with doctor's assessment (by interview)	Telephone interview at 4 weeks	Perceived recovery from undifferentiated symptoms
Orth *et al.* (1987)	Patient able to express concerns; doctor provides information (by audiotape)	Blood pressure	Better control of hypertension
Greenfield *et al.* (1988)	Patient control of consultation, expression of affect, provision of information at patient's request (by audiotape)	Health status questionnaire, blood sugar	Better perceived health status, better control of diabetes
Uhlmann *et al.* (1988)	Patient request fulfillment	Health status questionnaire, glycosylated hemoglobin	Better perceived health status, fewer insulin reactions, better control of diabetes

[a] Adapted from McWhinney (1989).

my is still respected within the patient-centered approach. Physicians would have to develop more effective coping mechanisms in order to live with the increased anxiety inherent in dealing with complex systems that are ripe with conflict. Physicians would need to supplement the sole use of objective validation criteria (such as autopsy results) with more subjective patient-defined outcomes. Additionally, a record system that will document aspects of the patient-centered approach has not been fully developed. Finally, physicians and patients wishing to utilize the patient-centered approach will be going against cultural and health care system precepts that support the biomedical model (Stein, 1990). This may mean a loss of respect or even anger from colleagues until this new approach is more widely accepted.

Despite these potential disadvantages, the patient-centered approach, since it subsumes the biomedical method within its purview and has so much potential for improving patient health, seems to offer many advantages over the biomedical method. In fact, to many clinicians it is even difficult to understand why such an approach has not already gained widespread favor. Perhaps as physicians become more comfortable with nontechnical aspects of clinical care, as governmental agencies and insurance agencies reimburse clinicians more fairly for nonprocedural skills, and as patients realize their own interdependence and how important psychological state is to illness, the patient-centered approach will gradually transform modern medical practice and be widely adopted by practicing clinicians.

CONCLUSIONS

Medicine's dominant method of clinical care is still the biomedical method. Despite the great strides medicine has made using this method, it has been severely criticized because some patients taken care of by physicians utilizing this method do not become significantly healthier despite this method's focus on disease states. Many physicians have come to realize that this is not only because health is much more than the absence of disease, but because the biomedical method does not allow physicians to come up with a diagnosis and an effective treatment in all situations, because the biomedical method provides no means for the physician to assess feelings and meanings surrounding the patient's illness, and, lastly, because the biomedical method does not allow physicians to explore contextual issues. Because of these shortcomings in the biomedical method, some physicians believe the method they use to care for patients will be undergoing a transformation in response to societal and patients' demands.

Although not enough work has been done by scholars and physicians to completely define a new method at this time, a new approach to clinical care is emerging. The philosophical characteristics of this approach will be somewhat different from those of the biomedical method. Autonomy and justice would be emphasized over beneficence and nonmaleficence as principles of practice. A person-oriented framework would be utilized, with physicians operating more from a collegial or contract model of the physician–patient relationship rather than an engineering or priestly model. Obligations of honesty and candor with patients would be emphasized.

Of all of the approaches that have recently been described and analyzed, the one that best fits the new philosophical framework described above is the patient-centered approach advocated by McWhinney and others. Under the patient-centered approach, the roles of the physician would be significantly expanded to include (1) aiding the patient in deciding what health is and how best to optimize it, (2) obtaining not only biomedical information from the patient but psychosocial and contextual information, (3) allowing the patient a role in the decision-making process through the formation and prioritization of goals, and (4) guiding the patient through an effective decision-making process to select therapeutic options that have the best chance of achieving the patient's health goals while respecting his or her values.

Medical decision making under the patient-centered approach would not only include multiple components (the data base, values, action constraints, decision theory, and ethical theory) but would also expand to include individual patient and physician factors as well as contextual information and issues arising from both the patient's and physician's context. Although the breadth of this clinical decision-making approach may be a disadvantage to some clinicians, physicians would not have to utilize the entire model for every patient but could select those factors that seem to have the most importance for the health of the patient. This would allow the physician and patient to come up with enough options that might improve the patient's health.

This new approach to care would also require much more from patients. Patients would not be able to achieve the complete dominance in the physician–patient relationship that they may want; some patients might have to adapt to a wider view of health than the traditional biomedical model would allow; and patients would be encouraged to allow the physician and perhaps others to help in improving their health. The approach would also demand a greater degree of responsibility on the part of patients as they participate in formulating goals and deciding on therapeutic options. These new responsibilities, rather than harming the patient, would empower patients to be more responsible for their health and thus would be conducive to individual growth and development.

Physicians adopting such an approach must be very careful to avoid burnout and excessive levels of frustration. Changing patient behavior and changing systems that affect patient behavior can be very difficult. The ethical implications of involving important parts of the patient's context in his or her health care may be difficult to broach at times. Physicians trained solely in using the biomedical method may find it difficult to develop the new knowledge, skills, and attitudes required under a patient-centered approach.

However, physicians using this approach have generally not found these problems insurmountable. Like-minded physicians have joined together in groups to alter systems that may be reinforcing unhealthy patient behaviors. Support from colleagues, consultation with health care providers skilled in systemic issues, and acknowledgment of systemic limitations to patients all help physicians deal with complex matters. Continuing medical education courses are available for physicians who need to upgrade their knowledge, skills, and attitudes with regard to the patient-centered approach. Likewise, ethical issues are not insurmountable as long as they are approached in an open fashion and consensus is reached among all parties concerned.

Studies reveal that the patient-centered approach appears to be efficacious with few side effects. Many physicians feel that strategies can be developed to cope with the potential side effects of the patient-centered approach and that the advantages of the patient-centered approach greatly outweigh its potential disadvantages. However, many aspects of the patient-centered approach still need to be adequately studied.

Medical practice is entering an exciting, turbulent time. Not only are patients becoming increasingly dissatisfied with old methods of clinical practice, but physicians too are seeing the disadvantages inherent in the biomedical method. Although a new clinical method has not fully asserted itself yet, many respected scholars and clinicians are undertaking further study and research on the patient-centered approach because they believe it will eventually yield the desired new method. Prior to a new method achieving dominance, however, clinicians in this chaotic time must continue to experiment with the various approaches to clinical care to find the one that best fits their clinical practice and the patients they are treating.

CASES FOR DISCUSSION

Case 1

David, a 16-year-old black male, came into his family physician's office with a 1-day history of pain in his lower abdomen, nausea, vomiting, and loss of appetite. Two hours ago, David's pain seemed to be located more in his right lower quadrant. On exam, David was noted to have a temperature of 101°F and be very tender in his lower abdomen, particularly in the right lower quadrant, where rebound tenderness was present. The physician then ordered two tests: (1) a white blood cell count, which returned elevated at 14.8 $\times$ 10^3 cells per hpf, and (2) a urine analysis, which was totally normal.

David's family physician made the diagnosis of appendicitis and referred David to a general surgeon, who recommended immediate surgery. On opening the abdomen, the general surgeon found an inflamed appendix, which was removed without complications. David recovered without difficulty and was discharged from the hospital 2 days later. At his 1-month follow-up visit with the general surgeon, David was back to normal.

1. Which method of clinical care were the family physician and general surgeon using in this case?
2. What are some of the strengths of that method?
3. What are some of the potential problems associated with this method?

Case 2

Mrs. F.Z. is a 68-year-old white female with mild Alzheimer's dementia who was admitted to an internal medicine teaching service of a busy tertiary care hospital with shortness of breath, right lower lobe pneumonia on chest x ray, and hypoxia on an arterial blood gas. On arrival on the ward, the patient was very confused and combative and so had to be restrained so that an intravenous line could be started. After the intravenous line was established, appropriate antibiotics were prescribed. Over the next 2 days the patient appeared to be getting better but was still occasionally confused and combative, and so restraints were kept in place.

On the third day Mrs. F.Z. became acutely short of breath. The resident taking care of Mrs. F.Z. immediately ordered a lung scan, which showed perfusion defects not matched with ventilation defects in the upper left lung field, consistent with a pulmonary embolus. In order to find a source for this embolus, the resident examined the patient's lower extremities and noted that the right calf was swollen and tender. The resident immediately started heparin therapy, which did seem to help the patient, but the patient did have to be placed on a larger amount of oxygen in order to decrease her shortness of breath.

One day later the patient refused to eat and complained of abdominal pain. Examination revealed no bowel sounds, bruising around the umbilicus, and hematuria on urinalysis. The resident then obtained an abdominal CT scan, which confirmed his diagnosis of retroperitoneal hematoma. Because of the hematoma formation, heparin therapy had to be stopped.

Two days later the patient still had not improved. On the afternoon of that day the patient became acutely short of breath again and was noted to be more swollen. The diagnosis of pulmonary embolus was again made based on classic findings on a lung scan with swelling secondary to renal failure from an embolus to a renal artery. Extremely poor oxygenation was noted on an arterial blood gas, so the patient was transferred to the intensive care unit, where she was intubated and placed on mechanical ventilation. Peritoneal dialysis was instituted for the patient's renal failure.

Over the next week the patient continued to do poorly, with many febrile episodes being noted. Despite a change in antibiotics, F.S.'s lung function continued to deteriorate such that she required larger and larger amounts of oxygen. Ten days after admission to the hospital, the patient died of respiratory arrest.

1. What method of clinical care was the resident using in this case?
2. What problem with this method does this case illustrate? Trace out how the resident's actions in this case contributed to the complications that arose.
3. How might this "cascade of unanticipated events" have been prevented?
4. How much do you estimate this hospitalization cost?

Case 3

A 54-year-old successful business executive, Nancy, presented to her family physician's office with a tired feeling, a chronic cough, which she attributed to her 40 pack-year history of smoking, and two recent episodes of hemoptysis. The physician obtained a chest x ray, which showed a large mass in the right hilum that later was diagnosed as an oat cell carcinoma by bronchoscopy. Both the oncologist and the family physician assured Nancy that cure was possible given new radiation therapy and drug treatment protocols that had been recently developed. Nancy gladly consented to these protocols, as she wanted to continue her work as a business executive.

However, after 9 months of painful radiation and chemotherapy, Nancy was becoming more and more depressed. She had to devote increasing amounts of time away from her business for her health care, and rather than becoming stronger she was becoming progressively weaker. Nancy began to suspect that her doctors were not telling her the truth and so began reading about oat cell carcinoma in medical textbooks she obtained from her local library. She was devastated to learn that the median survival of patients with oat cell carcinoma was only 1 to 2 years, and even the latest radiation therapy and chemotherapy protocols have not altered that survival. Nancy could not understand why her doctors had not been honest with her, but she did not confront them, becoming more and more depressed as it became obvious that therapy was not going to cure her.

Despite Nancy's depression, her physicians continued to reassure her that she could maintain an active life as long as she submitted to therapy. Eventually, Nancy became so depressed that she began contemplating suicide. One week later Nancy was found dead in her garage in which all the doors had been closed and her car was left running.

1. What method of clinical care were the physicians in Nancy's case using?
2. What problem arose in this case because of the method the physicians were using?
3. How common is suicide among terminally ill patients? Could this have been prevented?
4. What additional knowledge or information would have been helpful in this case?

Case 4

Debbie, a 28-year-old female factory worker, comes into your office complaining of fatigue of 2 months' duration. In talking with Debbie you learn that she is happily married with two children and considers her family life to be very satisfying. However, 3 months ago she was shifted from assembly line work to piecework at the local shoe factory, resulting in a substantial loss to her income. In order to make ends meet both Debbie and her husband have to work, placing the children at a local day care center during their working hours. Despite this loss of income, Debbie has still not confronted her boss, who would not do anything about it anyway, as Debbie was the only one who could do piecework well. The family physician, having been in this small town for 5 years, knew the boss of the shoe factory where Debbie worked and realized how difficult it was for the boss to find skilled workers.

1. What method of clinical care is the physician operating under in this case?
2. Is it within the purview of the physician to discuss occupational issues with his patients?
3. How would you help Debbie in this case if you were the physician and you knew the boss of the factory? Would you confront the boss directly, or would you encourage Debbie to do so?
4. Would you treat Debbie with antidepressants in this case, psychotherapy, both, or neither?

Case 5

Barbara, a 33-year-old female, presented to the labor and delivery service of a busy hospital with a rupture of membranes at 37 weeks estimated gestational age. The obstetrician taking care of Barbara, knowing the results of the decision analysis in Case 15-5, decided to present Barbara with two options, either expective management or induction immediately, even though Barbara's cervix was not favorable for induction. Tom, her husband, was also present in the room when the obstetrician presented the two options and the risks and benefits of both. A heated discussion followed in which Barbara elected one option and Tom elected the other.

1. How might this case have been different if the physician operated under a traditional biomedical approach?
2. If Tom and Barbara already had five children and Barbara played a large role in child care such that if she were injured or died, Tom would be left taking care of the children, but Barbara felt it was her duty to give her child the best chance of being born healthy and so wanted an immediate induction, whereas Tom wanted to wait 24 h to see if Barbara would go into labor on her own, how would you help this couple resolve this issue? Does Tom have any say legally or ethically in any option that Barbara decides on?
3. Would Tom's feelings change, given the ethical theory he is inferred to be using in question 2, if this was their first child after a long infertility workup? Would presenting this scenario to Tom help in the couple's decision making?

RECOMMENDED READINGS

McWhinney, I. R. (1989). *A textbook of family medicine.* New York: Oxford University Press.

The clearest review of the patient-centered approach to date by one of its strongest advocates. The chapters illustrating the use of the patient-centered approach in the treatment of patients with sore throat, headache, fatigue, hypertension, and diabetes mellitus are outstanding and should be read by even the most seasoned clinician.

Ramsey, C. N. (1989). *Family systems in medicine.* New York: Guilford Press.

This book contains chapters by many experts in the field of family systems medicine describing the science behind their work. Although heavily theoretical in places, the book does cover a broad range of medical problems in enough detail to be valuable to the practicing physician.

Stein, H. F. (1990). *American medicine as culture.* Boulder, CO: Westview Press.

An outstanding analysis of the values and dynamics of medical practice. Two later chapters on the physician socialization process and the self of the physician should be mandatory reading for all practitioners of the art.

References

Abel, T. M., Metraux, R., & Roll, S. (1987). *Psychotherapy and culture* (revised/expanded edition). Albuquerque, NM: University of New Mexico.

Ader, R. (Ed.). (1981). *Psychoneuroimmunology.* New York: Academic Press.

American Board of Family Practice. (1989). Well Child Care, Reference Guide #10. Lexington, KY: American Board of Family Practice, p. 5.

American Dental Association. (1989). Survey of Dental Practice—Employment Practice Personnel. Chicago, IL: ADA, pp. 20–30.

American Cancer Society. (1980). ACS report on the cancer related health checkup. *CA—A Journal for Clinicians, 30,* 194–240.

American Hospital Association. (1986). Hospital Statistics. Chicago.

American Medical Association. (1848). *Code of ethics of the American Medical Association.* New York: H. Ludwig & Co.

American Medical Association. (1987). Physicians Characteristics and Distribution in the U.S. Chicago, IL: AMA, p. 89.

American Psychological Association. (1981). *Specialty guidelines for the delivery of services in clinical psychology, counseling psychology, industrial/organizational psychology, and school psychology.* Washington, DC: American Psychological Association Committees on Professional Standards.

American Society of Clinical Pathologists Board of Registry. (1989). ASCP Board of Registry to certify phlebotomists. *Laboratory Medicine, 20*(5), 297.

American Speech–Language–Hearing Association. (1989–90). *ASHA Membership Directory.* Rockville, MD: ASHA.

Ammirato, T. (1989). The mounting problem of patient noncompliance. *Urban Medicine, 4,* 5–7.

Amundsen, D. W., & Ferngren, G. B. (1983). Evolution of the physician–patient relationship: Antiquity through the renaissance. In E. E. Shelp. (Ed.), *The clinical encounter* (pp. 3–46). Dordrecht, Holland: D. Reidel.

Arthur, J., & Shaw, W. H. (1978). *Justice and economic distribution.* Englewood Cliffs, NJ: Prentice-Hall.

Balint, M. (1957). *The doctor, his patient, and the illness.* New York: International Universities Press.

Barrow, R. (1982). *Injustice, inequality, and ethics: A philosophical introduction to moral problems.* Totowa, NJ: Barnes & Noble Books.

Barrows, H. S., Norman, G. R., Neufeld, V. R., & Feightner, J. W. (1982). The clinical reasoning of randomly selected physicians in general medical practice. *Clinical and Investigative Medicine, 5,* 49–55.

Barsky, A. J. (1983). Non-pharmacologic aspects of medication. *Archives of Internal Medicine, 143,* 1544–1548.

Barsky, A. J. (1988). The paradox of health. *New England Journal of Medicine, 318,* 414–418.

Bass, M. J., Buck, C. W., Turner, L., Pickie, G., Pratt, G., & Robinson, H. C. (1986). The physician's actions and the outcome of illness in family practice. *Journal of Family Practice, 23,* 43–47.

Bateson, G. (1972). *Steps to an ecology of mind.* New York: Ballantine Books.

Bayles, M. D. (1989). *Professional ethics.* Bellmont, CA: Wadsworth.

Beauchamp, T. L., & Childress, J. F. (1989). *Principles of biomedial ethics.* New York: Oxford University Press.

Beauchamp, T. L., & McCullough, L. B. (1984). *Medical ethics: The moral responsibilities of physicians.* Englewood Cliffs, NJ: Prentice Hall.

Becker, L. A., Steinbauer, J., & Doherty, W. J. (1985). A biopsychosocial smoking cessation protocol. *Family Systems Medicine, 3,* 103–110.

Becker, M. C., Abrams, K. S., & Onder, J. (1974). Goal setting: A joint patient–staff method. *Archives of Physical Medicine and Rehabilitation, 55,* 87–89.

Beckman, H. B., & Frankel, R. M. (1984). The effect of physician behavior on the collection of data. *Annals of Internal Medicine, 101,* 692–696.

Behar, S., Schor, S., Kariv, I., Barell, V., & Modan, B. (1977). Evaluation of electrocardiogram in emergency room as a decision-making tool. *Chest, 21,* 486–491.

Benfield, D. G. (1979). Two philosophies of caring. *The Ohio State Medical Journal, August,* Vol. 75, 508–511.

Berglung, R. (Ed.). (1989). *The story of modern beef.* National Cattleman's Association. Englewood, CO.

Berrien, R. (1987). What future for primary care private practice? *New England Journal of Medicine, 316,* 334–337.

Black, P. M. (1983). Clinical problems in the use of brain-death standards. *Archives of Internal Medicine, 143,* 121–123.

Blair, S. N., Kohl, H. W. III, Paffenbarger, R. S., Clark, D. G., Cooper, K. H., & Gibbons, L. W. (1989). Physical fitness and all-cause mortality: A prospective study of healthy men and women. *Journal of the American Medical Association, 262,* 2395–2401.

Bloom, S. M. (1963). *The doctor and his patient.* New York: Russell Sage.

Blum, T. C., & Roman, P. M. (1986). Alcohol, drugs, and EAPs: New data from a national study. *The Almacan, May,* 20–23.

Blumhagen, D. (1982). The meaning of hypertension. In N. Chrisman & T. W. Maretzki (Eds.), *Clinically applied anthropology* (pp. 297–323). Dordrecht, Holland: D. Reidel.

Board of Trustees Report. (1986). A proposal for financing health care of the elderly. *Journal of the American Medical Association, 256,* 3379–3382.

Bowen, M. (1972). Towards the differentiation of self in one's own family of origin. In F. D. Andres and J. P. Lorio (Eds.), Georgetown Family Symposia: A Collection of Papers, Vol. 1 (1971–1972), Washington, D.C. Georgetown University Medical Center, Department of Psychiatry.

Boyer, L. B. (1983). Approaching cross-cultural phychotherapy. *The Journal of Psychoanalytic Anthropology, 6,* 237–245.

Breidenstein, B. C., & Williams, J. C. (1987). *Red meat: Nutrient composition and actual consumption* (pp. 1–21). Chicago: National Live Stock and Meat Board.

Breslow, L., & Buell, P. (1960). Mortality from coronary heart disease and physical activity of work in California. *Journal of Chronic Diseases, 11,* 421–444.

Breslow, W. L., & Somers, A. R. (1977). The lifetime health-monitoring program: A practical approach to preventive medicine. *New England Journal of Medicine, 296,* 601–608.

Brett, A. S., & McCullough, L. B. (1986). When patient's request specific interventions: Defining the limits of the physician's obligation. *New England Journal of Medicine, 315,* 1347–1351.

Brock, C. (1977). Consultation and referral patterns of family physicians. *Journal of Family Practice, 4,* 1129–1134.

Brody, H. (1982). The lie that heals. The ethics of giving placebos. *Annals of Internal Medicine, 97,* 112–118.

Brody, H. (1988). *Ethics in the future of family medicine: Cunningham lecture.* Oklahoma City: University of Oklahoma Health Sciences Center.

Brownell, K. D., Kelman, J. H., & Stunkard, A. J. (1983). Treatment of obese children with and without their mothers: Changes in weight and blood pressure. *Pediatrics, 71,* 515–523.

Bruhn, J. G. (1978). The doctor's touch: Tactile communication in the doctor–patient relationship. *Southern Medical Journal, 71,* 1469–1473.

Byrne, P. S., & Long, E. L. (1976). *Doctors talking to patients: A study of the verbal behavior of general practitioners consulting in their surgeries.* London: HMSO.

Cady, L. D., Jr., Gertler, M. M., Gottsch, L. G., & Woodbury, M. A. (1961). The factor structure of variables concerned with coronary artery disease. *Behavioral Science, 6,* 37–41.

Campbell, T. L. (1986). Family's impact on health: A critical review. *Family Systems Medicine, 4,* 135–328.

Carlson, L. A. (1960). Serum lipid in men with myocardial infarction. *Acta Medica Scandinavica, 167,* 399–413.

Carter, W. B., Inui, T. S., KuKull, W. A., & Haigh, U. H. (1982). Outcome-based doctor–patient interaction analysis II. Identify effective provider and patient behavior. *Medical Care, 20,* 550–566.

Cassel, J. (1976). The contribution of the social environment to host resistance. *American Journal of Epidemiology, 104,* 107–123.

Cassell, E. J. (1982). The nature of suffering and the goals of medicine. *New England Journal of Medicine, 306,* 639–645.

Cassileth, B. R., Lusk, E. J., Strouse, T. B., Miller, D. S., Brown, L. L., & Cross, P. A. (1984). Psychosocial status in chronic illness: A comparative analysis of six diagnostic groups. *New England Journal of Medicine, 311,* 506–511.

Charap, M. H. (1981). The periodic health examination: Genesis of a myth. *Annals of Internal Medicine, 95,* 733–735.

Charns, M. (1976). Breaking the tradition barrier: Managing integration in health care facilities. *Health Care Management Review, Winter,* Vol. 1, 55–67.

Cherkin, D. C., Rosenblatt, R. A., Hart, L. G., Schneeweiss, R., & LoGerto, J. (1987). The use of medical resources by residency-trained family physicians and general internists: Is there a difference? *Medical Care, 25,* 455–469.

Childress, J. F., & Siegler, M. (1984). Metaphors and models of doctor–patient relationships: Their implications for autonomy. *Theoretical Medicine, 5,* 17–30.

Christie-Seely, J., & Crouch, M. A. (1987). The history of the family in medicine. In M. A. Crouch & L. Roberts (Eds.), *The family in medical practice: A family system primer* (pp. 1–27). New York: Springer-Verlag.

Christman, N. J. (1977). The health seeking process: An approach to the natural history of illness. *Culture, Medicine and Psychiatry, 1,* 351–377.

Christman, N. J., Maretzki, T. W. (Eds.). (1982). *Clinically Applied Anthropology.* Dordrecht, Holland: D. Reidel.

Citrin, W. S., Kleiman, G. A., & Skyler, J. S. (1986). Emotions: A critical factor in diabetic control. In M. B. Davidson (Ed.), *Diabetes mellitus: Diagnosis and treatment* (pp. 487–510). New York: John Wiley & Sons.

Clouser, K. D. (1983). Veatch, May and models: A critical review and a new view. In E. E. Shelp (Ed.), *The clinical encounter* (pp. 89–103). Dordrecht, Holland: D. Reidel.

Cobb, B. (1958). Why do people return to quacks? In E. G. Jaco (Ed.), *Patients, physicians, and illness* (pp. 283–287). New York: Free Press.

Cole, P. (1980). Major aspects of the epidemiology of breast cancer. *Cancer, 46,* 865–867.

Comley, A. (1973). Family therapy and the family physician. *Canadian Family Physician, 19,* 78–188.

Committee on International Relations, & Stein, H. F. (1987). *Us and them: The psychology of ethnonationalism* (Group for the Advancement of Psychiatry Report No. 123). New York: Brunner/Mazel.

Conetta, R., Tamarin, F. M., Wogalter, D., & Brandstetter, R. D. (1987). Liquer lung. *New England Journal of Medicine, 316,* 348–349.

Cooper, K. H. (1982). Physical training programs for mass scale use: Effects on cardiovascular disease—facts and theories. *Annals of Clinical Research,* 14(32), 25–32.

Cotton, P. (1988). Mortality among elderly has risen under prospective payment. *Medical World News,* June 13, Vol. 29(11) pp. 13–16.

Cotton, P. (1989). Care-rationing hits at local level. *Medical World News, 30*(8), 21–24.

Coulehan, J. L., & Block, M. R. (1987). *The medical interview: A primer for students of the art.* Philadelphia: F. A. Davis.

Council on Ethical and Judicial Affairs. (1988). Ethical issues involved in the growing AIDS crisis. *AIDS, 259,* 1360–1361.

Crawford, R. (1980). Healthism and the medicalization of everyday life. *International Journal of Health Services,* 10, 365–388.

Crawford, R. (1985). A cultural account of health: Self control, release, and the social body. In J. McKinlay (Ed.), *Issues in the political economy of health care.* London: Tavistock.

Croog, S. H., Levin, S., Testa, M. A., Brown, B., Bulpitt, C. J., Jenkins, C. D., Klerman, G. L., & Williams, G. H. (1986). The effects of antihypertensive therapy on the quality of life. *New England Journal of Medicine, 314,* 1657–1664.

Cross, A. W., & Churchill, L. R. (1982). Ethical and cultural dimensions of informed consent. A case study analysis. *Annals of Internal Medicine, 96,* 110–113.

Crouch, M. A., & Davis, T. (1987). Using the genogram (family tree) clinically. In M. A. Crouch & L.

Roberts (Eds.), *The family in medical practice: A family system primer* (pp. 174–192). New York: Springer-Verlag.

Delafield, F. A. (1885). *A Handbook of post-mortem examinations and of morbid anatomy.* New York: Wood.

DeMause, L. (1984). *Reagan's America.* New York: Creative Roots.

Department of Health and Human Services. (1981). *Summary report of the Graduate Medical Education National Advisory Committee to the Secretary.* Department of Health and Human Services, Sept. 30, 1980. DHHS Pub. No. (HRA) 81-651. Washington, D.C.: U.S. Government Printing Office.

Devereux, G. (1980). *Basic problems of ethno-psychiatry.* Chicago: The University of Chicago Press.

De Vos, G. A., & Romanucci-Ross, L. (Eds.). (1975). *Ethnic identity: Cultural continuities and change.* Palo Alto, CA: Mayfield.

Dirckx, J. H. (1982). Speaking of illness. *Pharos, 45,* 22–26.

Dishman, R. K. (1987). Exercise adherence and habitual physical activity. In W. P. Morgan & S. N. Golston (Eds.), *Exercise and mental health* (pp. 57–83). Washington, DC: Hemisphere.

Doherty, W. J., & Baird, M. A. (1983). *Family therapy and family medicine.* New York: Guilford Press.

Doherty, W. J., & Baird, M. A. (1984). A protocol for family compliance counseling. *Family Systems Medicine, 2,* 333–336.

Doherty, W. J., & Baird, M. A. (1987). *Family-centered medical care.* New York: Guilford Press.

Drucker, P. F. (1954). *The practice of management.* New York: Harper.

Duff, P., Huff, R. W., & Gibbs, R. S. (1984). Management of premature rupture of membranes and unfavorable cervix in term pregnancy. *Obstetrics and Gynecology, 63,* 697–702.

Duffy, J. (1983). American medical ethnics and the physician–patient relationship. In E. E. Shelp (Ed.), *The clinical encounter* (pp. 65–85). Dordrecht, Holland: D. Reidel.

Edelstein, L. (1943). The Hippocratic Oath: Text, translation, and interpretation. *Bulletin of the History of Medicine, Supplement 1,* 3.

Egdahl, R. H., & Taft, C. H. (1986). Financial incentives to physicians. *New England Journal of Medicine, 315,* 59–61.

Eisenberg, L., & Kleinman, A. M. (Eds.). (1981). *The relevance of social science for medicine.* Boston: D. Reidel.

Elias, S., & Annas, G. J. (1986). Social policy considerations in noncoital reproduction. *Journal of the American Medical Association, 255,* 62–68.

Ellis, J. R. (1956). The medical student. *Journal of Medical Education,* Vol. 31: pp. 42–46.

Elstein, A. S., Shulman, L. S., & Sprafka, S. A. (1978). *Medical problem solving: An analysis of clinical reasoning.* Cambridge, MA: Harvard University Press.

Engel, G. L. (1977). The need for a new medical model: A challenge for biomedicine. *Science, 196,* 129–136.

Engel, G. L. (1980). The clinical application of the biopsychosocial model. *American Journal of Psychiatry, 137,* 535–544.

Engel, G. L. (1987). Physician-scientists and scientific physicians: Resolving the humanism–science dichotomy. *American Journal of Medicine, 82,* 107–111.

Engelhardt, H. T., Jr. (1983). The physician–patient relationship in a secular, pluralist society. In E. E. Shelp (Ed.), *The clinical encounter* (pp. 253–266). Dordrecht, Holland: D. Reidel.

Epstein, F. H. (1964). Hereditary aspects of coronary heart disease. *American Heart Journal, 67,* 445–456.

Epstein, F. H. (1965). The epidemiology of coronary heart disease, a review. *Journal of Chronic Diseases, 18,* 753–774.

Epstein, L. C., & Lasagna, L. (1969). Obtaining informed consent: Form or substance. *Archives of Internal Medicine, 123,* 682–688.

Eraker, S. A., Kirscht, J. P., & Becker, M. H. (1984). Understanding and improving patient compliance. *Annals of Internal Medicine, 100,* 258–268.

Farrow, L., Wartman, S. A., & Brock, D. (1988). Science, ethnics, and the making of clinical decisions: Implications for risk factor intervention. *Journal of American Medical Association, 259,* 3161–3167.

Feinstein, A. (1967). *Clinical judgment.* Baltimore: Williams & Wilkins.

Feldman, A. (1978). The family practitioner as psychiatrist. *American Journal of Psychiatry, 135,* 730.

Felig, P. (1983). Metabolic and endocrine disorders and exercise. In A. A. Bove Lowenthal (Ed.), *Exercise medicine: Physiological principles and clinical applications* (pp. 305–318). New York: Academic Press.

Fisch, R., Weakland, J. H., & Segal, L. (1982). *The tactics of change: Doing therapy briefly.* San Francisco: Jossey-Bass.

Fisher, R., & Ury, W. (1981). *Getting to yes: Negotiating agreement without giving in.* New York: Penguin Books.

Foster, G. (1976). Disease etiologies in non-Western medical systems. *American Anthropologist, 78,* 773–782.

Foster, G. M., & Anderson, B. G. (1978). *Medical anthropology.* New York: John Wiley & Sons.

Frame, F. S. (1986). A critical review of metabolic, behavioral and miscellaneous conditions. *Journal of Family Practice, 23,* 23–29.

Frame, P. S., & Carlson, S. J. (1975). A critical review of periodic health screening using specific screening criteria. *Journal of Family Practice, 22,* 29–36, 123–129, 189–194, 283–289.

Francis, V., Korsch, B. M., & Morris, J. M. (1969). Gaps in doctor–patient communication. *New England Journal of Medicine, 280,* 535–540.

Frank, I. N., Keys, H. M., & McCune, C. S. (1983). Urologic and male genital cancers. In P. Rubin (Ed.), *Clinical oncology: A multidisciplinary approach,* 6th ed. (pp. 198–222). Washington, DC: American Cancer Society.

French, R. M. (1979). Interpersonal relations. In *Dynamics of health care,* 3rd ed. (pp. 141–143). New York: McGraw-Hill.

Freymann, J. G. (1989). The public's health care paradigm is shifting: Medicine must swing with it. *Journal of General Internal Medicine, 44,* 313–319.

Gadow, S. (1980). Existential advocacy: Philosophical foundation of nursing. In S. F. Spicker & S. Gadow (Eds.), *Nursing images and ideals: Opening dialogue with the humanities* (pp. 70–101). New York: Springer Publishing Co.

Garner, H. G. (1988). *Helping others through teamwork.* Washington, DC: Child Welfare League of America.

Gettman, L. R., Pollock, M. L., & Ward, A. (1983). Adherence to unsupervised exercise. *Physician and Sports Medicine, 11,* 56–66.

Geyman, J. P., Brown, T. C., & Rivers, K. (1976). Referrals in family practice: A comparative study by geographic region and practice setting. *Journal of Family Practice, 33,* 163–167.

Gill, J. S., Zezulka, A. V., Shipley, M. J., Gill, S. K., & Beevers, D. G. (1986). Stroke and alcohol consumption. *New England Journal of Medicine, 315,* 1041–1046.

Ginzberg, E. (1988). Medical care for the poor: No magic bullets. *Journal of the American Medical Association, 259*(22), 3309–3311.

Glazer, N., & Moynihan, D. P. (Eds.). (1975). *Ethnicity: Theory and experience.* Cambridge, MA: Harvard University Press.

Goldman, A. H. (1989). *The moral foundations of professional ethics.* Totowa, NJ: Roman and Littlefield.

Goldstein, M. K. (1989). Physicians and teams. In R. Ham (Ed.), *Geriatric medicine annual* (pp. 265–275). Oradell, NJ: Medical Economics.

Gonzalez, M. L., & Emmons, D. W. (Eds.). (1986). *Socioeconomic characteristics of medical practice.* Chicago: American Medical Association.

Gordon, T., Castelli, W. P., Hjortland, M. C., Kannel, W. B., & Dawber, T. R. (1977). High density lipoprotein as a protective factor against coronary heart disease. *American Journal of Medicine, 62,* 707–714.

Gorlin, R., & Zucker, H. D. (1983). Physician's reactions to patients. *New England Journal of Medicine, 408,* 1059–1063.

Greenberg, R. N. (1984). Overview of patient compliance with medication dosing: A literature review. *Clinical Therapeutics, 6,* 592–599.

Greenfield, S., Kayslan, S. H., Ware, J. E., Yamo, E. M., & Frank, H. J. L. (1988). Patient's participation in medical care: Effects on blood sugar control and quality of life in diabetes. *Journal of General Internal Medicine, 3,* 448–457.

Grieco, M. S. (1988). Birth-marked? A critical review on analyzing organizational culture. *Human Organization, 47,* 84–87.

Grobstein, C. (Chairman), Cairns, J., Berliner, R. W., Broitman, S. A., Gampbell, T., Gussow, J. D., Kolonel, L. N., Kritchevsky, D., Mertz, W., Miller, A. B., Prival, M. J., Slaga, T., Wattenberg, L., Sugimura, T. (1982). *Executive summary: Diet Nutrition and Cancer* (Vol. 1, pp. 14–16). Washington, DC: Committee on Diet, Nutrition, and Cancer, Assembly of Life Sciences, National Research Council, National Academy Press.

Groves, J. E. (1978). Taking care of the hateful patient. *New England Journal of Medicine, 298,* 883–887.

Grundy, S. M., Brown, W. V., Dietschy, J. M., Ginsberg, H., Goodnight, S., Howard, B., LaRosa, J.

C., & McGill, H. C. (1989). AHA conference report on cholesterol: Workshop III—Basis for dietary treatment. *Circulation, 80,* 729–734.

Guyatt, G. H., Pugsley, S. O., Sullivan, M. J., Thompson, P. J., Berman, L. B., Jones, N. L., Fallen, E. L., & Taylor, D. W. (1984). Effects of encouragement on walking performance. *Thorax, 39,* 811-822.

Harwood, A. (1971). The hot–cold theory of disease: Implications for treatment of Puerto Rican patients. *Journal of the American Medical Association, 216,* 1153–1154.

Harwood, A. (1981). *Ethnicity and medical care.* Cambridge, MA: Harvard University Press.

Headache Study Group of the University of Western Ontario. (1986). Predictors of outcome in headache patients presenting to family physicians. *Headache, 26,* 285–294.

Hefferin, E. A. (1979). Health goal setting: Patient–spouse collaboration at Veterans Administration facilities. *Military Medicine, December,* Vol. 144:814–821.

Henry, J. (1963). *Culture against man.* New York: Random House.

Heyman, A., Karp, H. R., Heyden, S., Bartel, A., Cassel, J. C., Tyroler, H. A., Cornon, J., Hames, C. G., & Stuart, W. (1971). Cerebral vascular disease in the bi-racial population of Evans County, Georgia. *Stroke, 2,* 509–519.

Hill, A. B. (1965). The environment and disease: Association or causation? *Proceedings of the Royal Society of Medicine, 58,* 295–300.

Hill, C. E., & Mathews, H. (1981). Traditional health beliefs and practices among southern rural blacks: A complement to biomedicine. In M. Black & J. S. Reed (Eds.), *Social science perspectives on the south* (pp. 307–322). New York: Gordon & Breach.

Hippocrates. (1979). *Hippocrates of the epidemics.* Franklin, PA: The Franklin Library.

Hocking, B. (1987). Anthropologic aspects of occupational illness epidemics. *Journal of Occupational Medicine, 29,* 526–530.

Hoffman, L. (1981). *Foundation of family therapy.* New York: Basic Books.

Holder, A. R. (1987). Minors' rights to consent to medical care. *Journal of the American Medical Association, 257,* 3400–3402.

Hsiao, W. C., Braun, P., Dunn, D., Becker, E. R., DeNicola, M., & Ketchum, T. R. (1988a). Results and policy implications of the resource-based relative value study. *New England Journal of Medicine, 319*(13), 881–888.

Hsiao, W. C., Braun, P., Yntema, D., & Becker, E. R. (1988b). Estimating physician's work for a resource-based relative value scale. *New England Journal of Medicine, 319*(13), 835–841.

Hunt, W. A., Barnett, L. W., & Branch, L. G. (1971). Relapse rates in addiction programs. *Journal of Clinical Psychology, 27,* 455–456.

Hypertension Detection and Follow-up Program Cooperative Group. (1983). The effect of treatment on mortality in "mild" hypertension. *New England Journal of Medicine, 307,* 976–980.

Illich, I. (1975). The medicalization of life. *Journal of Medical Ethics, 1,* 73–77.

Johnson, S. M., Kurtz, M. E., Tomlinson, T., & Howe, K. R. (1986). Students' stereotypes of patients as barriers to clinical decision making. *Journal of Medical Education, 61,* 727–735.

Johnson, T. M., & Kleinman, A. (1984). Cultural concerns in consultation psychiatry. In F. G. Guggenheim and M. F. Weiner (Eds.), *Manual of Psychiatric Consultation and Emergency Care* (pp. 275–284). New York: Jason Aronson.

Jonas, A. P., & Bauer, L. (1989). *Clinical teaching skills workshop.* Sponsored by the Department of Family Medicine, University of Oklahoma Health Sciences Center, Oklahoma City, Oklahoma, May 19 and 20.

Jonas, S. (1986). *Health care delivery in the United States.* New York: Springer Publishing Co.

Jones, B. E. (1978). *The difference a D.O. makes.* Oklahoma City: Times-Journal Publishing Company.

Jonson, A. R. (1978). Do no harm. *Annals of Internal Medicine, 88,* 827–832.

Kannel, W. B., Castelli, W. P., Gordon, T., & McNamara, P. M. (1971). Serum cholesterol, lipoproteins, and the risk of coronary heart disease: The Framingham study. *Annals of Internal Medicine, 74,* 1–12.

Kannel, W. B., Dawber, T. R., Sorlie, P., Revotskie, N., & Wolf, P. (1976). Components of blood pressure and risk of artherothromobotic brain infarction: The Framingham study. *Stroke, 7,* 327–331.

Kannel, W. B., Kagan, A., Dawber, T. R., & Revotskie, N. (1962). Epidemiology of coronary heart disease. *Geriatrics, 17,* 675–690.

Kass, L. R. (1980). Ethical dilemmas in the care of the ill: I. What is the physician's service? II. What is the patient's good? *Journal of the American Medical Association, 244,* 1811–1816, 1946–1949.

Kassirer, J. P. (1989). Our stubborn quest for diagnostic certainty. *New England Journal of Medicine, 320,* 1489–1491.

Katcher, A. H., Brightman, B., Luborsky, L., & Ship, I. (1973). Prediction of the incidence of recurrence herpes labialis and systemic illness from psychological measurements. *Journal of Dental Research, 52,* 49–58.

Katon, W., Kleinman, A., & Rosen, G. (1982). Depression and somatization. *American Journal of Medicine, 72,* 127–135, 241–247.

Keefe, S. E. (1984). Real and ideal extended familism among Mexican Americans and Anglo Americans: On the meaning of "close" family ties. *Human Organizations, 43,* 65–70.

Kenkel, P. J. (1988). Multi-unit providers survey. *Modern Healthcare, 18*(23), 20–38.

Keys, H. M., Bakemeier, R. F., & Savlov, E. D. (1983). Breast cancer. In P. Rubin (Ed.), *Clinical oncology: A multidisciplinary approach,* 6th ed. (pp. 120–142). Washington, DC: American Cancer Society.

Kirchner, M. (1988). Will this formula change the way you get paid? *Medical Economics,* April 4, Vol. 65, 138–149.

Kleinman, A. M. (1978). Explanatory models in health care relationships. In the Proceedings of the 2nd International Health Conference in Reston, VA, October 16–18, 1974, *Health of the Family* (pp. 159–172). Washington, DC: National Council for International Health Symposium. Microfiche "Health Care #IS77.

Kleinman, A. M. (1980). *Patients and healers in the context of culture: An exploration of the borderland between anthropology, medicine, and psychiatry.* Los Angeles: University of California Press.

Kleinman, A. M. (1982). The teaching of clinically applied medical anthropology on a psychiatric consultation–liaison service. In N. J. U. Chrisman & T. W. Maretzki (Eds.), *Clinically applied anthropology: Anthropologists in health science settings* (pp. 83–115). Dordrecht, Holland: D. Reidel.

Kleinman, A. M., Eisenberg, L., & Good, B. (1978). Culture, illness, and care: Clinical lessons from anthropologic and cross-cultural research. *Annals of Internal Medicine, 88,* 251–258.

Kletke, P. R., Marder, W. D., & Silberger, A. B. (1987). *The demographics of physician supply: Trends and projections.* Chicago: American Medical Association.

Kluckhohn, F., & Strodtbeck, F. (1961). *Variations in value orientations.* Evanston, IL: Row Peterson.

Kolder, V. E. B., Gallagher, J. D., & Parsons, M. T. (1987). Court-ordered obstetrical interventions. *New England Journal of Medicine, 316,* 1192–1196.

Kopelman, L. M., Irons, T. G., & Kopelman, A. E. (1988). Neonatologists judge the "Baby Doe" regulations. *New England Journal of Medicine, 318,* 677–683.

Koran, L. M. (1975). The reliability of clinical methods, data and judgment. *New England Journal of Medicine, 293,* 642–646, 695-701.

Kralewski, J. E., Dowd, B., Feldman, R., & Shapiro, J. (1987). The physician rebellion. *New England Journal of Medicine, 316,* 339–342.

Kraus, A. S., & Lillienfeld, A. M. (1959). Some epidemiologic aspects of the high mortality rate in the young widowed group. *Journal of Chronic Disease, 10,* 207–217.

Kroenke, K., & Mangelsdorff, D. (1989). Common symptoms in ambulatory care: Incidence evaluation, therapy, and outcome. *American Journal of Medicine, 86,* 262–266.

Kubler-Ross, E. (1969). *On death and dying.* New York: Macmillan.

Kushner, K., & Meyer, D. (1989). Family physicians' preceptions of the family conference. *Journal of Family Practice, 28,* 65–68.

Kushner, K., Meyer, D., & Hansen, J. P. (1989). Patients' attitudes toward physician involvement in family conferences. *Journal of Family Practice, 28,* 73–78.

Kvale, J. N., & Dayringer, R. (1987). The transference phenomenon in the care of the elderly patient. *Family Medicine, 19,* 141–143.

Laennec, R. T. (1827). *A treatise on the diseases of the chest, and on mediate auscultation* (pp. 389–390). Translation by John Forbes from the 2nd French edition. London: T. and G. Underwood.

Land, C. E. (1980). Low-dose radiation: A cause of breast cancer. *CA, 46,* 868–873.

Lang, G. C. (1985). Diabetes and health care in a Sioux community. *Human Organization, 44,* 251–260.

Lazare, A., Eisenthal, S., & Wasserman, L. (1975). The customer approach to patienthood. *Archives of General Psychiatry, 32,* 553–558.

Lazarus, R. S. (1966). *Psychological stress and the coping process.* New York: McGraw–Hill.

LeBaron, S., Reyher, J., & Stack, J. M. (1985). Paternalistic vs. egalitarian physician styles: The treatment of patients in crisis. *Journal of Family Practice, 21,* 56–62.

Lewis, J. W., Beavers, R., & Gossett, J. T. (1976). *No single thread.* New York: Brunner/Mazel.

Lin, E. H.-B. (1983). Intraethnic characteristics and the patient–physician interaction. *Journal of Family Practice, 16,* 91–98.

Lo, B. (1987). Behind closed doors. Promises and pitfalls of ethics committees. *New England Journal of Medicine, 317,* 46–49.

Lo, B., & Johnson, A. R. (1980). Ethical decisions in the case of a patient terminally ill with metastatic cancer. *Annals of Internal Medicine, 92,* 107–111.

The Lockman Foundation. (1960). *New American Standard Bible. Leviticus* 3:17 (p. 101). Philadelphia: A. J. Holman Co.

Lowenthal, D. T., & Broderman, S. J. (1983). Exercise in renal and hypertensive disease. In A. A. Bove & D. T. Lowenthal (Eds.), *Exercise medicine: Physiological principles and clinical applications* (pp. 292–300). New York: Academic Press.

Macquire, A. (1978). Psychic possession among industrial workers. *Lancet, 2,* 376–378.

Madanes, C. (1981). *Strategic family therapy.* San Francisco: Jossey-Bass.

Mancuso, C. A., & Rose, D. N. (1987). A model for physicians' therapeutic decision making. *Archives of Internal Medicine, 147,* 1281–1285.

Mann, J. I., & Inman, W. H. (1975). oral contraceptives and death from myocardial infarction. *British Medical Journal, 2,* 245–248.

Manson, J. E., Colditz, G. A., Stampfer, M. J., Willett, W. C., Rosen, B., Monson, R. R., Speizer, F. E., & Hennekens, C. H. (1990). A prospective study of obesity and risk of coronary heart disease in women. *New England Journal of Medicine, 332,* 882–889.

Marteau, T. M., Johnston, M., Baum, J. D., & Bloch, S. (1987). Goals of treatment in diabetes: A comparison of doctors and parents of children with diabetes. *Journal of Behavioral Medicine, 10,* 33–48.

May, W. F. (1975). Covenant, contract, or philanthropy. *Hastings Center Report, 5,* 29–38.

May, W. F. (1983). *The physician's covenant: Images of the healer in medical ethics.* Philadelphia: Westminster Press.

McCarthy, C. M. (1988). DRGs—five years later. *New England Journal of Medicine, 318*(25), 1683–1686.

McCormick, R. A. (1974). To save or let die. The dilemma of modern medicine. *Journal of the American Medical Association, 29,* 172–176.

McDaniel, S., Campbell, T. L., & Seaburn, D. B. (1990). *Family-oriented primary care: A manual for medical providers.* New York: Springer-Verlag.

McDonough, J. R., Hames, C. G., Stulb, S. C., & Garrison, G. E. (1965). Coronary heart disease among negros and whites in Evans County, Georgia. *Journal of Chronic Diseases, 18,* 443–468.

McGoldrick, M., & Gerson, R. (1985). *Genograms in family assessment.* New York: W. W. Norton.

McWhinney, I. R. (1986). Are we on the brink of a major transformation of clinical method? *Canadian Medical Association Journal, 135,* 873–878.

McWhinney, I. R. (1989). *A textbook of family medicine.* New York: Oxford University Press.

Mechanic, D. (1983). *Handbook of health, health care, and the health professions.* New York: The Free Press.

Medical Practice Committee, American College of Physicians. (1981). Periodic health examination: A guide for designing individualized preventive health care for the asymptomatic patient. *Annals of Internal Medicine, 95,* 729–732.

Mendelson, J. H., & Mello, N. K. (1985). *The diagnosis and treatment of alcoholism,* 2nd ed. New York: McGraw–Hill.

Mengel, M. B. (1987a). Lower abdominal pain in an adolescent. In W. J. Doherty & M. A. Baird (Eds.), *Family-centered medical care: A clinical casebook* (pp. 189–193). New York: Guilford Press.

Mengel, M. B. (1987b). A patient with alopecia areata. In W. J. Doherty & M. A. Baird (Eds.), *Family-centered medical care: A clinical casebook* (pp. 228–231). New York: Guilford Press.

Mengel, M. B. (1987c). Physician ineffectiveness due to family of origin issues. *Family Systems Medicine, 5,* 176–190.

Mengel, M. B., & Mauksch, L. B. (1989). Disarming the family ghost: A family of origin experience. *Family Medicine, 21,* 45–49.

Mengel, M. B., Connis, R. T., Gordon, M. J., & Taylor, T. R. (1988). The relationship of family dynamics and social support to personal, emotional, and social functioning in diabetic patient on the insulin pump. *Family Systems Medicine, 6*(3), 317–344.

Merrill, T. S. (1989). Oregon rationing plan ranks Medicaid services. *Family Practice News, 19*(9), 1, 17.

Micetich, K. C., Steinecker, P. H., & Thomasma, D. C. (1983). Are intravenous fluids morally required for a dying patient? *Archives of Internal Medicine, 143,* 975–978.

Miles, S. H. (1988). Paternalism, family duties, and my Aunt Maude. *Journal of the American Medical Association, 259,* 2582–2583.

Miller, L. J. (1986). Informed consent: IX. *Journal of the American Medical Association, 244,* 2661–2662.

Millon, T., Green, C., & Meagher, R. (Eds.). (1982). *Handbook of clinical health psychology.* New York: Plenum Press.

Minuchin, S. (1974). *Family and family therapy.* Cambridge: Harvard University Press.

Minuchin, S., Baker, L., Rosman, B., Liebman, R., Milman, L., & Todd, T. C. (1975). A conceptual model of psychosomatic illness in children: Family organization and family therapy. *Archives of General Psychiatry, 32,* 1031–1038.

Minuchin, S., Rosman, G. L., & Baker, L. (1978). *Psychosomatic families.* Cambridge: Harvard University Press.

Mold, J. M., & Stein, H. F. (1986). The cascade effect in the clinical care of patients. *New England Journal of Medicine, 314*(8), 512–514.

Mollmann, M., Bonnevie, O., Gudbrand, H. E., & Wulff, H. R. (1975). Diagnostic study of patients with upper abdominal pain. *Scandinavian Journal of Gastroenterology, 10,* 805–809.

Monjan, A. A., & Collector, M. I. (1977). Stress-induced indulation of the immune response. *Science, 196,* 307–308.

Montagne, J. P., Moss, A. A., & Margulis, A. R. (1978). Double-blind study of single and double contrast upper gastrointestinal examinations using endoscopy as a control. *American Journal of Roentgenology, 130,* 1041–1045.

Moore, M. A. (1985). Current management of hypertension. *Archives of Family Practice, 32*(6), 129–136.

Morales, W. J., & Lazar, A. J. (1986). Expectant management of rupture of membranes at term. *Southern Medical Journal, 79*(8), 955–958.

Morisky, D. E., Levine, D. M., Grein, L. W., Shapiro, S., Russell, R. P., & Smith, C. R. (1983). Five year blood pressure control and mortality following health education for hypertensive patients. *American Journal of Public Health, 73,* 153–162.

Morton, J. M., Poulter, C. A., & Pandya, K. J. (1983). Alimentary tract cancer. In R. Rubin (Ed.), *Clinical oncology: A multidisciplinary approach,* 6th ed. (pp. 154–178). Washington, DC: American Cancer Society.

National Center for Health Statistics. (1989). *Health in the United States.* DHHS Publ. No. (PHS) 90-1232. Washington, DC: U.S. Government Printing Office.

National Cholesterol Education Program Expert Panel. (1988). Report on detection, evaluation, and treatment of high blood cholesterol in adults. *Archives of Internal Medicine, 148,* 36–69.

National Recreation and Park Association. (1989). Information Booklet: "Professional Preparation" in Therapeutic Recreation. Alexandria, VA.

Nga, N. (February 23, 1988). *Vietnamese relocation.* Department of Family Medicine Grand Rounds, University of Oklahoma Health Sciences Center, Oklahoma City.

Nichols, M. J. (1984). *Family therapy: Concepts and methods.* New York: Gardner Press.

Noddings, N. (1989). *Caring: A feminine approach to ethics and moral education.* Berkeley, CA: University of California Press.

Novak, D. H., Detering, B. J., Arnold, R., & Farrow, L. (1989). Physician's attitudes toward using deception to resolve difficult ethical problems. *Journal of the American Medical Association, 261,* 2980–2985.

Nuckolls, K. B., Cassel, J., & Kaplan, B. H. (1972). Psychosocial assets, life crisis, and the prognosis of pregnancy. *American Journal of Epidemiology, 95,* 431–441.

Ockene, J. K., Benfar, R. C., Nuttall, R. L., Hurwitz, I., & Ockene, I. S. (1982). Relationships of psychosocial factors to smoking behavior change in an intervention program. *Preventive Medicine, 11,* 13–28.

Ohnuki-Tierney, E. (1984). *Illness and culture in contemporary Japan.* New York: Cambridge University Press.

Oklahoma State Medical Association. (1986). *Professional liability—medical malpractice: A medical–legal guide for physicians.* Oklahoma City: OSMA.

Oldridge, N. B. (1982). Compliance and exercise in primary and secondary prevention of coronary heart disease: A review. *Preventive Medicine, 11*(1), 56–70.

Orth, J. E., Stiles, W. B., Schwerwitz, L., Hennrikus, D., & Vallbona, C. (1987). Patient exposition and provider explanation in routine interviews and hypertensive patients' blood pressure control. *Health Psychology, 6,* 29–42.

Osler, W. (1985). *Counsels and ideals from the writings of William Osler.* Birmingham, AL: Gryphon Editions, Classics of Medicine Library.

Paffenbarger, R. S., Hyde, R. T., Wing, A. L., & Hsien, C. C. (1986). Physical activity, all-cause mortality, and longevity of college alumni. *New England Journal of Medicine, 134*(101), 605–613.

Palazzoli, M. S., Boscolo, L., Cecchin, G., & Prata, G. (1978). *Paradox and counter paradox.* New York: Jason Aronson.

Parry, K. K. (1984). Concepts from medical anthropology for clinicians. *Physical Therapy, 64,* 929–933.

Pauker, S. G., & Kassirer, J. P. (1980). The threshold approach to clinical decision making. *New England Journal of Medicine, 302,* 1109–1116.

Pauker, S. G., & Kassirer, J. P. (1980). The threshold approach to clinical decision making. *New England Journal of Medicine, 302,* 1109–1116.

Peabody, F. W. (1927). The care of the patient. *Journal of the American Medical Association, 88,* 877–882.

Pellegrino, E. D. (May 1977). The ethics of team care: Some notes on the morality of collective decision-making. In *American Cancer Society Proceedings of the Second National Conference on Cancer Nursing* (pp. 51–55). Washington, DC: American Cancer Society.

Pellegrino, E. D. (1983a). The healing relationship: The architectonics of clinical medicine. In E. E. Shelp (Ed.), *The clinical encounter* (pp. 153–172). Dordrecht, Holland: D. Reidel.

Pellegrino, E. D. (1983b). What is a profession? *Journal of Allied Health, August* Vol. 12, 168–172.

Pellegrino, E. D. (1987). Altruism, self-interest, and medical ethics. *Journal of the American Medical Association, 258,* 1939–1940.

Pellegrino, E. D., & Pellegrino, A. A. (1988). Humanism and ethics in Roman medicine: Translation and commentary on a text of Scribonius Largus. *Literature and Medicine, 7,* 22–38.

Pellegrino, E. D., & Thomasma, D. (1988). *For the patient's good: The restoration of beneficence in health care.* New York: Oxford University Press.

Pendleton, D., Scholfield, T., Tate, P., & Havelock, P. (1984). *The consultation: An approach to learning and teaching.* Oxford: Oxford Medical Publications.

Penna, R. P., & Sherman, M. S. (1985). *Pharmacy degrees conferred over time.* Bethesda, MD: American Association of Colleges of Pharmacy.

Percival, T. (1803). *Medical ethics: A code of institutes and precepts adapted to the professional conduct of physicians and surgeons.* Manchester, England: S. Russell.

Perkoff, G. T. (1985). The boundaries of medicine. *Journal of Chronic Disease, 38,* 271–278.

The Perrier Study. (1979). *Fitness in America* (pp. 1–59). New York: Louis Harris and Associates.

Pieroni, R. E. (1981). Folk medicine of the Black elderly. *Quarterly Contact [National Caucus and Center on Black Aged, Inc.], 4,* 7.

Pinner, M., & Miller, B. F. (Eds.). (1952). *When doctors are patients* (p. 108). New York: W. W. Norton.

Platt, F. W., & McMatch, J. C. (1979). Clinical hypocompetence and the interview. *Annals of Internal Medicine, 91,* 898–902.

Pocock, S. J. (1983). *Clinical trails: A practical approach.* New York: John Wiley & Sons.

Pollitt, K. (1982). The politically correct body. *Mother Jones, May,* Vol. 7 66–67.

Poynter, F. N., & Bishop, W. J. (1951). *A seventeenth-century country doctor and his patients: John Syncotts, 1592?–1662* (p. 59). Lufton: Bedfordshire Historical Record Society.

Priebe, W. M., Laurington, R. D., & Beck, I. T. (1982). Is epigastric tenderness a sign of peptic ulcer diseases? *Gastroenterology, 82,* 16–19.

Primosch, R., & Young, S. (1980). Pseudo battering of Vietnamese children (*Cao gio*). *Journal of the American Dental Association, 101,* 47–48.

Quill, T. E. (1983). Partnership in patient care: A contractual approach. *Annals of Internal Medicine, 98,* 228–234.

Rabin, D., Rabin, P. L., & Rabin, R. (1982). Compounding the ordeals of ALS: Isolation from my fellow physicians. *New England Journal of Medicine, 307,* 506–509.

Ramsey, C. N. (1989). The science of family medicine. In C. N. Ramsey (Ed.), *Family systems in medicine* (pp. 3–17). New York: Guilford Press.

Ramsey, P. (1970). *The patient as person: Explorations in medical ethics.* New Haven: Yale University Press.

Rawls, J. (1971). *A theory of justice.* Cambridge, MA: Harvard University Press.

Reinhardt, U. E. (1981). The GMENAC forecast: An alternative view. *American Journal of Public Health, 71*(10), 1149–1157.

Reiser, S. J. (1978). *Medicine and the reign of technology.* Cambridge: Cambridge University Press.

Reiser, S. J., & Anabar, M. (Eds.). (1984). *The machine at the bedside: Strategies for using technology in patient care.* Cambridge: Cambridge University Press.

Relman, A. S. (1980). The new medical–industrial complex. *New England Journal of Medicine, 303,* 963–970.

Relman, A. S. (1987). The changing climate of medical practice. *New England Journal of Medicine, 313,* 333–334.

Richardson, M. (1988). Mental health services: Growth and development of a system. In S. J. Williams & P. R. Torrens (Eds.), *Introduction to health services,* 3rd ed. (pp. 255–277). New York: John Wiley & Sons.

Riegelman, R. K. (1985).The hidden holes in the history. *Postgraduate Medicine, 70,* 40–45.

Ring, M. E. (1985). *Dentistry. An illumined history.* New York: Harry N. Abrams.

Roberts, J. M. (1951). Three Navaho households. In *papers of the Peabody Museum of American Archaeology and Ethnology,* Vol. II, No. 3, Cambridge, MA: Harvard University Press.

Robertson, W. O. (1985). *Medical malpractice: A preventive approach.* Seattle: University of Washington Press.

Rogers, C. (1961). *On becoming a person.* Boston: Houghton Miffin.

Rogers, D. E., & Blendon, R. J. (1977). The changing American health scene: Sometimes things get better. *Journal of the American Medical Association, 237,* 1710–1714.

Rolland, J. (1984). Toward a psychosocial typology of chronic and life-threatening illnesses. *Family Systems Medicine, 2*(3), 245–262.

Roper, W. L., Winkenwerder, W., Hackbarth, G. M., & Krakaner, H. (1988). Effectiveness in health care: An initiative to evaluate and improve medical practice. *New England Journal of Medicine, 319,* 1197–1202.

Rose, G., & Shipley, M. J. (1980). Plasma lipids and mortality: A source of error. *Lancet, 1,* 523–526.

Rosenfeld, M., & Thornton, R. F. (1978). *A national study of the practice of pharmacy.* Washington, DC: American Pharmaceutical Association.

Rosenman, R. H., Jenkins, C. D., Brand, R. J., Friedman, M., Straus, R., & Wurm, M. (1975). Coronary heart disease in the Western Collaborative Group Study: Final follow-up experience of 8½ years. *Journal of the American Medical Association, 233,* 872–877.

Rosoff, A. J. (1987). Legal aspects of medical practice and community medicine. In B. J. Cassens (Ed.), *Preventive medicine and public health* (pp. 267–284). New York: John Wiley & Sons.

Ross, J. L., & Phipps, E. (1986). Physician–patient power struggles: Their role in noncompliance. *Family Medicine, 18,* 99–101.

Rothberg, J. S. (1981). The rehabilitation team: Future direction. *Archives of Physical Medicine and Rehabilitation, 62,* 407–410.

Rubenstein, L. (1983). The clinical effectiveness of multidimensional geriatric assessment. *Journal of the American Geriatric Society, 31*(12), 758–761.

Sackett, D. L., Haynes, R. B., & Tugwell, P. (1985). *Clinical epidemiology: A basic science for clinical medicine.* Boston: Little, Brown.

Sacks, O. (1984). *One leg to stand on.* London: Gerald Duckworth.

Sanne, H. (1973). Exercise tolerance and physical training of non-selected patients after myocardial infarction. *Acta Medica Scandinavica, 551 Supplementum,* 1–214.

Satir, V. (1972). *People making.* Palo Alto, CA: Science and Behavior Books.

Sawa, R. J. (1988). Incorporating the family into medical care. *Canadian Family Physician, 34,* 87–93.

Scheper-Hughes, N., & Lock, M. M. (1987). The mindful body: A prolegomenon to future work in medical anthropology. *Medical Anthropology Quarterly, 1,* 6–41.

Scheper-Hughes, N., & Stein, H. F. (1987). Child-abuse and the unconscious. In N. Scheper-Hughes (Ed.), Child survival: *Anthropological approaches to the treatment and the maltreatment of children.* Dordrecht, Holland: D. Reidel.

Schloss, E. P. (1988). Beyond GMENAC—another physician shortage from 2010 to 2030? *New England Journal of Medicine 318,* 920–922.

Schmidt, D. D. (1978). The family as the unit of medical care. *Journal of Family Practice, 7,* 303–313.

Scholendorff v. The Society of New York Hospital. 211 NY 125 (1914). 105 N. E. 92.

Schwartz, G. E., & Weiss, S. M. (1978). Yale conference on behavioral medicine: A proposed definition and statement of goals. *Journal of Behavioral Medicine, 1,* 3–12.

Schwartz, W. B., Sloan, F. A., & Mendelson, D. N. (1988). Why there will be little or no physician surplus between now and the year 2000. *New England Journal of Medicine, 318,* 892–897.

Schwenk, T. L., Marquez, J. T., Lefever, R. D., & Cohen, M. (1989). Physician and patient determinants of difficult physician–patient relationship. *Journal of Family Practice, 28*(1), 59–63.

Seldin, D. W. (1981). The boundaries of medicine. *Transactions of the Association of American Physicians, 94,* 75–84.

Selikoff, I. J., & Hammond, E. C. (1978). Asbestos associated diseases in United States shipyards. *Cancer, 28,* 87–99.

Selvini, M. P., Boscola, L., Ceccin, B., & Prata, G. (1980). Hypothesizing–circularity–neutrality: Three guidelines for the conductor of the session. *Family Process, 19,* 3–12.

Selye, H. (1976). *The stress of life,* revised ed. New York: McGraw–Hill.

Shastid, T. H. (1944). *My second life* (p. 890). Ann Arbor: George Wahr.

Sheldon, M. (1982). Truth telling in medicine. *Journal of the American Medical Association, 247,* 651–654.

Shorter, B. (1985). *Bedside manners: The troubled history of doctors and patients.* New York: Simon and Schuster.

Siegler, M. (1977). Critical illness: The limits of autonomy. *Hastings Center Reports, 7,* 12–15.

Siegler, M. (1981). Searching for moral certainty in medicine: A proposal for a new model of the doctor–patient encounter. *Bulletin of the New York Academy of Medicine, 57,* 56–69.

Siegler, M. (1982). Confidentiality in medicine: A decrepit concept. *New England Journal of Medicine, 307,* 1518–1521.

Sims, J. M. (1889). *The story of my life.* New York: Appleton.

Sisson, J. C., Schoomaker, E. B., & Ross, J. C. (1976). Clinical decision analysis: The hazard of using additional data. *Journal of the American Medical Association, 236,* 1259–1263.

Smilkstein, G. (1980). The cycle of family function: A conceptual model for family medicine. *Journal of Family Practice, 11,* 223–232.

Smith, M. C., & Knapp, D. A. (1987). *Pharmacy, drugs, and medical care,* 4th ed. Baltimore: Williams & Wilkins.

Smith, R. C. (1984). Teaching interviewing skills to medical students: The issue of countertransference. *Journal of Medical Education, 59,* 582–588.

Smith, R. C. (1986). Unrecognized responses and feelings of residents and fellows during interview of patients. *Journal of Medical Education, 61,* 982–984.

Smucker, D. R. (1988). Obstetrics in family practice in the state of Ohio. *Journal of Family Practice, 26,* 165–168.

Snow, L. F. (1974). Folk medical beliefs and implications for care of patients. *Annals of Internal Medicine, 81,* 82–96.

Snow, L. F. (1983). Traditional health beliefs and practices among lower class black Americans. *Western Journal of Medicine, 139,* 820–828.

Solowiejczyk, J. N., & Baker, L. (1981). Physician–patient communication in chronic illness. *Diabetes Care, 4,* 427–429.

Sox, H. C., Blatt, M. A., Higgins, M. C., & Marton, K. I. (1988). *Medical decision making.* Boston: Butterworths.

Spiegel, J. (1971). *Transactions: The interplay between individual, family, and society.* New York: Science House.

Spitzer, W. D. (1979). Report of the task force on the periodic health examination. *Canadian Medical Association Journal, 121,* 1193–1254.

Starr, P. (1982). *The social transformation of American medicine.* New York: Basic Books.

Steckle, S. B., & Swain, M. A. (1977). Contracting with patients to improve compliance. *Hospitals, 51,* 81–84.

Stein, H. F. (1980). The problem of cultural persistence, and the differentiation of self in one's culture. *Family, 8,* 3–12.

Stein, H. F. (1982). Ethanol and its discontents: Paradoxes of inebriation and sobriety in American culture. *Journal of Psychoanalytic Anthropology, 5,* 355–377.

Stein, H. F. (1985a). Alcoholism as metaphor in American culture: Ritual desecration as social integration. *Ethos, 13,* 195–235.

Stein, H. F. (1985b). An argument for more inclusive context in clinical intervention: The case of family medicine. In H. F. Stein & M. Apprey (Eds.), *Context and dynamics in clinical knowledge* (pp. 78–91). Charlottesville, VA: University Press of Virginia.

Stein, H. F. (1985c). *The psychodynamics of medical practice.* Berkeley, CA: University of California Press.

Stein, H. F. (1987a). The annual cycle and the cultural nexus of health care behavior among Oklahoma wheat farming families. In H. F. Stein & M. Apprey (Eds.)., *From Metaphor to meaning: Papers in psychoanalytic anthropology* (pp. 156–177). Charlottesville, VA: University Press of Virginia.

Stein, H. F. (1987b). Farmer and cowboy: The duality of the midwestern male ethos—a study in ethnicity, regionalism, and national identity. In H. F. Stein & M. Apprey (Eds.), *From metaphor to meaning: Papers in psychoanalytic anthropology* (pp. 178–227). Charlottesville, VA: University Press of Virginia.

Stein, H. F. (1987c). Review of R. A. Koenigsberg, *The psychoanalysis of racism, revolution and nationalism* (New York: The Library of Social Science, 1977/1986). *Canadian Review of Studies in Nationalism, 14,* 345–347.

Stein, H. F. (1987d). Where is "the case"? A psychoanalytic–ethnographic inquiry into the boundary of pathology in a spinal cord-injured woman. *Journal of Psychoanalytic Anthropology, 10,* 361–383.

Stein, H. F. (1987e). Whatever happened to countertransference: The Subjective in Medicine. In H. F. Stein & M. Apprey *Context and dynamics in clinical knowledge* pp. 1–55. Charlottesville: University Press of Virginia.

Stein, H. F. (1990a). *American medicine as culture.* Boulder, CO: Westview Press.

Stein, H. F. (1990b). In what systems do alcohol/chemical addictions make sense? Clinical ideologies and practices as cultural metaphors. *Social Science and Medicine, 30,* 987–1000.

Stein, H. F., & Apprey, M. (1985). *Context and dynamics in clinical knowledge.* Charlottesville: University Press of Virginia.

Stein, H. F., & Apprey, M. (1987). *From metaphor to meaning: Papers in psychoanalytic anthropology.* Charlottesville, VA: University Press of Virginia.

Stein, H. F., & Apprey, M. (1990). *Clinical stories and their translation.* Charlottesville: University of Virginia press.

Stein, H. F., & Hill, R. F. (1977). *The ethnic imperative: Examining the new white ethnic movement.* University Park, PA: Pennsylvania State University Press.

Stein, H. F., & Mold, J. W. (1988). Stress, anxiety, and cascades in clinical decision making. *Stress Medicine, 4,* 41–48.

Stein, H. F., & Pontious, J. M. (1985). Family and beyond: The larger context of non-compliance. *Family Systems Medicine, 3,* 179–189.

Steinbrook, R., & Lo, B. (1988). Artificial feeding—solid ground, not a slippery slope. *New England Journal of Medicine, 318,* 286–290.

Stetten, D., Jr. (1981). Coping with blindness. *New England Journal of Medicine, 305,* 458–460.

Stewart, M. A., McWhinney, I. R., & Buck, C. W. (1979). The doctor–patient relationship and its effect on outcome. *Journal of the Royal College of General Practice, 29,* 77–84.

Stunkard, A., & McLaren-Hume, M. (1959). The results of treatment for obesity: A review of the literature and report of a series. *Archives of Internal Medicine, 103,* 79–85.

Szasz, T. S., & Hollender, M. H. (1987). A contribution to the philosophy of medicine: The basic model of the doctor–patient relationship in encounter between patients and doctors. In J. E. Stoekle (Ed.), *Encounters between patients and doctors* (pp. 165–178). Cambridge, MA: MIT Press.

Tapp, J. T., & Warner, R. W. (1985). The multisystems view of health and disease. In N. Schneiderman & J. T. Tapp (Eds), *Behavioral medicine: The biopsychosocial approach.* Hillsdale, NJ: Lawrence Erlbaum Associates.

Tarlov, A. R. (1983). Shattuck lecture—the increasing supply of physicians, the changing structure of the health-services system, and the future practice of medicine. *New England Journal of Medicine, 308,* 1235–1244.

Taylor, H. L., Klepeter, E., Keys, A., Parlin, W., Blackburn, H., & Puchner, T. (1962). Death rates among physically active and sedentary employees of the railroad industry. *American Journal of Public Health, 52,* 1697–1707.

Taylor, T. R., Gordon, M. J., & Ashworth, C. D. (1984). A systems perspective on clinical management. *Behavioral Science, 29,* 233–247.

Tierney, W. M., Siu, L. H., & McDonald, C. J. (1986). Delayed feedback of physician performance versus immediate reminders to perform preventive care. *Medical Care, 24,* 659–666.

Tipton, R. M. (1983). Clinical and counseling psychology: A study of rules and functions. *Professional Psychology, 14,* 837–846.

Toombs, S. K. (1987). The meaning of illness: A phenomenological approach to the patient–physician relationship. *Journal of Medical Philosophy, 12,* 219.

Uhlmann, R. F., Inui, T. S., Pecorado, R. E., & Carter, W. B. (1988). Relationship of patient request fulfillment to compliance, glycemic control, and other health care outcomes in insulin-dependent diabetes. *Journal of General Internal Medicine, 3,* 458–463.

U.S. Department of Commerce. (1980). *Statistical abstracts of the United States, 1980.* Washington, DC: U.S. Government Printing Office.

U.S. Department of Health and Human Services. (1984). *The health consequences of smoking: Chronic obstructive lung disease. A report of the surgeon general.* Rockville, MD: Department of Health and Human Services, DHH(PHS) 84-50205.

Van Houtte, P., Salazer, O. M., Phillips, C. E., & Asbury, R. F. (1983). Lung cancer. In P. Rubin, R. F.

Bakemeier, & S. K. Krackov (Eds.), *Clinical oncology: A multidisciplinary approach* (pp. 142–153). Washington, DC: American Cancer Society.

Veatch, R. M. (1972). Models for ethical medicine in a revolutionary age. *Hastings Center Report, 2,* 5–7.

Veatch, R. M. (1983). The physician as stranger: The ethics of the anonymous patient–physician relationship. In E. E. Shelp (Ed.), *The clinical encounter* (pp. 187–202). Dordrecht, Holland: D. Reidel.

Veith, I. (1949). *The yellow emperor's classic of internal medicine.* Baltimore: Williams & Wilkins.

von Bertalanffy, L. (1968). *General system theory.* New York: Braziller.

Wagner, M. V., Chin, V. P., Peters, C. J., Drexler, B., & Newman, L. A. (1989). A comparison of early and delayed induction of labor with spontaneous rupture of membranes of term. *Obstetrics and Gynecology, 74,* 93–97.

Walters, L. (1988). Ethical issues in fetal research: A look back and a look forward. *Clinical Research, 36,* 209–214.

Ware, J. E. (1984). Conceptualizing disease impact and treatment outcome. *Cancer, 53*(Supplement), 2316–2322.

Watkins, C. E., Lopez, F. G., Campbell, V. L., & Himmell, C. D. (1986). Counseling psychology and clinical psychology: Some preliminary comparative data. *American Psychologist, 41*(6), 581–582.

Weikel, W. J., & Palmo, A. J. (1989). The evolution and practice of mental health counseling. *Journal of Mental Health Counseling, 11*(1), 7–25.

Weinberger, M., Greene, J. Y., & Mamlin, J. J. (1981). The impact of clinical encounter events on patient and physician satisfaction. *Social Science and Medicine, 15E,* 239–244.

Weinberger, M. H., Cohen, S. J., Miller, J. Z., Luft, F. C., Grim, C. E., & Fineberg, N. S. (1988). Dietary sodium restriction as adjunctive treatment in hypertension. *Journal of the American Medical Association, 259,* 2561–2565.

Weiss, B. D. (1986). The effect of malpractice insurance costs on family physician's hospital practice. *Journal of Family Practice, 23,* 55–58.

Welin, L., Svardsudd, K., Wilhelmsen, L., Larsson, B., & Tibblin, G. (1987). Analysis of risk factors for stroke in a cohort of men born in 1913. *New England Journal of Medicine, 317,* 521–526.

White, K. L. (1988). *The tasks of medicine: Dialogue at Wickenburg.* Menlo Park, CA: The Henry J. Kaiser Family Foundation.

Whittaker, C. A., and Keith, D. V. (1981). Symbolic–experimental family therapy. In A. S. Gurman & D. P. Khiskern (Eds.), *Handbook of family therapy.* New York: Brunner/Mazel pp. 187–225.

Whitley, J. M. (1984). Counseling psychology: A historical perspective. *Counseling Psychologist, 12,* 3–109.

Williams, M. E., & Williams, T. F. (1986). Evaluation of older persons in the ambulatory setting. *Journal of the American Geriatric Society, 34,* 37–43.

Williams, R. R., Sorlie, P. D., Feinleib, M., McNamara, P. M., Kannel, W. B., & Dawber, T. R. (1981). Cancer incidence by levels of cholesterol. *Journal of the American Medical Association, 245,* 247–252.

Winawer, S. J., Flehinger, B. J., Buchalter, J., Herbert, E., & Shike, M. (1990). Declining serum cholesterol levels prior to diagnosis of colon cancer: A time-trend, case-control study. *Journal of the American Medical Association, 263,* 2038–2085.

Wing, R. R., & Jeffery, R. W. (1979). Outpatient treatment of obesity: A comparison of methodology and clinical results. *International Journal of Obesity, 3,* 261–279.

World Health Organization. (1947). The constitution of The World Health Organization. *WHO Chronicle, 1,* 29.

Wright, R. A. (1987). *Human values in health care: The practice of ethics.* New York: McGraw-Hill.

Wynder, E. L. (1972). Etiology of lung cancer: Reflections on two decades of research. *CA, 32,* 1332–1339.

Wynder, E. L. (1980). Dietary factors related to breast cancer. *CA, 46,* 899–904.

Zborowski, M. (1969). *People in pain.* San Francisco: Jossey-Bass.

Author Index

Subject Index